Special Consultant

Dr Jean Emberlin, director of the Pollen Research Unit at the University of North London, acted as special consultant on those sections of the book concerned with pollen dispersal and pollen seasons. She is a botanist and aerobiologist, and one of the directors of the European Aeroallergen Network.

About the authors

Dr Jonathan Brostoff is a Physician in charge of the Allergy Clinic at the Middlesex Hospital in London and Reader in Clinical Immunology at University College London Medical School. After training as a general physician he became interested in inhalant and food allergy. He has spent many years studying the way the immune system works and how it produces allergic diseases such as hayfever, asthma, eczema and food allergy. He is currently engaged in programmes of research in these areas. Dr Brostoff is recognized as a leading international authority on allergy and is co-author of several principal textbooks on this subject.

Linda Gamlin trained as a biochemist and worked in research for several years, before turning to journalism. She specializes in writing about the immune system, allergy and other health matters.

HAYFEVER

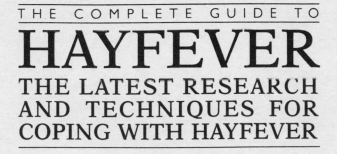

THE COMPLETE GUIDE TO
HAYFEVER
THE LATEST RESEARCH AND TECHNIQUES FOR COPING WITH HAYFEVER

DR JONATHAN BROSTOFF
AND LINDA GAMLIN

First published 1993
This edition first published 1998

Published by Parragon Publishing
in arrangement with
Bloomsbury Publishing Plc
38 Soho Square, London W1V 5DF

British Library Cataloguing in Publication Data
A CIP catalogue record for this book is available
from the British Library

ISBN 0 75252 428 3

Printed in Great Britain by Clays Ltd, St Ives plc

Contents

Acknowledgements

Many people have given freely of their time in helping us with the research for this book, and we are immensely grateful to them. We would particularly like to thank Dr A. Armentia-Medina, Mina Barge, Dr Diana Bass, Peter Bateman, Dr Ian Burgess, David Burnie, Sheila Burnie, Stuart Collier, Dr Matthew Colloff, Dr Roland Davies, Dr Eugenio Dominguez-Vilches, Dr Keith Eaton, Dr Michael Emanuel, Dr Nils Eriksson, Dr Penny Fitzharris, Dr William Frankland, Dr Tony Ganderton, Dr Richard Godfrey, Derek Hall, Dr R.J. Harris, Professor John Heslop-Harrison, Dr Stephen Holgate, Andrew Jones, Dr Richard Lawson, Dr George Lewith, Dr Colin Little, Dr Christina Luczynska, Dr Jonathan Maberly, Dr Len McEwen, Dr Charlie McSharry, Quintin McKenzie, Dr John Mansfield, Dr Bruce Mitchell, Dr John Morrison-Smith, Dr Harry Morrow-Brown, Dr Masaharu Muranaka, Gerard Nelson, Shigeki Ohyama, Professor Eldryd Parry, Dr John Pettitt, Pavel Pietrzak, Dr Tom Platts-Mills, Morrika Rae, Dr Kyllikki Remes, Dr Tim Rich, Mohammed Saleem, Ludmilla Semenova-Ducksbury, Dr Bonnie Sibbald, Don Skelton, Simon Small, Dr Ian Smith, Dr David Strachan, Lynne Strugnell, Colin Taylor, Dr Morton Teich, Dr Gilles Vincent, Dr Victoria von Witt, Dr Tony Walter, Dr Alan Wheeler, Professor Bruno Wüthrich, Professor V. Zavazal.

Finally, we would like to thank Fraser May for his excellent work on the illustrations.

Chapter One

WHAT IS HAYFEVER?

Sex causes hayfever. Most people are surprised to discover this, because they had no idea that plants, whose lives seem fairly dull and uneventful, actually engage in sex. But the fact is that they do, and that the sexual exploits of plants set millions of people sneezing and sniffing every year. (Very occasionally, the sexual exploits of human beings spark off hayfever-like symptoms in the participants, or an attack of asthma, or both. This unusual reaction is discussed on pp231–2.)

Plant sex is no different from any other sort of sex, in that it involves an interaction between male and female. But being rooted firmly to the ground makes it difficult for plants to pursue their mate, so they do it all at a distance, in a detached and dispassionate fashion that is rather like artificial insemination. Mating takes place without any meeting. Pollen – a fine powder which is the plants' equivalent of semen – is dispatched from one plant to another while the plants themselves stay put. A tiny pinch of pollen dust contains thousands of microscopic pollen grains, and each of these carries inside it a potent male cell, equivalent to the sperm cell of an animal.

For plants such as roses and buttercups, the pollen is transported by a six-legged artificial inseminator – a bee, butterfly or other insect. The plant depends on the insect pollinator, which is lured into its flowers by a free meal of syrupy liquid – nectar. As the insect feeds, it brushes against the pollen-producing organs, called anthers, and inadvertently collects pollen on its head or body. At the next flower, some of this pollen brushes on to the female parts of the flower. Assuming the two flowers are compatible, the pollen will fertilize the egg cells in the flower, and each of these will develop into a seed.

As a way of improving the efficiency of this system, most flowers have both male and female parts – they are hermaphrodites – so they can dispatch pollen to other plants, and receive it as well. In the majority of plants there are special mechanisms that prevent them from fertilizing themselves.

BEES OR BREEZE? THE POLLINATION OPTIONS

Pollination by insects was used by the very earliest flowering plants, which were evolving their first colourful petals and sugary nectar as the dinosaurs plodded by, over 100 million years ago. Those early flowers were something like modern-day magnolias and were probably pollinated by small beetles.

In time, some flowering plants developed other ways of being pollinated. Insects, as it turned out, had certain drawbacks. They did not fly far enough to pollinate plants that were widely scattered, and they were fussy about the weather – if it was too cold, they stayed at home. A few plants developed larger flowers and more nectar, attracting active warm-blooded animals such as bats and small birds to act as their pollinators. But this only worked in certain parts of the tropics, where there were flowers available all year round to keep these large and hungry pollinators well fed.

What other options were available for a plant that needed to dispense with insect pollinators? There was only one realistic possibility: the wind. Many flowering plants gradually evolved in this direction, notably the grasses, all of which are wind-pollinated. In time, they lost the showy, colourful petals that had been used to attract insects. They also stopped producing nectar to feed the insects, and sweet scents to beguile them.

All these measures saved the plants a great deal of energy, so dispensing with insects was worthwhile. However, there was one huge disadvantage to set against these energy savings – an insect carries pollen straight to other flowers, while the wind simply blows it anywhere.

The solution that evolution came up with was to saturate the air with pollen – to release millions of pollen grains from every flower. Among modern plants the champion pollen producer, the giant ragweed, can generate 8,000 million pollen grains in just five hours, a staggering rate of production that brings misery to ragweed-sensitive patients.

As wind pollination evolved, natural selection also favoured pollen grains that were extremely light in weight, so as not to settle rapidly but to remain suspended on the breeze for hours. This greatly increases the chance of the right pollen grain reaching the right flower. Unfortunately, it also maximizes the chance of it reaching the nose of a hayfever victim.

In a sense, by developing wind pollination in flowering plants, the forces of evolution were just 'reinventing the wheel'. A separate group of plants, an older and more primitive group, had been using wind pollination for millions of years; in fact, they had never tried any other method. These were the coniferous trees, such as pines, firs and spruces, which still grow in many

WHAT DOES HAYFEVER MEAN?

The term **hayfever** can be used in two different ways. The most common meaning, and the one used in this book, is an allergic reaction to pollen – any sort of pollen.

However, when the word was coined in the nineteenth century by the general public (and later taken up, rather reluctantly, by the medical profession), it was intended to mean an unusual reaction to hay. Since hay is a mixture of grass and wild flowers, and it is the grass pollen that causes the symptoms in this mixture, hayfever, strictly speaking, means a reaction to grass pollen. A few doctors and researchers still use the word in this restrictive sense. This is particularly true in Britain and northern Europe, where, in any case, allergy to pollen means allergy to grass pollen for the great majority of sufferers.

For those using hayfever in this restrictive sense, another word is needed to cover pollen allergy generally. The word **pollinosis** (or 'pollenosis') is sometimes used, but this has not caught on as widely as 'hayfever', even though it is far more scholarly and precise.

A third possibility, sometimes used by doctors, is **seasonal allergic rhinitis** or **SAR**. Apart from being excessively long-winded, this term is rather confusing, since it lumps pollen allergy together with seasonal mould-spore allergy (see p194), while excluding perennial mould-spore allergy.

parts of the world today. Their pollen is produced in such huge amounts that, close to a pine forest, it can form a slick of yellow scum on the surface of puddles. But despite their abundance, conifer pollens are not common culprits in hayfever (see box, pp6–7).

FEAR OF FLOWERS?

The differences between insect-pollinated and wind-pollinated flowers are not just a matter of academic interest – they are very important to anyone with hayfever. Pollen grains that are carried by insects are slightly sticky to ensure that they become attached to their insect pollinator. This also makes them stick to each other, so that they form clusters of pollen grains which are then easily visible. (You may see the pollen among the petals of flowers, or stuck to the 'fur' on a bee.) By contrast, the pollen of grasses and most other wind-pollinated plants is virtually invisible because it comes in minute, separate grains which disperse rapidly. On a sunny day, if you watch a nettle flower or a birch catkin that is catching the sun but is positioned against a dark background, you may just see a puff of pollen escaping, but you have to look very carefully, as it disperses in seconds.

Being relatively large, heavy and sticky, the pollen grains of insect-pollinated plants do not become airborne easily, and only small amounts are inhaled. Such flowers are far less likely to cause hayfever than wind-pollinated flowers, because the amount of pollen in the air is insufficient to sensitize most people.

The sort of flowers that are picked and placed in vases are almost all insect-pollinated: the scents and showy petals that appeal to us are exactly those that evolved to attract insects. Virtually any large-petalled flower, from a daisy to an orchid, comes in this category.

Some people make the mistake of thinking that such flowers – pretty, scented, conspicuous flowers – cause their hayfever. They can even develop floriphobia, a deadly fear of flowers! In fact, it is the plants you scarcely notice, the self-effacing ones with tiny, dull green flowers that are really to blame. Likewise, it is the pollen you *cannot see* that is likely to be causing your hayfever. The golden powder produced by garden flowers is probably harmless to you.

So much for the public misconception about insect-pollinated flowers. *But there is a widespread medical misconception about them too*. This is that insect-pollinated flowers *never* cause hayfever, and that none of their pollen becomes airborne. This view is equally mistaken, yet it is the firm belief of many doctors. A study in Britain found pollen from dandelions, buttercups and elderberries all floating in the air, along with pollen from plants of the carrot, cabbage and rose families. Scientists in India found that 12 per cent of airborne pollen was from insect-pollinated plants. When two American researchers set out to find well-verified cases of hayfever to insect-pollinated plants, they came up with hundreds of case reports, involving over 40 different species of plant.

There are two main situations in which insect-pollinated plants produce hayfever. The first involves those unfortunate, highly sensitive individuals who can become allergic to a pollen even though the amounts in the air are small. The second occurs when people are exposed to huge quantities of a particular insect-dispersed pollen, either at work or around the home.

The first situation produces some rare cases of allergy to plants such as honeysuckle, hydrangea, rose, sweet pea or dahlia. Usually, these patients are highly prone to allergy, and react to other pollens as well, but occasionally there is just one offender and it is an insect-pollinated plant. **Cross-reactions** between related plants may be important here. For example, ragweed belongs to the same botanical family (the Compositae or Asteraceae) as dandelions. Children who are ragweed-sensitive may suffer a bad attack of hayfever after rolling in grass that is full of flowering dandelions. This is uncommon, but several cases have been reported in North America where ragweed hayfever is rife. In other parts of the world, such as Britain, where dandelion is equally common, but ragweed is rare, children roll among the dandelions with impunity – sensitivity to dandelion pollen is unknown.

The second situation, when people are exposed to large numbers of a particular insect-pollinated plant, produces far more cases of hayfever, because it is not just those who are highly prone to allergy that succumb.

In some regions of Russia, fields of golden sunflowers stretch as far as the eye can see, and there are many cases of allergy to sunflower pollen. Wherever a large area of farmland is devoted to a particular insect-pollinated crop, the potential for sensitization may be there. Big orchards of apples, cherries or plums can produce hayfever in a few of the local residents, while in California, Florida and Israel – all major producers of oranges – sensitivity to orange pollen is found. (In this case, an interesting discovery has been made about how the pollen becomes airborne: over-laden bees flying away from the orange trees drop some of their pollen on the way back to the hive.)

Could the same be happening with oil-seed rape, the oil and fodder crop that is adding squares of brilliant yellow to the British and European landscape, courtesy of Common Market subsidies? Its pollen is found in the air around rape fields, and many people believe they suffer hayfever when close to these fields. Whether this is really a response to oil-seed rape itself is still under discussion. Nor is it certain whether the rape pollen, or some other substance given off by the plants, is to blame (see p120).

Those whose work brings them into close daily contact with a particular insect-pollinated plant – plant breeders, farm workers, flower growers and florists, for example – also encounter enough pollen to increase their risk of hayfever. Chrysanthemums are a common problem for florists, and mimosa (which may be pollinated by insects or wind) causes a lot of hayfever among commercial flower growers in Italy. Farmers and farm labourers who grow alfalfa, lucerne or clover may be exposed to the pollen all year round because it remains in the dried fodder that they feed to their animals during the winter months. Hayfever in response to these pollens has been reported from many parts of the USA and from South Africa.

A study of gardeners, plant specialists and nursery workers in Germany discovered eight cases of hayfever to cyclamen, three to begonias and one to

THE CONIFER PUZZLE

All conifers are wind-pollinated, yet they cause hayfever far less often than wind-pollinated flowering plants. In Scandinavia, where forests of spruce and pine cover vast areas (and where the pollen cloud is so dense that it can blow across the North Sea to Britain), it is not these trees that generally cause hayfever. The guilty trees are the delicate little birches which grow among the conifers or along the forest edges: birches belong to the flowering plant group. Only a tiny minority of Scandinavians are sensitive to pine pollen.

There are occasional reports of pine hayfever from some Mediterranean countries and from North America, but again these are relatively rare, with very few people being affected. The only true pine that produces hayfever to any appreciable extent is the eastern white pine of New England in the USA, and even this affects only 10 per cent of those with spring hayfever. As for spruces, firs, larches and cedars, hayfever in response to these trees is unknown. The same is true of yews. The possible reasons for the lack of hayfever in response to these conifers will be discussed later in this chapter.

There are some notable exceptions to the rule about conifers, however. Certain types *do* cause hayfever, particularly the cypresses and junipers (a group of closely related conifers), the white cypress pine (which is not a true pine at all, but a native Australian conifer), and the Japanese red cedar (a relative of the American redwoods). Other trees in the

lilies. A weeping undertaker at a funeral may be one of an unusually sentimental nature, but it is also possible that his red, watery eyes are a response to the Easter lilies about the casket. They cause one of the more esoteric forms of occupational hayfever.

Plant breeders are a particularly vulnerable group of workers because their job involves actually handling pollen, as they cross-pollinate one plant with another. One plant breeder found that he had to repeatedly change the type of crop he worked on, as he became sensitive to almost any plant after a year or two. Having started as a carrot breeder, he was forced to move on to beans, redwood family, such as the bald cypress, may sometimes cause hayfever.

Of these, the only one to cause a major outbreak of hayfever – the sort of widespread outbreak that grasses, ragweeds or other flowering plants can produce – is the Japanese red cedar. This has, in the past 40 years, produced a dramatic hayfever epidemic in Japan. There is some intriguing research from California which suggests that people of Asiatic origin are more likely than Caucasians to react allergically to conifer pollen – cypresses and junipers in this case, but their **allergens** (see p11) are similar to those of Japanese red cedar. This ethnic difference may help to explain the unprecedented scale of the Japanese epidemic, although other factors undoubtedly play a part.

Sometimes people are aware of being affected by pine pollen, although medical tests show no real allergic reaction to it. This seems to be particularly true in New Zealand and Australia, where introduced pines have been planted for timber. The most plausible explanation for this is that the sheer volume of pine pollen in the air, and its relatively large size, may make it an irritant to the nose. (A grain of pine pollen is over twice the size of other airborne pollens, and should not, by rights, become airborne at all, but it has two large air bladders which keep it buoyant.) Another possible cause of the symptoms is an irritant chemical, called benzoic acid, that is released by some pine pollen.

then to cabbages, and then to a succession of other crops. (All these crops are insect-pollinated.) Research programmes already begun had to be conducted at long distance, using assistants, as he could no longer enter the glasshouses where the offending crops were growing.

In conclusion, then, how should you proceed if your hayfever seems to be brought on by sniffing a rose, although your doctor says this is nonsense? Firstly, consider the other possibilities. The most likely explanation is that you are sensitive to grass or some other wind-pollinated plant that pollinates at the same time as roses are in flower. When sniffing a rose, you may inhale a little rose pollen that acts as an irritant and aggravates, or precipitates, the reaction to grass. Once hayfever has set in, the membranes of the nose become over-sensitive and can be affected by all kinds of minor irritants. Even the scent of the rose (or other flowers) can rank among those irritants and apparently trigger off an attack of hayfever (see p231). In these cases, the rose is just an innocent bystander, and floriphobia is an inappropriate reaction. Ask the doctor for a skin-prick test to the common windborne pollens, and this may reveal the true culprit.

A true sensitivity to the rose (or other insect-pollinated plant) is far less likely, but it is possible. Unfortunately, neither skin-prick tests nor hypo-sensitization treatments (see Chapter Nine) are likely to be available, since extracts of such pollen are not available commercially. But an enterprising allergist should be able to produce 'home-made' extracts, for either diagnosis or treatment. The standard drug treatments are just the same as for wind-pollinated plants, so you do not necessarily need to be sure which plant is causing your symptoms.

THE RACE TO POLLINATE

So far, we have considered how pollen gets from one plant to another, but not looked at what happens to the pollen on arrival at its destination. This is crucial, because knowing how pollen grains 'behave' in normal circumstances can help us to understand what causes hayfever. A pollen grain that lands in the nose goes through a sequence of actions which, in the right place, would help it to father a seed. In your nose or eyes, it is doing the right thing but in the wrong place.

The right place to be for a pollen grain is on the **stigma** of another flower. The stigma protrudes from the centre of most flowers and is the only entrance way to a hidden cavity, deep inside the flower, which contains the egg cell. However, it is not an open entrance. The pollen has to work to get its male cell through the stigma to the egg, and this is the key to its 'behaviour' when it reaches a stigma – or a nose.

In wind-pollinated flowers, the stigma is often feathery to maximize its chance of catching any pollen floating past in the air, and slightly moist, so that pollen tends to stick to it. The moisture of the stigma tells the pollen grain that it has hit its target.

From that moment, the pollen grain is in a hurry. Only one pollen grain can fertilize each egg cell, and there may be other pollen grains elsewhere on the stigma, racing to be the first there.

Microscopes reveal pollen grains as incredibly beautiful little objects, with intricately sculpted surfaces. Like most things in nature, this exquisite piece of 'decoration' actually serves a purpose, playing a part in the race for fertilization, as we shall see.

Pollen grains

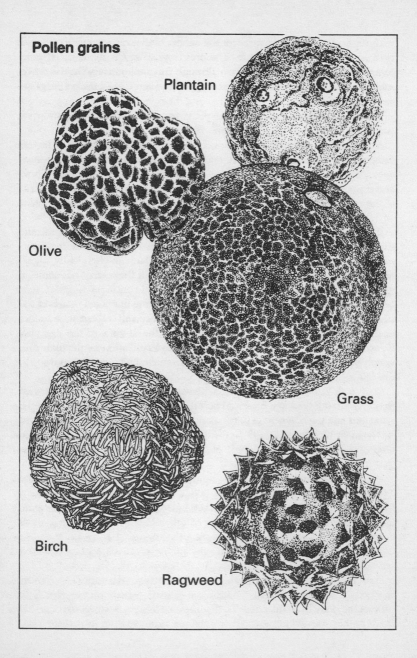

Plantain

Olive

Grass

Birch

Ragweed

The egg cell, which is the prize for the winner of that race, is safely enclosed by a solid mass of green tissue. The only way to reach the egg cell is to penetrate the stigma, forcing a way through the apparently solid tissue. To achieve this, and to get there before competing pollen grains, the pollen grain has to react promptly.

Within a few seconds of landing on the stigma, the pollen grain discharges chemicals, specific types of **proteins** that are characteristic of the plant species. And this is where the intricately sculpted pollen coat comes in. The proteins to be discharged first are held in the crevices of the pollen grain's outer coat, lightly sealed in by a fatty layer, ready for a quick release. These first proteins act as chemical passwords, revealing the identity of the pollen to the receiving plant. Only if the pollen comes from the right sort of plant will the stigma allow it to compete for the egg.

If it passes this first test, the pollen grain's next task is to penetrate the stigma by literally growing into it. To achieve this it produces more chemicals, special types of protein known as **enzymes**, that can chemically 'chew' holes in the fabric of the stigma. Hot on the heels of these enzymes comes a special cell that grows out of the pollen grain, and continues to grow, very fast and straight, pushing its way through the enzyme-damaged tissues of the stigma towards the egg cell. If successful, this pioneering cell creates a tunnel leading from the pollen grain straight down the stigma to the egg cell. Known as the pollen tube, this is the highway to fertilization for the male cell, which now emerges from the pollen grain to make its triumphal journey to the egg.

Only a few lucky pollen grains will achieve such fulfilment. The vast majority are doomed to a brief and pointless existence, floating about on the wind and landing nowhere in particular. Some of these end their days caught on the inner membranes that line the human nose: the nose exists in order to filter air before it gets to the lungs, and pollen grains are among the particles that it removes.

Unfortunately, most pollen grains cannot tell the difference between a nose and a stigma. Both are moist, and the pollen grain that lands in a nose reacts just as if it had landed on a stigma – it promptly discharges the proteins from its outer coat, followed by a battery of other chemicals, including those enzymes whose rightful job is to penetrate the stigma.

This could be part of the reason why pollen provokes such a powerful reaction from some human noses – its behaviour, as 'interpreted' by the human body, is highly suspect. Hayfever is, in effect, an attack on pollen by the body's defensive system, or **immune system**, whose proper role is to protect the body from infection. To the immune system, a small particle that lands in the nose and immediately discharges proteins from its surface could very well be a living invader, intent on penetrating the body. The pollen's behaviour is actually quite harmless, but it could seem suspiciously like that of a parasitic intruder, and so trigger a violent immune reaction.

Although many other substances cause an allergic reaction in some noses (substances as diverse as mould spores and dried-up cat saliva) none can match pollen in the sheer numbers of people affected. Pollen provokes more allergies than any other substance and this could well be due to the apparently aggressive behaviour of the pollen grain on landing in the nose. However, as we shall see in Chapter Four, pollen was disregarded by the immune system of most human beings before 1800, and hayfever has only become common during the twentieth century. Somehow, the noses of our ancestors could distinguish pollen from parasites.

How did they do it and why have things changed? These are questions to which there are no definite answers yet, but Chapter Four will consider the most likely possibilities.

KNOW YOUR ENEMY – HOW THE IMMUNE SYSTEM DOES IT

The immune system will be explained in greater detail in Chapter Three, but one crucial fact should be mentioned here. If the immune system is to fight off a parasite, or any other disease-causing microbe, it must be able to recognize that microbe. More importantly, it must distinguish it from the body's own cells and from the many harmless substances it encounters. It generally does so by recognizing particular chemicals carried on the invader's surface.

These are chemicals with individual and highly recognizable features, the chemical equivalent of a distinctive aquiline nose, a mole on the chin, or unusually bushy eyebrows – features that make a particular face quite unmistakable. These distinctive recognition features are called **epitopes**, and the chemicals that carry them are known as **antigens**.

Hayfever is an **allergy**, a particularly violent type of immune reaction that is mistakenly directed against a harmless item such as pollen, dust or food. (There will be more on allergies in Chapter Three.) Allergic reactions only affect certain people, and they are different from other immune reactions in many ways, but in one respect they are the same – they depend on the body specifically recognizing particular antigens. In this case, however, the antigens are often referred to as **allergens**, to emphasize the fact that they help to cause allergies.

It takes a special sort of chemical to act as an allergen, and only a tiny minority of proteins fit the bill, which is some small comfort for those prone to allergy. Medical researchers believe that the shape and chemical details of the proteins play a part in determining which ones act as allergens, but they are still trying to discover exactly what it is that makes them special.

UNDERSTANDING PROTEINS

The majority of antigens are made of **protein**, a word that is worth explaining because it is so widely misunderstood. Most people think of protein as something they must have in their diet. This is entirely correct, but there is much more to proteins than that. They are a wonderfully diverse group of chemicals that are the mainstay of all living bodies. They allow animals to move about (muscle proteins), they make up the skin, hair and nails (keratin), carry oxygen in the blood (haemoglobin), and support and shape every organ of the body.

Most importantly, they get things done, chemically speaking. The proteins known as **enzymes** act as catalysts in the body, chemical entrepreneurs that turn one substance into another, build things up if they are needed, and break them down if they are not. Without enzymes, there would be no life, and plants use them just as much as animals do.

In the case of hayfever, proteins are of prime interest as **allergens**, the provokers of allergic reactions. Such reactions are the work of the **immune system**, which exists to defend the body against disease.

Because proteins are highly individual and distinctive chemicals, they are particularly useful to the body's immune system, acting as markers or 'identity badges'. For example, the proteins on the outer coat of a *Salmonella* bacterium are very different from those on the coat of a harmless bacterium living normally in the gut, and the immune system uses these proteins to tell the difference. A cell in the nose that is infected with influenza virus has typical influenza proteins on its surface, which are not normally there, and the immune system responds to these by destroying the infected cell. In both these cases the proteins are acting as **antigens** – molecules that stimulate the immune system. An allergen is simply an antigen that provokes allergic reactions by the body, rather than any other type of immune reaction.

THE THREE FACTORS IN HAYFEVER

So far, we have identified three characteristics that can make pollen into a hayfever provoker: being spread by the wind, discharging its proteins rapidly in the nose, and having allergenic proteins.

The last of these factors is undoubtedly the most crucial. Of the quarter of a million flowering plants, it is only a small minority – as few as 1 per cent – that contain allergenic proteins. And within those offending pollen grains, there are often only two or three proteins that act as major allergens, out of the 20–40 proteins which they release into the nose.

The first factor, being spread by the wind, is also important, as we have already seen (p2). Pollen that is carried by insects rarely causes hayfever, except in situations where people are exposed to unusually large amounts

SNEEZE-FREE GRASSES

Since most plants are both male and female (see pp1–2), they could, in theory, fertilize themselves. A few plants have in fact become self-pollinators, producing pollen but keeping it within the flower, where it pollinates the same flower's egg cells. Although some of this pollen does escape inadvertently, there is not a great deal of it floating about in the air, and it is therefore unlikely to produce hayfever.

Several cereal crops are among the self-pollinators, including wheat, barley, oats and rice. Since these are grasses (like all cereal crops), anyone allergic to grass pollen might expect to react badly to fields of these crops. They can relax, however, in the knowledge that self-pollinators release very little pollen unless there is substantial disturbance to the plants, which can break the flowers open. Only the most sensitive individuals, or those who work closely with such plants, are likely to react.

Not all cereal crops are self-pollinating. Rye cross-pollinates, as does millet. Maize is cross-pollinating, but the pollen causes relatively few problems (see p14). Sorghum is largely self-pollinated, but can release quite large amounts of pollen. Sugar cane, another grass, is a cross-pollinator and allergenic, but in many areas where it is grown (e.g: the Caribbean islands) it is harvested before it flowers.

every day. Even among wind-pollinated plants, however, there are some that fail to produce hayfever because their pollen does not travel far enough or remain airborne for long enough. Maize (also called corn or sweetcorn) is a good example. Although it is wind-pollinated, and has allergenic proteins like most members of the grass family, maize is not often a cause of hayfever. This is probably because its pollen grains are relatively large and do not travel far in the air. The enormous stigmas of the maize flower – the silky 'tassels' that extend from the top of the corn cob – are probably so efficient in picking up pollen grains that dense clouds of pollen in the air are unnecessary.

The remaining factor of the three is the seemingly 'aggressive' behaviour of pollen grains in rapidly discharging proteins when they encounter a moist surface, such as the lining of the nose. It is likely that, combined with allergenic proteins, this characteristic makes pollen a powerful challenge to the immune system. Some pollen grains do not behave in this way, notably those of pines, which have a thick, waxy covering and a built-in delay that prevents them from starting to grow a pollen tube immediately. Their reticent attitude towards releasing proteins may help to make these pollen grains less allergenic, but other factors probably play a large part as well, particularly the nature of their proteins.

Chapter Two

THE SYMPTOMS OF HAYFEVER

One of the greatest honours of a successful medical career is to have a disease named after you. For many years the medical profession used the term 'Bostock's catarrh' for hayfever, in memory of John Bostock, a London physician who, in 1819, reported the strange case of a patient with 'a periodical affection of the eyes and chest'. The patient was Bostock himself, and he attributed his symptoms (which were highly unusual in those days) to the heat and sunshine of summer.

His failure to identify the real cause lost Bostock his chance of medical immortality. By the 1820s, a fair number of the public were similarly afflicted, mainly those of the upper classes, and they became convinced that the new disease was 'produced by the effluvium from new hay'. To suffer from this novel disease was a sign of good breeding; it became something of a fad, and the public, or the newspapers perhaps, thought up the term 'hayfever'. Doctors of the day rejected the explanation, deplored the fashionable nature of the disease, and disliked the name. But it happened that the public was right about hay, while Bostock and his colleagues were wrong, so the name 'hayfever' stuck.

Although many doctors now use 'pollinosis' for this disease (see p3), the term 'hayfever' is not entirely inappropriate because some patients actually do feel feverish and sweat easily during the pollen season. However, their temperatures are usually normal, and feverishness is not the most typical symptom of hayfever: the major reactions to pollen occur in the nose and eyes.

An attack of hayfever often begins with an unpleasant, itchy sensation in the mouth, nose, throat and eyes. This is a sign that the allergic reaction to the pollen (described more fully in Chapter Three) has begun. Shortly after this, symptoms begin in the nose, with volleys of sneezes, a runny nose, or a completely blocked nose.

Sneezing is a natural reflex that serves to remove bothersome particles from the nose by expelling them violently. The production of large amounts of mucus serves a similar end – it is intended to flush the unwanted items out of the nose. The fact that the symptoms persist suggests that neither response is of much use in expelling pollen, probably because each new breath brings in a fresh supply. Thus the sneezing and the runny nose are part of a frustrated and futile effort to eject pollen from the nose.

A blocked nose occurs for different reasons. In this case, the degree of **inflammation** in the nose is so great that the delicate membranes swell up and block the air passages. 'Inflammation' is a term used to describe the reaction which occurs whenever there is an intense immune response in a particular area of the body. This reaction is usually characterized by swelling and redness (hence 'in flames'). Inflammation in the nose produces no obvious redness, but the swelling is very apparent to those who find that they can no longer breathe with their mouth closed!

A blocked nose can make it difficult to sleep, and constant breathing through the mouth may lead to dryness of the tongue and throat. For some hayfever sufferers, there is also a loss of the sense of smell. (This seemingly trivial symptom can prove fatal if there is something ablaze in the kitchen and you are watching television, oblivious to the smell. Fitting smoke detectors in the home is a good idea for anyone whose sense of smell is lost, either permanently or temporarily.)

SYMPTOMS IN THE EYE

Hayfever often involves the eyes just as much as the nose, and it is the eye symptoms that can help to distinguish it from the common cold, and to some extent from allergies to other airborne substances such as mould spores and house dust. Given the way air flows around the body, particles of different sizes and shapes move around us in different ways, and settle out of the air at different points on the body's surface. The size of pollen grains makes them especially likely to flow close to the eye as we walk or run about, and to stick to its moist surface.

When the eyes react allergically to pollen, they first tend to water copiously. In the normal, healthy eye, tear fluid is secreted all the time and flows across the surface of the eye, then drains away down a tiny tube, called the tear duct, that leads from the inner corner of the eye to the nose. In doing so, it sweeps away dust and bacteria, keeping the eye clean and disease-free. The reaction to pollen during the hayfever season is simply an exaggerated version of this normal cleansing process.

PHILIP

Philip developed hayfever very early in life, when he was only six years old. His parents were aware that he sneezed a lot in the summer and always had a runny nose, but they had no idea that there was anything wrong with his eyes as well. When Philip was referred to a consultant allergist by his family doctor, the allergist noticed that Philip blinked a great deal. The family had always put this down to shyness. As well as a nose spray, the allergist prescribed eye drops for Philip, containing a drug that prevents the allergic reaction from occurring. After using the drops for a while, Philip reported that his eyes felt 'not so itchy', although he had never mentioned that there was anything wrong with them before. His blinking decreased noticeably.

Philip is not unusual in suffering symptoms in the eye. An allergic reaction to pollen often involves the eyes, although most people think of hayfever as mainly affecting the nose. Just occasionally, patients have symptoms in the eye alone.

As Philip showed, small children may not always think to tell an adult exactly what is wrong with them, or they may not know how to describe their symptoms clearly. Parents and doctors alike need to question children carefully and sometimes observe them closely (as this allergist did) in order to find out exactly what is wrong with them.

One of the consequences of a blocked nose, or a nose that is producing a great deal of watery mucus, is that the tear duct runs into a dead end, or an already flooded channel. Either way, the tear fluid cannot seep away, so an overflow occurs at the top of the tear duct. Since there may well be more tears from the eye anyway, the overflow can become a steady stream of tears down the face. The effect is similar to a heavy storm on a house whose drainpipes are already choked with leaves.

Watery eyes, however, are only a minor symptom. In some people there is also **conjunctivitis**, inflammation of the outer surface of the eyeball, the **conjunctiva**. The effect is to produce soreness, redness and severe itching of the eyes. *Occasionally conjunctivitis is the only sign of hayfever, with no symptoms in the nose at all.*

Anyone who wears contact lenses and also suffers from hayfever is likely to find the lenses especially uncomfortable during the pollen season. Some people have to revert to glasses for a few weeks at the height of the season. However, certain types of lens, or certain cleaning solutions, may be aggravating the sore eyes, and a change may make it possible to keep wearing lenses all year round. A good optician should be able to advise you on this point. Bear in mind that glasses can help to keep pollen out of the eyes (see p121), so abandoning lenses for a while may have a double benefit.

Some people are unfortunate enough to suffer far more serious eye problems, ranging from swollen eyelids to very severe inflammation in the eye that can lead to blistering or ulceration. Needless to say, severe inflammation requires prompt medical treatment as there is a risk of blindness.

NO NOSE IS AN ISLAND TO ITSELF

If your nose is inflamed and unhappy, the chances are that it will affect some other organ. The nose, after all, is connected to the mouth, the lungs, the ears and the sinuses. Its malaise can spread to all these organs.

The sinuses

The sinuses are air-filled cavities within the bones of the skull, which serve no other purpose than to make it a lighter burden for the neck to bear. No cavity in the body can afford to be unprotected, so the sinuses are lined with delicate membranes that connect up with those lining the nose. The membranes are there to supply blood and immune cells to the sinus cavities.

Since these cavities are rather isolated, peaceful cul-de-sacs that usually remain free of infection or inflammation, most people are unaware that they even exist. When they do become infected or inflamed, however, they can cause a gnawing pain in the face which makes the location of the sinuses all too clear. And if the problem does not clear up of its own accord, but requires medical attention, their relative inaccessibility within the skull becomes something of a disadvantage because they are not open to direct treatment. Antibiotics taken by mouth, which are carried to the membranes of the sinus cavities in the blood, are the usual form of treatment.

Most cases of **sinusitis** stem from an infection that begins in the nose and spreads outwards. However, allergic reactions in the nose can also spread to the sinuses, producing a headache over the eyes, if the frontal sinuses are involved, or an aching in the cheeks if the maxillary sinuses are affected.

There is one very simple treatment that is worth trying for sinusitis. First, take a deep breath in. Then hold your nose, shut your mouth and blow hard. This creates high pressure in the nasal cavity, which may open up the blocked passages to the sinus cavities.

THE OVER-DOSED CHILD

Children with recurrent attacks of sinusitis have often been given repeated courses of antibiotics by their doctor. Tackling their allergy problems can relieve the sinusitis, but the child may still be generally unwell. Common symptoms are tiredness, colic and a pale face with dark rings under the eyes. They may also have itchiness around the anus. These symptoms seem to be a result of the antibiotics, which have disturbed the **gut flora**, the beneficial bacteria that are normally found in a healthy person's intestine. It is probably an overgrowth of yeasts (one-celled fungi) in the gut that causes the problem – these yeasts are present in everyone, but their numbers are kept in check by the bacteria present. Children with these symptoms are often helped by a course of the anti-fungal drug nystatin. This is a very safe drug with virtually no side-effects.

Children with allergies to pollen or house-dust mite (see p172), or both, are sometimes afflicted with recurrent bouts of sinusitis. Often these children are treated with a course of antibiotics each time, and the antibiotics achieve some partial success, suggesting that an infection is playing its part in the symptoms. However, experience in allergy clinics shows that when these children's allergies are dealt with, their regular bouts of sinusitis often disappear. It cannot be good to dose children with antibiotics regularly and unnecessarily, so if allergy treatment can remove the symptoms instead, this is surely preferable.

The ear

Most people only discover their **Eustachian tube** twice a year – on the way to their summer holiday and on the way back. It is a small piece of plumbing that functions perfectly well until you ascend or descend in an aeroplane.

The Eustachian tube runs from the middle ear (the chamber behind the eardrum) down to the nasal cavity. The function of this tube is to drain any fluid from the ear, and to allow air to get from the nose into the middle ear. This ensures that the air pressure in the middle ear is equalized with that outside the eardrum. If the pressure is higher on one side than the other, the eardrum bulges away from the high pressure, causing intense pain. Normally this does not occur because every time you swallow or yawn the

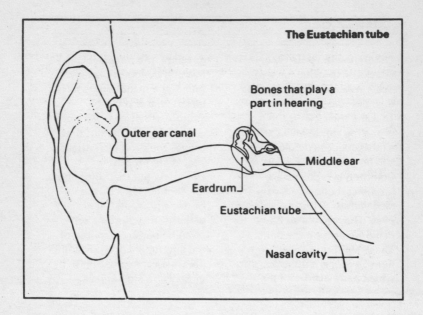

The Eustachian tube

Bones that play a part in hearing

Outer ear canal

Middle ear

Eardrum

Eustachian tube

Nasal cavity

Eustachian tube is opened wide and air can rush into the middle ear from the nose, or out from the middle ear through the nose.

When you go up in an aeroplane, however, the pressure in the cabin falls slightly, and this affects the outer part of the ear immediately. The middle ear has to 'catch up' by expelling air through the nose, thus lowering its pressure. As the plane descends, the reverse process is needed. Chewing gum or sucking a sweet speeds up the process, as the repeated swallowing opens the Eustachian tube every few seconds. Falling asleep during ascent or descent can result in severe earache, as swallowing occurs much less frequently and the pressure gets little chance to equalize.

So much for the Eustachian tube in flight; how does it react in hayfever? Problems arise when the build-up of mucus in the nose is so great that it works its way up into the Eustachian tube and blocks it off. Air can no longer get into the middle ear, so pressure cannot be equalized, which may cause 'popping' or a 'stuffy feeling' in the ears, or mild earache. A few people notice that their hearing is not quite as good as usual. For hayfever sufferers, the symptoms are unlikely to get any worse than this, but a few children with hayfever suffer from 'glue ear' (see p176) as a secondary effect. Usually this occurs when they have other allergies as well, to substances such as house dust, which are present all year round.

Itching in the ears is another unpleasant symptom, and it is of little comfort to most sufferers to discover that it is probably illusory! There is no allergic reaction in the ears themselves to produce itching. It seems to arise because the nerves leading from the nose to the brain run alongside those leading from the ears. If the interconnections between these particular nerves are less than perfect, there could be a 'crossed wire' on the way to the brain, with the result that an itchy sensation in the nose can be attributed, by the brain, to itchiness in the inner ear. (Occasionally, intense itchiness in the ears is the only symptom of rhinitis, apart from a slightly runny nose. Such patients usually turn out to be allergic to house-dust mites, but they may need a skin-prick test, see p78, to be sure.)

The lungs and airways

One simple way in which the nose can affect the airways is through **post-nasal drip**. The mucus in the nose builds up to such an extent that some trickles from the back of the nose, down the throat and into the **trachea**, the tube that leads to the lungs. This mucus has to be coughed up later, which is why some hayfever sufferers find that they constantly need to clear their throats. However, the mucus does not generally cause any serious problems. Occasionally, the sheer quantity of it being coughed up and then swallowed can upset the stomach.

Deeper down in the chest, the trachea branches into two tubes, the **bronchi**, which lead to the lungs. It is the bronchi that produce attacks of **asthma**, and asthma is sometimes a response to pollen, although there are many other potential causes.

In the walls of each bronchus there are layers of muscle which can contract suddenly, making the bronchus much narrower so that it lets through less air. When this happens, asthmatics find it difficult to exhale and their breath, whistling through the narrowed bronchi, produces a characteristic 'wheezing' sound. Because they cannot exhale properly, they cannot inhale either, and they feel short of breath and uncomfortably tight in the chest. (During more severe attacks, asthmatics may feel as though they are suffocating, but such attacks are rare with pollen asthma.) In most cases, the asthma attack passes as the bronchi relax, but a severe asthma attack can be fatal and should always be taken seriously. Advice on dealing with asthma is given in Chapter Five.

Pollen does not need to actually reach the bronchi in order to bring on pollen-induced asthma: this can simply be a **reflex reaction** to pollen in the nose. A reflex is an automatic reaction produced by the nerves linking two parts of the body. Presumably the reflex exists so that the nose can alert the bronchi to the arrival of unwanted substances in the air, which the bronchi

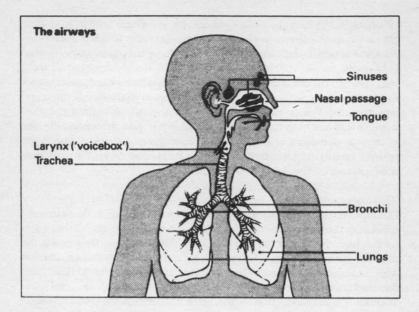

The airways

Sinuses

Nasal passage

Tongue

Larynx ('voicebox')

Trachea

Bronchi

Lungs

can help to keep out of the lung if they contract a little. In an asthmatic attack, however, the contraction of the bronchi has gone way beyond any useful function.

The automatic link between nose and bronchi reveals how important it can be to treat rhinitis. Doctors have found that by treating the symptoms in the nose (with a nasal spray, for example) they can make asthmatic attacks less severe or less frequent, or both. Given the serious nature of asthma, this is undoubtedly worthwhile.

Even those hayfever sufferers with no signs of asthma often show an interesting change in the bronchi during the pollen season. Their bronchi are described as 'hyperresponsive', which means that they will contract far more readily if submitted to a standard medical test with a substance known to cause bronchial contraction. Whether this hyperresponsive state can produce symptoms is unknown, but it might if the hayfever sufferer were exposed to an irritant such as sulphur dioxide (see p320), ozone (see p319) or cold air.

Although a reflex reaction from the nose can produce asthma, for many pollen-sensitive asthmatics there is also a direct effect of pollen allergens on the bronchi. This raises an interesting question because most airborne pollen grains are too large for them to reach the bronchi (see p23), except in small numbers. Air has to travel through the nose or mouth and down the trachea before it reaches the bronchi, and most pollen grains never get that far. These relatively large particles are filtered out by the nose, and, even if someone has a badly blocked nose and is breathing entirely through the mouth, most settle in the trachea.

So how can pollen allergens reach the bronchi? In 1972 American researchers working on ragweed discovered that in releasing pollen, plants may also release much smaller particles that contain pollen allergens. The part of the flower which produces the pollen, known as the **anther**, may disintegrate as the pollen is shed. Since the anther contributed the proteins found in the pollen grain wall, it is not surprising to discover that it still contains some of those proteins. As it disintegrates, tiny particles containing these proteins – one of which is a powerful ragweed allergen – are scattered on the breeze. These particles are only a quarter the size of the ragweed pollen grain – five thousandths of a millimetre, compared to twenty thousandths of a millimetre. When inhaled, they reach the bronchi unhindered.

For a long time it was thought that these pollen-like fragments might be unique to ragweed, but researchers in Australia have now discovered equally allergenic particles coming from rye grass plants. And in 1991 scientists found that Japanese red cedar also produces tiny fragments, far smaller than pollen itself, containing some of the pollen allergens. It now seems likely that many plants release allergenic pollen fragments, as well as pollen itself.

Those who have both hayfever and pollen asthma find that the asthma attacks usually begin later in the pollen season than the hayfever symptoms, suggesting that repeated exposure is needed. However, the asthma may also continue long after the pollen season has ended because the sensitivity in the airways, once established, tends to perpetuate itself. Often, asthma that begins as a response to pollen, continues throughout the year and eventually becomes a permanent part of life. An attack can then be brought on by all sorts of allergens and irritants, not just pollen. This tendency for asthma to self-perpetuate makes a powerful argument for using the available treatments during the pollen season, rather than letting hayfever and pollen asthma 'run their course'.

Asthma is well known as a disorder that can be influenced by many different factors, some physical and some psychological. Often, the allergen alone merely makes an attack likely, while some other factor must come into play for the attack to start. In the case of pollen-induced asthma, for example, it sometimes takes a bout of vigorous exercise, as well as the presence of pollen in the air, to trigger an asthma attack. Psychological factors might also play a part (see p72).

RAY

Ray had suffered from hayfever since he was a boy, and simply accepted the problem, rarely taking any medicines for it. In his mid-thirties he and his wife decided to move out of the city and bought a dilapidated cottage in the country. They moved in at the height of a beautiful summer and began clearing away the accumulated dirt of many years. Dust filled the air – and Ray's nose. He began to sneeze a little and within a few days he had a strange and unfamiliar feeling of tightness in his chest. During the following weeks, harvesting began in the surrounding fields, with several huge combine-harvesters working away all day and night. Ray noticed that, when outdoors, his eyes began to stream and the tightness in his chest became more noticeable. A few more days passed and Ray found it harder to breathe, so he reluctantly went to see the doctor. The diagnosis was asthma, and since that time Ray has had to carry an inhaler containing a bronchodilator (see p106) in his pocket wherever he goes.

Ray's case shows how someone who is already sensitized to pollen may be vulnerable to developing asthma. With Ray it was a massive dose of house dust, followed by the dust and mould spores generated during a cereal harvest. Since cereals are grasses, the dust that their dried leaves produce may well contain some of the same allergens (see p11) as grass pollen – allergens to which Ray was already sensitive.

UNUSUAL REACTIONS TO POLLEN

There are some unusual reactions to pollen that do not involve the eyes, nose or airways. Some are quite serious, but fortunately these are very rare.

Reactions in the digestive system include an upset stomach or, in a few instances, colitis, an inflammation of the large bowel. These conditions could be produced by pollen that settles on food and is eaten, or by pollen that is inhaled and caught in the saliva, then swallowed.

Reactions in the skin include the allergic form of eczema, and another allergic reaction known as urticaria, or nettle rash, because it produces large, itchy bumps on the skin. In these reactions, bare areas of skin could be

ELIZABETH

Elizabeth had suffered hayfever in the spring since she was nine years old, and hayfever in the late summer since she was fifteen. When she was twenty-one, she developed an unpleasant itchy rash on her hands during August. This died down of its own accord at the end of September, and only a trace of the rash remained during the winter and spring. The following August it flared up again, and this was repeated in the third year. The doctor tried skin-prick tests (see p78), but these gave many positive results; Elizabeth reacted to house dust, mould spores, feathers, wool, skin particles from cats and dogs, various foods and many different pollens. It was impossible to tell which of these allergens might be causing the problem, and the doctor remained puzzled.

By chance, Elizabeth discovered the cause herself. The following summer she happened to take a holiday in late August in a mountainous area, far from her home town. Here her rash cleared up, at the same time as her hayfever vanished. The vegetation in the mountains was quite different from that at home, and one of the weeds whose pollen had produced a major reaction on skin-prick testing did not grow there. Clearly, this weed pollen was producing both hayfever and the rash on her hands.

acquiring a dusting of pollen and reacting directly to this. Alternatively, pollen antigens that have entered the bloodstream (through tiny blood vessels in the nose) could reach the skin by this indirect route.

When urticaria occurs on the ankles after walking through grass, it is clear that direct contact is triggering off the allergic response. While the pollen in the grass may be the prime culprit, its effects may be worsened by the juice that oozes from crushed grass leaves, because the leaves and stems of a plant often share allergens with its pollen. This is why some people with grass-pollen hayfever are so badly affected by mowing a lawn, even though the grass is not in flower. The action of the mower blades turns the grass juice into an **aerosol** of tiny airborne droplets that are inhaled by anyone near the mower. A few people experience allergic reactions when cutting privet hedges, and again the reaction may be to the juice of the crushed leaves, as well as the pollen.

Among the very rare reactions to pollen are kidney disorders. As already mentioned, allergens from inhaled pollen pass into the bloodstream from the nose. The blood then carries them to all parts of the body, including the kidneys. Here the blood is purified in a process that involves it passing through very fine tubes. A strong immune reaction to pollen in the blood can affect the tiny blood vessels (**capillaries**) that lie around those tubes, and stop the filtering process from functioning fully. The symptoms include puffiness, especially around the face and hands, and cloudy urine which is also unusually plentiful.

Very occasionally, hayfever sufferers also report joint pains (**arthralgia**) during the pollen season. In these cases, the underlying mechanism is probably the same as that in kidney disease: the immune reaction to pollen in the blood produces an inflammatory reaction in the blood capillaries of the joints, which results in joint pain.

Migraine is another symptom that sometimes accompanies hayfever, but this too is rare. Usually people find that their migraines occur throughout the year, but are more frequent in the pollen season. Some effect on the blood vessels, due to the immune response to pollen, is probably responsible for this reaction.

RELATED CONDITIONS

Hayfever is just one form of **rhinitis**, the technical term for inflammation (*-itis*) in the nose (*rhin-*). The more precise term **allergic rhinitis** is usually employed, to make it clear that this reaction is due to an allergy rather than to a cold or any other cause. Various forms of **non-allergic rhinitis** are also known, and some of these are discussed in Chapter Thirteen.

Not all allergic rhinitis is due to pollen. Several other airborne allergens can produce these irritating reactions in the nose, the most common ones being house dust (or rather the allergens it contains, mainly those produced by mites), and particles from cats or other pets. In all these cases the symptoms are generally less violent than in hayfever, but this is small compensation for the fact that they may well last all year round.

Apart from pollen, the only allergens to produce strictly seasonal symptoms are mould spores, the tiny airborne 'seeds' of moulds and other fungi. In temperate climates these become much more abundant in autumn, when fallen leaves and dead plants are infested with moulds. Some mould-sensitive patients are only affected then, but others may experience symptoms all year round, especially if they live in damp houses, where moulds abound.

Chapter Twelve looks in more detail at the various allergens, other than pollen, that can cause allergic rhinitis.

Chapter Three

WHAT GOES WRONG IN HAYFEVER?

In the early 1980s a boy in Houston, Texas, suddenly became famous throughout the world. He was photographed by newspapers and magazines, and filmed by television crews as he played, ate and slept inside a large plastic 'bubble'. The boy had spent his entire life, since early infancy, inside the bubble, sealed off from normal human contact. He could not even breathe the air that most people breathe because he had been born without a fully functioning **immune system** (the system that defends our bodies from disease). The air going into the bubble was treated to remove bacteria and viruses. Food was sterilized before being passed in through a special protected entry-port. The boy in the bubble was healthy, but only because his world had been made unnaturally safe.

At the age of twelve, surgeons attempted to transplant bone marrow from a relative. Bone marrow is the major source of immune cells in the body and such transplants can sometimes re-create a functional immune system. Unfortunately, the operation failed and the boy died.

The case of this little boy, and other children like him, suddenly makes us uncomfortably aware of how dangerous the natural world really is. The fact that we are normally oblivious to these dangers is a testament to the efficiency of our immune systems in dealing with the constant threats from disease-causing microbes.

The immune system comes into play even before we are born, although it is aided, at that stage, by immunity provided by the mother. At birth, a baby still carries some of this **passive immunity** acquired from its mother, and continues to be protected for many months. During this time, the baby's own immune system is maturing and taking stock of the world around it. An important part of that process is learning which items entering the body need to be attacked, because they cause disease, and which do not. Among those that do not need to be attacked are **pollen grains** (see Chapter One). There are also many other harmless items that the immune system must learn to ignore, including food molecules (the chemical constituents of food), dust particles, fragments of mites and insects, and other items in the air.

If the immune system *does* attack these harmless items, and if it does so vigorously enough to produce unpleasant symptoms in the person concerned, the reaction is known as an **allergy**. (The word simply means 'altered reactivity'.) The classical allergies include hayfever, asthma, food allergy and two skin disorders, eczema and urticaria (although these are not always allergic in origin). Allergy to pollen can play a part in *all* these reactions, although it is mainly associated with hayfever.

To understand allergy, it helps to know a little about how the immune system normally works. But first a word of warning: if the immune system were a movie, it would have a cast of thousands and a very, *very* complicated plot. Most filmgoers would leave before the end. What follows is a simplified account, with many of the key players omitted, and the rest of the immune system explained as clearly as possible. Even so, it is not an easy read, and if you wish to pass quickly on to the next chapter feel free to do so – the rest of the book can still be readily understood. We believe that it is worth trying to explain immunity and allergy because such knowledge can help people in understanding their illness and in making more informed decisions about their treatment. We hope, therefore, that you will read this chapter and find it interesting, but it is not essential.

THE FIGHT AGAINST DISEASE

The immune system consists of millions of free-ranging cells which permeate the whole body – guerrilla fighters in the war against disease. The blood-stream provides an important transport route for these **immune cells**, but once they reach the parts of the body where they are needed, they must leave the bloodstream by squeezing through gaps in the blood vessel walls. The immune cells pass through the tissues of the body and may become involved in any skirmishes with invaders that are going on there.

The fluid that bathes these tissues is constantly draining into special channels called **lymphatic vessels**, and as it does so it takes the immune cells, living or dead, along with it.

Lymphatic vessels permeate the body, and are connected into larger lymph vessels – a collection and transport network known as the **lymphatic system** that most people are quite unaware they possess. The colourless fluid

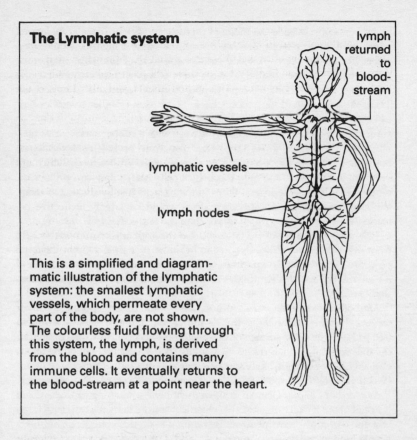

The Lymphatic system

lymph
returned
to
blood-
stream

lymphatic vessels

lymph nodes

This is a simplified and diagram-
matic illustration of the lymphatic
system: the smallest lymphatic
vessels, which permeate every
part of the body, are not shown.
The colourless fluid flowing through
this system, the lymph, is derived
from the blood and contains many
immune cells. It eventually returns to
the blood-stream at a point near the heart.

which flows through it, with its precious load of immune cells, is called
lymph.

Having been collected from the most distant parts of the body, the lymph is
eventually channelled into a single large lymph vessel, called the thoracic
duct, which pours lymph back into the bloodstream at a point near the heart.
En route to this point, the immune cells pass through **lymph nodes**. These are
concentrations of specialized immune cells that 'vet' the guerrilla fighters to
see what invaders they have encountered (they are carrying identifiable
fragments of those invaders), and then react accordingly.

It is in the lymph nodes that many **antibodies** are produced, although they
can be generated in other parts of the body as well. Of the many useful
weapons deployed by the immune system, antibodies are probably the best

known to people outside the medical profession. They are special molecules which bind to other molecules in a discriminating and highly selective way, rather like tracker dogs – one dog goes for the scent of cannabis, another for the scent of explosives, another for the scent of a particular criminal. In the same way, each antibody has a particular chemical target, called its **antigen**. These targets are used to pinpoint bacteria, viruses, or other microbes that can cause disease.

An antibody is like one of those toy arrows with a rubber sucker at its tip – all it can do is stick to its target, not penetrate or kill it. Nevertheless, antibodies can stop infections in a variety of ways. With viruses, which are very small and need to invade the body's cells before they can proliferate, antibodies may be able to stop them in their tracks just by sticking to them. With bacteria, however, antibodies alone would be largely ineffective because the bacteria are so much larger than the antibodies (see pp36–7).

Help is needed to defeat the bacteria, and the antibodies summon this help from other cells and molecules in the immune system, ones that have the power to kill. Frequently, hundreds of antibodies stick to the outer surface of a bacterial cell and this stimulates action by the immune system's assassination teams.

Antibodies would not work unless they were highly specific for their targets, the antigens. An antigen is an individual chemical, usually a protein (see p12), on the outer surface of the invading microbe. However, molecules on the outside of other items, including pollen grains, can also act as antigens. If they did not, hayfever and other allergies would simply not occur. (When an antigen provokes an allergic reaction it is known as an **allergen**.)

As noted in Chapter One, an antigen must have something distinctive and unusual about it – an unmistakable chemical feature known as an **epitope**, by which it can easily be recognized. By homing in on this epitope, an antibody should bind to one type of antigen only, and therefore to one type of microbe only. (In practice, things are not always quite that simple and cross-reactions can occur. This is something that we will come back to later as it is an important factor in allergy.)

To combat all the many infectious microbes in the world, the body produces a vast range of different antibodies – millions of them. These antibodies are not 'tailor-made' for the antigen as you might expect, but are 'off the peg'. Very early in life, the millions of different types of antibody are generated randomly on a 'just in case they're needed' basis. (In this sense, they are quite unlike the tracker dogs mentioned earlier, which are *trained* to go for particular targets. The antibody comes into the world with the chemical nature of its target already fixed.) Most of the antibodies we generate are useless because they never meet an antigen that they can bind to. Others do encounter such an antigen and, if this turns out to be an antigen that requires an immune response, the body begins producing that antibody in large quanitities. (During this production process, the antibody may change a little so that it becomes an even better match for the allergen. It is rather like buying an off-the-peg suit, but having the sleeves shortened and the waist taken in a bit to give a perfect fit.)

This system may seem rather wasteful and badly organized, with so many antibodies being generated and then not used. But it has the merit of being able to respond instantly to any new threat that comes along. Among the millions of different antibodies waiting around for something to happen, there is bound to be at least one which binds to antigens on the new invader.

THE TWO ENDS OF THE ANTIBODY MOLECULE

An antibody molecule is shaped like a catapult. At the tips of the two arms (where the elastic should be tied on) are the sites that bind to antigen – two binding sites per antibody molecule, specific for the same sort of epitope. The other end of the molecule – the handle of the catapult – interacts with various immune cells and molecules.

Not all antibodies are the same in the 'handle' region. There are about eight different forms that the antibody 'handle' can take, giving eight different **isotypes**. The characteristics of the 'handle' region are of crucial importance because they determine which immune cells or molecules the antibody reacts with. This, in turn, determines what effect the antibody has on the rest of the immune system.

When the antibody has bound its antigen at one end, that fact is communicated to whatever is bound at the other end, which may be a potent killing cell, or a molecule with the power to cause inflammation, or some less violent immune agent that deals with things far more quietly. As a result of the differences in the 'handle' region, some antibody isotypes raise hell when they encounter their antigen, while others contain the problem with a minimum of fuss.

The isotype that causes allergy is, unfortunately, one of the hell-raisers. It is known as immunoglobulin E, or **IgE** for short, and its handle end can bind to many different immune cells. However, it has a special affinity for some of the most disruptive and damaging cells in the body, the **mast cells** and **basophils**.

THE MIGHTY MAST CELL

Mast cells and basophils are basically very similar, but they patrol different territories in the body: basophils circulate in the blood, while mast cells are found fixed to the tissues of the body, including the membranes inside the

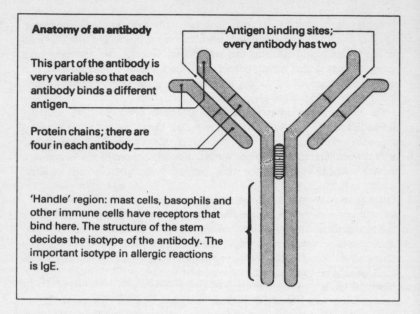

Anatomy of an antibody

Antigen binding sites; every antibody has two

This part of the antibody is very variable so that each antibody binds a different antigen

Protein chains; there are four in each antibody

'Handle' region: mast cells, basophils and other immune cells have receptors that bind here. The structure of the stem decides the isotype of the antibody. The important isotype in allergic reactions is IgE.

nose and airways. Since mast cells play the major role in hayfever, we will deal only with them from this point onwards, but basophils basically react in much the same way.

A single mast cell can carry as many as 100,000 IgE molecules on its surface. To trigger a reaction by the mast cell, several IgE molecules on its surface have to bind to the same antigen – they must be cross-linked by that antigen molecule. While IgE molecules are the major trigger for mast cells, however, they are not the only ones. Different triggers probably produce different levels of reaction in the mast cell.

Mast cells are packed full of large, round granules. Each granule contains a cocktail of powerful chemicals that can produce dramatic effects on the body when released. Among these chemicals are **histamine** and **leukotrienes**. The first of these will already be familiar to many hayfever sufferers because drugs that block the effects of histamine, called **antihistamines**, are widely used for hayfever. (Histamine is also found in the sting of a nettle plant, which injects it under the skin by means of sharp, hollow hairs. The hot, itchy bump that a nettle sting produces is an indication of what histamine can do to the tissues of the body.)

Within a few years, 'anti-leukotrienes' may join antihistamines in the fight against allergy. In the past, drug companies have not taken much interest in

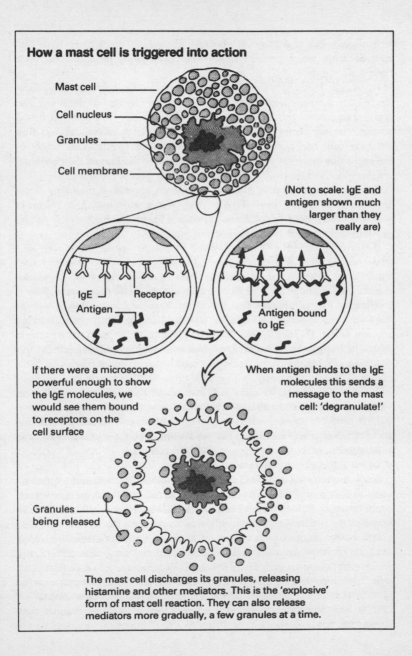

How a mast cell is triggered into action

Mast cell

Cell nucleus

Granules

Cell membrane

(Not to scale: IgE and antigen shown much larger than they really are)

IgE Receptor

Antigen

Antigen bound to IgE

If there were a microscope powerful enough to show the IgE molecules, we would see them bound to receptors on the cell surface

When antigen binds to the IgE molecules this sends a message to the mast cell: 'degranulate!'

Granules being released

The mast cell discharges its granules, releasing histamine and other mediators. This is the 'explosive' form of mast cell reaction. They can also release mediators more gradually, a few granules at a time.

leukotrienes, but that may be about to change, as researchers have discovered drugs which prevent leukotrienes from being produced, or block
their action in the body.

Histamine, leukotrienes and other chemicals in the mast cells are collectively known as **mediators** because they mediate changes in the body. The
main change they produce is an increase in the size of the tiniest blood
vessels, the capillaries. The capillaries also become more leaky so that
immune cells can pass in and out of them more easily. This produces
inflammation in the area where the mast cells have discharged their contents
– it may look red and swollen if it is in a visible part of the body.

The mast-cell mediators also act as distress signals, summoning more
immune cells to the scene. Finally, they make surrounding membranes
produce more mucus, hence the runny nose of hayfever (although this can be
partially due to other causes as well, see pp226–7).

If there are enough of these mast-cell mediators on the loose, they will
make certain types of muscle contract, including the muscles that surround
the **bronchi**, the tubes leading to the lungs. Contraction of these muscles
narrows the bronchi, and the hollow core can be made narrower still by a
swelling of the membranes that line them. This swelling is due to inflammation. Extra mucus may also be produced inside the bronchi, making
matters worse. These three reactions can all contribute to an asthma attack,
when the bronchi become so narrow that breathing is difficult (see p21).

A mast cell has dozens of granules stored inside it, and it can let off these
chemical bombs gradually, a few at a time, or all at once in a massive
'explosion'. In general, far more is known about the spectacular explosions
(which involve IgE as the trigger) than about the gradual piecemeal reactions
(which probably involve other triggering mechanisms). Exactly what role
these different reactions have is not yet known, especially in the case of the
milder reactions, but we can make educated guesses.

Given the evidence now available, it seems likely that the two types of
reaction are directed at different groups of invaders. The massive explosions
seem to play a major part in combating large parasites such as tapeworms,
round worms and liver-flukes. Unlike bacteria, which are small enough to be
engulfed by a suitable immune cell, these worms and flukes are veritable
giants being attacked by an army of Lilliputian immune cells (see p36).
Because of their great size, they need some special and rather drastic immune reactions to combat them. If mast cells lining the intestine release all
their histamine and other chemicals simultaneously, the violent muscular
spasms that follow, along with the inflammation and prolific mucus secretion, may be enough to dislodge many of the parasitic worms that have
made their home there.

The gentler bit-by-bit release of granules probably plays a part in entirely different immune reactions, perhaps in those directed against bacteria, or in the specialized defensive actions launched against viruses. A steady trickle of the mast cell's chemical contents may serve to summon other immune cells to the vicinity and keep them active there. This is largely speculative at present, but it seems plausible. For one thing, it would explain why there are so many mast cells in the eyes, nose and airways. Their presence is definitely a puzzle if mast cells are only involved in combating worms and other large parasites. None of these parasites enters the body through the eyes or nose – most come in with food, or burrow through the skin, or are transmitted by biting insects. Mast cells in the eyes, nose and airways must be there to combat some other type of invader, probably bacteria.

What seems to happen in hayfever is that the mast cells produce the violent, explosive reaction in the wrong place (the nose rather than the gut) and in reaction to the wrong items (pollen rather than parasites). This presumably happens because the normal control mechanisms, the restraints that keep the mast cells in check, have somehow broken down. To understand these control systems we must first return to IgE, the antibody involved in allergy.

CHECKS AND BALANCES

All immune reactions have to be controlled, and while researchers have discovered a great deal about how this is done, many details remain unclear. This, then, is 'the story so far' – an incomplete picture which we hope will be filled in by more medical research.

Antibodies are manufactured by special cells called **B cells**. B cells spend most of their lives waiting for their moment of glory to arrive, and when it *does* arrive – their particular brand of antibody is suddenly needed – they divide rapidly and produce hundreds of young B cells, all capable of mass-producing antibodies.

Each B cell, and all its offspring, produce antibodies that bind to a particular antigen because they all have the same sort of antigen-binding site (see p32). In general, they bind that antigen, and that antigen only. (There are exceptions to this, where another antigen is similar and a **cross-reaction** occurs – see p45.) By controlling the activities of particular B cells, therefore, the production of particular antibodies can be regulated.

If an item (such as a pollen grain) has been classified as 'safe' by the immune system, then various sorts of control are possible. One is to block the production of *any* antibodies to the antigens on that item. Another is to only produce antibodies of particular isotypes (see p31). By opting for the 'minimum fuss' isotypes, the immune system can clear the item out of the body

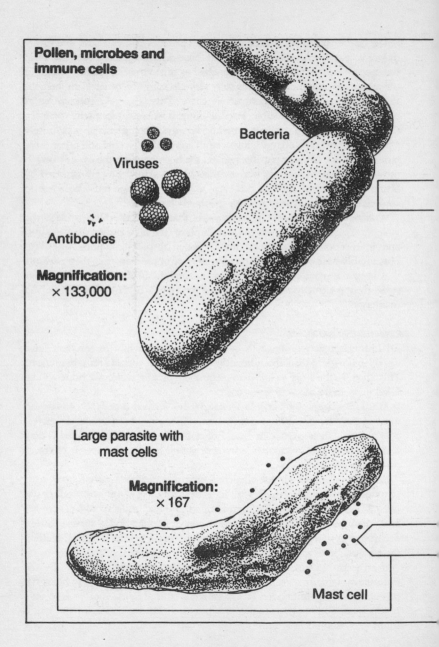

Pollen, microbes and immune cells

Bacteria

Viruses

Antibodies

Magnification: × 133,000

Large parasite with mast cells

Magnification: × 167

Mast cell

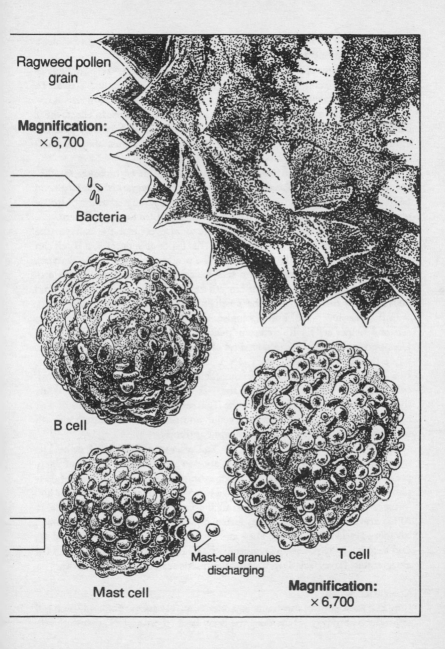

Ragweed pollen grain

Magnification:
×6,700

Bacteria

B cell

Mast cell

Mast-cell granules discharging

T cell

Magnification:
×6,700

(which may be necessary if it is plentiful) without instigating any violent, damaging reactions to it.

Both these forms of control work at the level of the B cell. The main way in which B cells are controlled is through another set of cells called **T cells**. To interact with a B cell, the T cell must be specific for the same antigen – it has receptors on its surface that are just as specific as antibodies. In effect, the T cell binds to the same antigen as the B cell (although it often goes for different epitopes on the antigen) and then issues chemical 'commands' that tell the B cell whether to start up antibody production or not.

One set of T cells, called **T helper cells**, issues the 'go' commands. Another set of T cells, called **T suppressor cells**, issues 'stop' commands. The B cell can be frozen into inaction in two ways, by the lack of a 'go' signal or the presence of a 'stop' signal, so there are two separate possibilities for control here.

T helper cells and T suppressor cells can also control the isotype (the 'handle' end) of the antibodies produced. This is possible because a B cell can change the type of 'handle' it puts on to the antibodies (change the isotype), while keeping the antigen-binding sites exactly the same. Thus, it can produce hell-raising antibodies or minimum-fuss antibodies for its antigen, and does so under the direction of the T helper cells or T suppressor cells.

In the past few years, immunologists have discovered that there are two sets of T helper cells, with different 'policies' on antibody production, rather like opposing political parties. One set of T helpers, the T_H2 set, favours IgE, while the other set, called the T_H1 set, favours less violent antibodies. The two opposing sets of helper cells issue their messages in the form of chemicals. The main chemical issued by the T_H2 set is called **interleukin 4**, while the main chemical message from the T_H1 set is **interferon gamma**. If T_H2 cells, rather than T_H1 cells, are involved in an immune reaction then IgE will be produced rather than a less damaging antibody.

But who or what decides to involve T_H2 cells rather than T_H1 cells? The answer requires us to introduce yet another set of cells, called **antigen-presenting cells**, or **APCs**. One of the appealing things about APCs is that their name tells you exactly what they do: chew up the antigen into fragments and 'present' it to other immune cells in such a way that they can 'recognize' it. APCs are plentiful in the nose, airways, skin and any other site where invaders are likely to arrive. They are the front line of the immune system, and they have the power to favour either T_H1 or T_H2 cells. The nature of the antigen they have picked up somehow influences which set they favour.

CONTROLLING IgE

Suppose these control mechanisms are not entirely successful, and some IgE is produced anyway – how does the body cope? Fortunately, there are fail-safe mechanisms which can neutralize the IgE. One is the production of a free-ranging chemical called **S-Fc epsilon RII**, which can bind to the 'handle' end of IgE and so prevent it binding to mast cells. Recent studies in Japan have shown that those prone to allergy have lower levels of S-Fc epsilon RII in their blood.

Another form of control is the production of **anti-idiotypic antibodies**. These are the immunological equivalent of highly specific anti-missile missiles (the sort of thing President Reagan had in mind for the 'Star Wars' programme). They spike the guns of an antibody by binding to its antigen-binding sites. In other words, if an IgE antibody is being made that is specific for a pollen antigen, the immune system can form *another* antibody which takes the place of the pollen at its binding sites. This prevents the pollen itself from binding.

Some patients with ragweed allergy undergoing **hyposensitizaion** (in which a series of injections of pollen extract are used to make the patient tolerant of pollen – see p135) begin producing anti-idiotypic antibodies to their ragweed IgE. This could be a factor in reducing their symptoms, although it is certainly not the only one (see below).

Whether this form of control operates normally in people who do not suffer from allergies, or those who lose their hayfever symptoms as they get older, remains to be seen. Certainly, those who spontaneously recover from hayfever in later life may still have high levels of IgE to pollen antigens, so something is acting to prevent that IgE from causing trouble. Similarly, if you take 100 people off the street and test them for high levels of IgE in their blood (or IgE to specific allergens, such as pollen or house dust), you usually find that over 30 of them have enough IgE to produce allergic symptoms. They are said to be **atopic**. Yet fewer than half of those 30 atopic people would actually suffer from allergies. Something is preventing the potentially damaging IgE molecules from doing any harm. If researchers could find out exactly what, they might be closer to preventing allergic reactions.

There are many other mechanisms involved in the allergic response and the control of allergy: we have mentioned only the major ones here. One thing which is clear from modern research is that the question 'What goes wrong in allergy?' is a pretty stupid question, because every patient is different. It is rather like asking, 'What makes a person turn to crime?' – you may be able to identify certain factors that are likely to produce criminal behaviour, but there is no single explanation that applies to everyone.

One person may get an allergy because a certain control mechanism has broken down and a backup mechanism isn't working all that well either. In a second allergic patient, both these mechanisms may be fine, but something else is at fault, something so fundamental that other control mechanisms

ATOPY AND ALLERGY

Someone who is **atopic** is producing enough IgE to develop allergies. The majority get through their lives without any sign of allergy, but about a third develop an allergy, usually as children or teenagers.

The curious thing about these people is that they may develop one allergy as babies (atopic eczema for example, or an allergy to cows' milk), lose it as they grow older, then develop a new allergy later (asthma or hayfever perhaps). The allergic tendency is there, but the allergy itself 'wanders about' from one site in the body to another. The offending allergen may change, or may stay the same.

In the same way, allergies run in families, but while a mother might have asthma, her son has eczema and food allergy, while his son later gets hayfever. It is the allergic predisposition – atopy – that is inherited, not a particular form of allergy.

cannot cancel it out. These differences explain why some people do well on one treatment, but not so well on another.

Hyposensitization treatments (see above) throw an interesting light on these control systems. Researchers have looked at the people who respond well in the hope of finding out how the treatment works. (This may or may not show how allergies are prevented naturally in healthy people.) To their surprise and consternation, they have found that all these 'cured' hayfever sufferers are actually reacting in different ways under the surface. Some show a fall in IgE levels, others do not. Most show an increase in pollen-specific antibodies of the 'minimum fuss' isotypes, but not all do. A proportion show anti-idiotypic antibodies to their pollen-specific IgE. Some have more pollen-specific T suppressor cells. Others have mast cells that are less hasty in releasing mediators after their treatment. A patient may show any mixture of these reactions.

Most intriguing of all are the patients who respond well to hyposensitization but have *no changes in their immune system as far as researchers can tell.* Nothing that doctors can currently measure has changed in these patients. This is a clear sign of just how ignorant we still are about allergic responses. Something must have changed to make these patients better, but whatever it is remains a mystery. Much is now known, but much remains to be discovered.

PRIMING

One of the unfortunate things that happens in hayfever is the reaction known as 'priming'. When an allergic reaction starts up in the nose, all sorts of chemicals are released, as already discussed. Many of those chemicals act as messengers to other cells, bringing them to the scene of the action. Among the cells that make for the nose are young cells that can develop into mast cells, and this increases the mast cell numbers. Basophils (the cells that circulate in the blood and are very similar to mast cells) also flood in. They too can produce histamine and other mediators when they encounter the pollen allergens. The result is that there are even more highly damaging immune cells available to react to the next day's intake of pollen, so that symptoms generally get worse as the pollen season progresses. Priming seems to occur in about 50 per cent of hayfever patients.

Cells known as **eosinophils** also move into the nose, particularly during the late-phase reaction (see below). They too can contribute to keeping hayfever going, even when the pollen count is falling, and can help to make the symptoms more severe.

As well as having more histamine-producing cells (mast cells and basophils), the hayfeverish nose also becomes more sensitive to histamine and reacts more strongly to it. This is probably just part of its generally increased sensitivity, since it will also take far more objection to cigarette smoke and other pollutants than it usually does (see p231). This increased sensitivity adds to the priming effect.

THE LATE-PHASE REACTION

Patients with hayfever make very good 'guinea pigs' for immunologists because they are not exposed to their allergen all year round. If a researcher can find a set of willing hayfever patients and arrange to test them with their pollen in mid-winter, he or she can see exactly what happens when they are given just one brief exposure to their allergen.

If the original diagnosis was correct, within minutes of inhaling a dose of pollen, they will all be sneezing, blowing their noses and wiping their eyes. The measurements are taken, a box of tissues provided, and in a while the symptoms pass . . . But something odd happens a few hours later: some of the 'guinea pigs' find themselves blowing their noses again, with an uncomfortable blocked-up feeling. This can begin two hours later, or as much as twelve hours later, and it affects up to half the people tested. What these patients have experienced is a **late-phase reaction**. Like the initial reaction, it too passes in time. Normally, during the pollen season, hayfever sufferers are unaware of the late-phase reaction because it simply merges with the initial reaction to a new dose of pollen being inhaled.

During the late-phase reaction, many immune cells are attracted to the nose, especially two groups known as **eosinophils** and **neutrophils**. The eosinophils, in particular, are thought to cause inflammation in the nose during the late-phase reaction.

A late-phase reaction also occurs in asthmatic patients, and it has been much more fully studied in asthma. The bronchi are generally slower to react to pollen than the nose, because fewer pollen antigens reach them (see pp22–3). But once asthmatic attacks have begun, the late-phase reaction that follows each attack helps to make the bronchi inflamed, sensitive and over-reactive, so that the smallest dose of allergen or irritant will set off a new attack. The late-phase reactions of the separate attacks eventually run together in an unbroken pattern of over-sensitivity. For this reason, asthmatic symptoms often continue long after the pollen season has ended.

Occasionally, pollen-induced asthma turns into year-round asthma as a result of these self-perpetuating reactions. Treating the asthma at an early stage, before the pattern of repeated attacks and repeated late-phase reactions is established, has obvious benefits. It can prevent the bronchi from becoming habitually inflamed and over-sensitive.

GENES AND AGE

An allergic response to a harmless substance such as pollen depends, first and foremost, on making IgE to that substance. As we have already seen, not everyone who is atopic (who makes enough IgE to suffer from allergy) actually develops allergies. Other control systems must also have failed for this to happen. In most studies, about a third of atopics are found to show allergic symptoms, but the number can be higher than this in certain circumstances.

It has been known for many years that allergies 'run in families'. Modern research has been able to show that, where some members of a family have allergies, several others are atopic but symptom-free. Clearly, the underlying tendency to allergy is inherited.

Not all members of a family will have high IgE levels, however. There are usually some 'anti-allergy genes' in the family mix, as well as the 'pro-allergy genes' that produce high IgE, and some children are lucky enough to get only the good ones.

If two people marry who *both* suffer from allergies, the outlook for their children is less promising. They are both putting in some 'pro-allergy genes', so there are more in the mix, and the chance of their children acquiring them is therefore quite high. But even people with allergies are probably carrying good versions of the relevant genes, as well as the 'pro-allergy' ones – the 'pro-allergy' version may be masking the effects of the good one. With luck, one or more of their children will get the good versions only.

Given two children who are both atopic, why does one go on to develop allergies when the other does not? (This can happen even with identical twins who have exactly the same genes and are brought up in the same household.) The last chapter of this book looks at this question more fully and considers how vulnerable children can be protected from developing hayfever and asthma. Briefly, some aspects of the environment do seem to make a difference, especially in the first year of life, but exactly how important they are is still being debated.

Although the crucial environmental influences may operate in the first year of life, it is very unusual for hayfever actually to appear then. Usually it begins many years later. Why this should be is not fully understood, but it seems clear that, in immunological terms, the scene is set for hayfever in infancy, or early childhood, whereas the actual appearance of hayfever depends on certain changes in other departments of the immune system – changes that only come on several years later. The immune system clearly changes as we mature, and these changes affect the appearance (and disappearance) of hayfever. The positive aspect to this is that most people also grow out of hayfever as they get older.

As a broad generalization, most people with hayfever begin having symptoms in their teenage years or early twenties, but some start earlier, during childhood. Very few people first develop hayfever in their thirties or forties, although this is not unknown. For those who develop hayfever as children or teenagers, there is a good chance that they will 'grow out of it' in their twenties, or later. As already noted, they do not necessarily lose their high IgE levels, so clearly some other form of control is coming into play.

Exactly what this control might be is still unknown, but an interesting observation on AIDS patients may throw some light on this. Several cases are now known of patients who had suffered from hayfever or other allergies in childhood, but had then grown out of them many years before contracting the AIDS virus. Within a few months of the onset of AIDS symptoms, their allergies returned, although it was not always the same type of allergy that they had experienced in childhood. One man of thirty-six, who had suffered asthma in his teens, developed eczema and hayfever as AIDS began. Others who have suffered hayfever as teenagers, develop asthma or food allergy as they succumb to AIDS. This sort of pattern fits in well with the 'wandering' nature of atopy (see p40).

The virus which causes AIDS is known to disable the T helper cells. We have already seen how the T helper subsets, T_H1 and T_H2, differ in their 'policies' on IgE production. In the case of AIDS patients, it seems to be the

PAUL

Neither of Paul's parents had any signs of allergy, but it ran in both their families – several aunts, uncles and cousins had asthma, hayfever or urticaria (nettle rash). The young couple assumed that because they were free of allergies, their children would be too, but they were wrong.

Both were carrying some genes for allergy, even though the effects were masked. Of their four children, only Paul was affected, and he developed eczema and asthma as a baby. The eczema did not last long and at the age of five the asthma disappeared, but hayfever then began. Every year Paul sneezed and blew his nose throughout the first eight weeks of summer. The doctor diagnosed hayfever to grass pollen. This continued until Paul was twelve, when the family moved from an unspoiled rural area into a large city with fairly high levels of air pollution. Within a few months his asthma had returned, and the following summer his hayfever was worse than ever before. Both continued until Paul was in his mid-twenties.

Paul was unfortunate in suffering from so many different allergic disorders, and starting asthma and hayfever at such an early age, but in many ways he is a good example of an atopic – someone with an allergic disposition.

As his case illustrates, that disposition can express itself in several different parts of the body, and may show up in different places (nose, bronchi, skin or digestive system) at different phases of a person's life.

lack of T_H1 cells that is causing the allergy problem. T_H2 cells, you will recall, influence B cells by producing interferon gamma, a chemical messenger which discourages the production of IgE. By treating AIDS patients with interferon gamma, which is available as a drug, their allergic problems can be brought under control. (Interferon gamma is of no use to most people with allergies, however.)

Perhaps hayfever sufferers who find themselves spontaneously 'cured' as they grow older, are experiencing a natural shift in their helper cells. If a shift occurred, away from T_H2 cells and towards T_H1 cells, this would reduce their production of IgE and thus their allergic tendencies.

CASTOR BEANS AND OTHER BADDIES

The immune system has to 'decide' when producing IgE might be a good idea (in response to a liver fluke or tapeworm, for example), and when it is definitely a bad idea (in response to pollen). How this decision is taken we do not know, but medical researchers have found that they can play a part in that decision, at least in the laboratory. By adding certain substances to an injection containing an antigen they can persuade the immune system to produce IgE to that antigen. The substances that have this effect are known as **IgE-specific adjuvants**. Presumably they mimic certain effects of large parasites in some way, thus promoting IgE production.

One of the most powerful IgE-specific adjuvants is found in castor beans, the raw material from which castor oil is made. During oil production, a dust comes out of the milling machinery and fills the air all around. It has unpleasant effects on many people working at the oil mills, or living nearby. Dockers who handle castor beans may also be affected. Allergies to the dust are remarkably common, and it can also induce allergies to other substances, suggesting that the castor-bean dust contains both a powerful allergen and an IgE-specific adjuvant. Castor-bean dust often affects people with no previous signs of allergy.

Platinum salts are likewise known to favour IgE reactions to antigens, *and* act as antigens themselves. However, this only affects workers in platinum-using factories. Small amounts of tobacco smoke may also promote the production of IgE, although at high doses it seems to suppress IgE reactions. If these two factors cancel out, it would explain why smokers do not show any greater or lesser susceptibility to allergies. The children of smokers are more vulnerable to asthma, but that may well be due to the irritant properties of the smoke, rather than its effects on IgE.

Some IgE-specific adjuvants are simply particles that attract and hold proteins. These particles pick up protein antigens that originated elsewhere, resulting in a large antigen-coated particle which apparently stimulates the immune system to produce IgE. This effect can occur with a variety of particles, including carbon particles, the 'soot' produced by burning various fuels. The possible link between pollution and hayfever is one we will return to in the next chapter.

CROSS-REACTIONS

Most people have had the experience of seeing someone they know, saying hello – and then realizing, with great embarrassment, that they have made a mistake. The reason for the mistake is usually clear – the stranger's nose, mouth or some other feature is similar to that of an acquaintance or friend. Exactly the same thing can happen to antibodies. Just as one nose can resemble another, so one epitope (see p11) can resemble another, chemically speaking. If two epitopes are reasonably similar, then one antibody may bind to both of them. If those epitopes are on different chemical molecules (different antigens) then a **cross-reaction** has occurred. Usually the antibody has multiplied in the body as a response to one antigen, but then reacts to a second one as well.

In terms of fighting disease, cross-reactions often make sense. Many microbes occasionally undergo a **mutation** – a change in their hereditary material. This can change the antigens in their outer coats, helping them to escape immune attack, so it pays if antibodies ignore minor alterations. Cross-reactions may also help the immune system if it has to tackle a related microbe, a similar type to one that has already been encountered and successfully defeated. It will already have a plentiful stockpile of B cells which make a suitable antibody for this new intruder.

Cross-reactions become a problem when they occur in allergic reactions because they can make a patient sensitive to a second item, as well as to their original allergen. As one might expect, many cross-reactions in hayfever are between related plants. Because they are related, their pollen antigens can be chemically similar, and they may share key epitopes. This type of cross-reaction is very common in the grass family (Gramineae or Poaceae), where patients are often sensitive to pollen from several different species of grass. There are some other plant families where such cross-reactions are common (see pp154–9).

If a chemically similar antigen is found in food, as well as in pollen, then this too may produce a cross-reaction because the relevant IgE molecule can be produced anywhere in the body, not just in the nose. The most common reaction is a tingling or itching sensation in the mouth, but sometimes a more violent and potentially dangerous immune reaction occurs (see p166). Many cross-reactions between pollen and foods have now been documented and a list of all those currently known is given on pp163–5.

Finally, one very curious cross-reaction should be mentioned. To understand this particular medical tale, you must remember that all living things are descended from a single ancestor, a little nondescript blob of a thing that squidged about in the sea over 1,000 million years ago. Although we may have come a long way since then, some of our most basic life processes are still the same, which means that some of the chemical 'nuts and bolts' are also unchanged.

Among those nuts and bolts is a protein called **profilin**, a chemical heirloom so useful and precious that almost every living thing on Earth has hung on to it. Molecular biologists gave it the name profilin because it is produced so prolifically by animals and plants (it might equally well have been called 'ubiquitin', but someone had already claimed that name for another of these heirloom molecules).

Profilin is found inside human cells, and in amoebae, yeasts, slime moulds, mice and cows. As you may have guessed by now, profilin is also found in pollen. In 1991 researchers in Austria discovered that it was one of the minor allergens in birch pollen, provoking an IgE response in 10 per cent of those who are sensitive to birch pollen. When they took IgE from these patients, it bound equally well to human profilin as to birch-pollen profilin. Other tests showed that human profilin could probably trigger off allergic responses in these patients.

The discoveries about profilin raise the intriguing possibility of patients being 'allergic to themselves', or to some small part of themselves, at least. The idea of the immune system turning on the body itself – the biological equivalent of a military coup – is not unheard-of. There are many diseases caused solely or partly by such **autoimmune reactions**, including rheumatoid arthritis and one form of diabetes. Cross-reactions are thought to play a part in some of these, notably in rheumatoid arthritis, where molecules produced by some bacteria are similar to those produced in inflamed joints.

Whether an autoimmune reaction is actually occurring in the case of profilin is not known. Perhaps one of the body's control mechanisms intervenes and prevents a reaction to home-grown profilin. Certainly, if the body is reacting to its own profilin, there are no obvious symptoms in these patients as a result – only the symptoms of hayfever.

The Austrian researchers who discovered the profilin cross-reaction speculate that the body's own profilin may help to perpetuate hayfever: its presence all year round may maintain the level of IgE against pollen profilin. Profilin is also found in some other pollens, so this reaction may be important there too.

WHY US?

When people fall ill they often ask indignantly 'Why me?' In the case of hayfever, it would be quite reasonable for *Homo sapiens* as a whole to demand 'Why us?' Hayfever is very uncommon among other animals.

It is not that animals do not show allergic reactions at all – they do. Food allergies are known in dogs, pigs and cows, mainly when they are fed an unnatural food such as soya, but sometimes in response to natural foodstuffs as well. Dogs sometimes develop itchy skin conditions in reaction to allergens they eat or inhale. Here pollen *may* play a part, one of the rare instances of a natural allergic reaction to pollen – but it does not generally produce symptoms in the nose. (Dogs *may* sneeze if they inhale a large dose of pollen when sniffing around in vegetation, but this is rarely a true allergic reaction, rather a simple response to the irritant effects of the pollen when inhaled in such quantities.)

According to Professor Brunello Wüthrich, who studies hayfever in Switzerland, the Swiss cow is sometimes afflicted by hayfever. However, this has not been observed in other countries. The only animals to show a condition resembling hayfever with any regularity are horses, notably thoroughbred horses. They sometimes also suffer from allergic reactions to the mould spores found in stored hay.

Efforts to induce hayfever in rats and mice, for the purposes of studying the disease and testing new treatments, have entirely failed. There is no allergic reaction to pollen unless it is inhaled along with a powerful adjuvant (see p45) that promotes the production of IgE. Medical researchers turned to other experimental animals, but with little success. The only suitable animals that proved at all susceptible to hayfever were certain breeds of dog, and even they would not easily develop symptoms in the nose.

It seems that most airborne allergens are tolerated well by animals, so there is nothing exceptional about pollen in this respect. Why animals should have this particular immune reaction under firm control, when a great many humans do not, is a profound medical mystery. The next chapter looks at this mystery from another viewpoint – a historical one.

Chapter Four

A MODERN DISEASE

'At first I did not know what I had, and neither did any other doctor I encountered in the next two or three years. I gradually recognized that it was not an ordinary cold and that the symptoms were much worse on the golf course or even during a nice day rowing on Loch Lomond . . .' These are the recollections of Dr John Morrison Smith, who developed hayfever in the late 1930s, while at medical school in Glasgow. 'I do not remember seeing a case of hayfever as a student or being aware of any of my contemporaries suffering similarly . . . I do not believe any relative of mine for two or three generations in the past suffered from hayfever, but two of my own children have been affected by it . . .'

That was just over fifty years ago. The idea of a succession of Scottish doctors being baffled by hayfever symptoms today is unthinkable.

Medical statistics tell much the same story as Dr Morrison Smith's family history: hayfever has been steadily rising throughout the past 200 years. Before 1800 it seems to have been unknown. Today, in most developed countries, one teenager in six suffers from the disease.

From time to time, people cast doubt on the statistics showing that hayfever has increased dramatically: as we all know, there are 'lies, damned lies and statistics'. The sceptics suggest that people simply did not bother about such minor ailments in the past, and did not visit the doctor with them, so hayfever never figured in the medical records. Another line of argument is that people just dismissed hayfever as a summer cold. Dr Morrison Smith's account makes such theories seem extremely unlikely. Here was a young medical student on the lookout for an explanation of his unusual symptoms, which, unlike a cold, were worse on a fine day in the countryside, and persisted for two months. If hayfever was as widespread then as it is now, how could he have missed it in his friends, relatives and fellow students? Fortunately, one of the earliest hayfever sufferers was also a doctor who made a point of trying to find others with the same complaint. Dr John Bostock (see p15) had suffered from his summertime symptoms, which included itchy eyes, a constantly running nose and paroxysms of sneezing, since the age of eight, but he first reported them to the medical world in 1819, when in his forties. He continued to study the disease after 1819, and within nine years he had collected twenty-eight fellow sufferers. (Today you could find that number of hayfever sufferers in a few hours if you simply stopped passers-by on a busy street.) Bostock made extensive enquiries among other doctors and reported that, 'One of the most remarkable circumstances respecting this complaint is its not having been noticed as a specific affection, until within the last ten or twelve years.'

Another oddity struck Bostock: all the patients he had collected were from 'the middle or upper classes of society, some indeed of high rank'. A tireless investigator, by the standards of his time, Bostock decided to make sure this observation was correct: 'I have made inquiry at the various dispensaries in London and elsewhere, and I have not heard of a single unequivocal case occurring among the poor.' Medical historians today are able to confirm this particular report because dispensaries kept records and published them. At a dispensary in a very poor district of northwest England, the sale of medicines for 'catarrh' (the general name used for a blocked or runny nose) was high in winter but low throughout the summer.

As the nineteenth century progressed, the disease became better known, but was still far from common. In 1837 a distinguished physician observed, 'I have now seen several unequivocal instances of it – very few persons in comparison with the entire community are susceptible.' The link with the upper classes was still there: '. . . you may read almost every year in the newspapers that one of our English Dukes has gone to Brighton to escape the hay fever,' he continued. The disease had became fashionable and newsworthy.

Soon afterwards, a case of summer catarrh was recorded in Bordeaux, in the south of France, where it was attributed to sunlight. In 1852 Dr J. Swett, unaware of any of the reports from Britain or France, described two forms of summer catarrh in the USA, one a reaction to grasses, the other to ragweed. Unlike Bostock, who blamed heat and sunlight, Swett shrewdly came to the correct conclusion about the cause of the disease at once. In Britain it was the public who identified the origin of the illness (see p15).

By 1859 hayfever was known in Germany as well, and a Professor Phoebus of the University of Giessen, who collected information on the problem from both Britain and Germany, was able to report that there were finally some

HAYFEVER PIONEER: CHARLES BLACKLEY

Charles Harrison Blackley was a physician working in Manchester, and, like Bostock before him, was a sufferer from hayfever. Between 1859 and 1871 he carried out a series of experiments on the possible cause of hayfever. Among the causes that had already been suggested were benzoic acid, perfumes and odours, ozone, heat and light. Each of these he tried in turn, but none produced the characteristic symptoms. Dust collected from a roadside did, however, and when he inspected it under the microscope he found that it contained grass pollen.

Blackley then collected grass pollen during the summer, stored it for several months, and inhaled some on a winter's day. The effect was immediate and dramatic, confirming the public hunch about the cause of hayfever (see p15). Blackley collected other pollens – from garden flowers, weeds and trees – and found that he reacted to them all (his hayfever must have been particularly bad).

Other experiments included flying a kite with a sticky glass microscope slide attached, and then observing the slide under a microscope. This showed that pollen floated about high up in the atmosphere.

Blackley also invented a pollen trap and made the world's first pollen counts. For one man, working alone, he achieved a remarkable amount, and put the study of hayfever on a serious scientific footing.

sufferers who were 'not of the higher members of society'. Hayfever, after sixty years or so, had reached the lower middle classes, but it took a few decades more to really conquer the proletariat. In the 1870s the English physician Charles Blackley found that hayfever was almost wholly confined to educated and professional people, and suspected that there was a 'predisposition which mental culture generates'. He thought that the rise in standards of education might be part of the reason for the spread of hayfever.

The numbers were growing all the time. The United States Hayfever Association was founded in the 1870s and had almost 200 members. By 1903 there were thousands applying to join. A medical journal published in London in 1907 described hayfever as 'a very common complaint'.

In 1925 the disease was sufficiently well known for Noël Coward to discard

Oranges and Lemons as the title of his new comedy about an eccentric English family entertaining guests during a summer weekend at their country house, and call it instead *Hay Fever*. (The connotations of 'midsummer madness' must still have been there in the 1920s, a distant memory of the time when English dukes galloped off to Brighton to escape their aristocratic malady.)

Attentive readers will have noticed what seems like a contradiction here. By 1925 hayfever is sufficiently well known to serve as the title of a play in London. Yet almost fifteen years *later*, as a young medical student sneezes his way across Loch Lomond, no local doctor can identify his symptoms. This paradox cannot easily be explained, but it is certainly the case that hayfever affected some countries, and some districts, far earlier than others. Clearly the disease took longer to gain ground in Scotland, although today it is as common there as anywhere else in Britain.

TOWN AND COUNTRY

Reliable data are hard to find, but it does seem that, during its early days, hayfever was something of an urban disease. In the 1870s Charles Blackley observed that hayfever was virtually unknown among the farming community. Another author, writing in 1871, remarked that 'in Ireland hay-fever is seldom heard of '.

Fortunately, there is some solid evidence from Switzerland, where a doctor carried out a careful survey in 1926 and found that cases were ten times as common in the town as in the country. Roughly one urbanite in every hundred was affected, compared with only one per thousand in rural areas.

When a similar survey was carried out in Switzerland in 1985, 10 per cent of the population suffered from hayfever, and there was no difference between the town and the countryside. Nor is there any difference between urban and rural populations in Britain today.

In some countries, hayfever is still a little more common in towns, but the tenfold difference recorded in the 1920s is never seen now. In southern Spain for example, olive pollen sets many of the citizens of Cordoba sneezing, while those working in the olive groves on the hillsides beyond the city (where pollen counts reach far higher levels) are less likely to be affected. In Norway, Sweden and Finland hayfever is still more common in the urbanized and industrialized areas. The same is also true of many east European countries, notably Czechoslovakia, where very high levels of hayfever and other allergies are found among children in industrialized areas. Italian city dwellers are twice as likely to have hayfever as those in the country. (There are some exceptions to this rule. Occasionally rural populations today have more hayfever than nearby towns, but this is generally in hot, arid countries such as Israel, where there is extensive irrigation to create farms. What happens is that the plants flourish and pollinate as vigorously as they would in a damp climate, but there is no rainfall to wash the pollen from the air. As a result, it builds up to massive levels.)

Today, in undeveloped regions of the world such as rural Africa, it does seem that hayfever is still unknown, or very rare, although no one has made a proper scientific study of this. In India hayfever is quite common.

Just as the old link between hayfever and urban living still lingers on in places, so there is still a ghost of the old link with social class. In some studies, but not all, hayfever is more common among the educated and upper classes. A recent study in the USA found it to be more common among those with higher incomes, and among the better educated. In Switzerland there is apparently a huge class difference – hayfever is three times as common among professional people as it is among manual labourers. This is not the case in Britain, but researchers *have* found that upper-class people with hayfever tend to get diagnosed more accurately than those in the lower classes, whose hayfever is more frequently mistaken for an infection. Could the differences between classes seen today in countries such as Switzerland therefore be illusory, or exaggerated? This is difficult to say, but the enquiries made by Bostock and others in the nineteenth century can make us confident that the class difference was there in the past.

Before we attempt to explain the strange and sudden rise of hayfever – a rise that still seems to be continuing – there are two other important pieces of evidence that must be included. One is the rarity of hayfever among animals, described in the previous chapter (see pp47–8). The other comes from a mammoth medical survey, which included 17,414 children.

During one week in March 1958, every child born in Britain became part of medical science. These children were studied at birth, and again at the ages of seven, eleven and twenty-three, when they or their parents were asked about a huge variety of symptoms. Many different aspects of their living conditions and social status were also recorded. This sort of information is like a treasure trove for medical scientists, who can, with the aid of modern computers, scan the data for possible links and associations. One researcher has done just that for hayfever but he found very few important links. Being born in the town or the country made no difference, nor did social class, nor did smoking by the parents (although this is known to affect asthma).

The one factor that did correlate remarkably well with hayfever was family size. An only child was much more likely to have hayfever than one with several brothers and sisters. Explaining away such a finding seems simple enough at first sight. Minor illnesses tend to attract less attention and concern among large families than they do in the cosseted only child, and parents with few children might have noticed hayfever more readily. Yet the difference was equally pronounced at the age of twenty-three, when the young adults were reporting their own symptoms.

There is another possible explanation here. We know that susceptiblity to hayfever and other allergic diseases is genetically inherited (see p42). Perhaps atopic parents – those predisposed to allergy – simply have fewer children? Other evidence suggests that this is unlikely. What is more, if this explanation were true, allergies in general would show the same association with family size as hayfever. While eczema does show the same pattern as hayfever, asthma does not.

When the figures were looked at again, it became clear that family size was only part of the story anyway. Being the firstborn or the baby of the family also made a huge difference. Those least likely to develop hayfever were the youngest children from large families. Someone with four older brothers or sisters, for example, had only one-quarter the chance of developing hayfever as someone with no older brothers or sisters. (To have four *younger* brothers and sisters also reduced the chance of hayfever, compared to the chance for an only child, but not nearly as much.) The differences persisted long after the children were grown up – in fact they were more pronounced at age twenty-three than they had been at eleven. Another large group of children, born in 1970, have shown the same puzzling pattern.

PIECING THE PUZZLE TOGETHER

If this were a detective story, now would be the moment for Sherlock Holmes, Maigret or Philip Marlowe to step forward and explain all these strange facts, which do not at first sight fit together. Unfortunately, this is not a detective story, but we can still make a mental list of the suspects and carefully assess the evidence for and against them, as any competent sleuth would.

It would be a mistake, however, to expect to find a single guilty culprit. What, after all, could single out nineteenth-century aristocrats and the eldest children of twentieth-century families, favour town dwellers at first but not later, and cause hayfever in human beings but not in most animals? The sheer contrariness of these facts makes it unlikely that there is just one villain, one simple causative factor behind the hayfever epidemic.

SUSPECT NUMBER ONE: CHANGES IN THE POLLEN

Some change in the pollen – either its quantity or its type – has been a popular culprit ever since the nineteenth century. People blamed the Corn Laws, the greater amount of hay being grown to feed the horses of urban populations, grasses grown on 'rich soils' and anything else which looked like a possible scapegoat. However, these explanations were, and are, extremely implausible. The pollen count may change from time to time as agricultural practices change, but there has always been a fair amount of grass pollen in the air – enough, certainly, to spark off hayfever if the human population was susceptible to it. Indeed, it was on the grassy plains of Africa that human beings evolved, and our ancestors' exposure to grass pollen then must have been massive. Breathing plenty of pollen, particularly grass pollen, is an age-old part of human life.

In Britain in the past twenty years, with the switch from hay to silage, which involves harvesting grasses before they flower, the pollen count has been steadily declining. Yet the cases of hayfever have continued to rise.

Looking at hayfever around the world, there are certainly specific instances of new pollens causing outbreaks of hayfever. In the southern states of the USA, for example, various imported species grown in gardens have begun to cause severe hayfever symptoms. In India epidemics of hayfever have been sparked off by introduced weeds, such as Santa Maria feverfew. The spread of ragweed in various parts of the world also brings more hayfever in its wake (see p130). But these are specific and isolated instances: in general, changes in pollen cannot be blamed for hayfever. Like grasses, many of the major allergens are from plants with which we have happily coexisted for thousands of years.

SUSPECT NUMBER TWO: A GENETIC CHANGE IN HUMAN BEINGS

The tendency to allergy is inherited (see p42), and the genes producing that tendency must have been in the human population for thousands of years. We can state this confidently because the medical writers of Ancient Greece gave clear descriptions of food allergy and asthma. They did not, however, mention anything remotely resembling hayfever, nor were there any convincing descriptions of it until Bostock's account. (There are sporadic reports of something called the 'rose cold' in earlier times, which produced sneezing and was apparently brought on by roses. Its sufferers 'held the smell of roses in deadly hatred'. Some have suggested that this was actually hayfever, but it seems more likely to have been vasomotor rhinitis, which can be sparked off by strong scents – see p231.)

The noses of our ancestors, even those ancestors who were atopic, apparently had the wisdom to tolerate pollen. They do not seem to have extended this tolerance to other airborne allergens, however. Reports from AD 41 tell of a violent allergy to horses seen in the son of a Roman Emperor, and there are later reports from Germany of allergies to horses, dogs and mice. Baker's asthma, a reaction to inhaled flour, was also known. Given the close contact that most people had with horses in the past, and the powerful nature of horse allergens (see p212), then *more* historical accounts of horse allergy might be expected – perhaps such reactions were less common than now, but they were certainly not unknown, as hayfever apparently was.

Could there be another genetic mutation which, when added to the genes for atopy, make the nose intolerant of pollen? If such a mutation had appeared in the late eighteenth century, this would perhaps explain the sudden appearance of hayfever. It is a nice idea, but it does not hold water. New genes spread very slowly. Calculations show that it would be impossible for a mutant gene to spread so rapidly through the population as to affect 10 or 15 per cent of the population in the space of 200 years.

WHAT SORT OF CULPRIT ARE WE LOOKING FOR?

With the two obvious suspects eliminated from the inquiry, we can be more precise about the sort of culprit we are seeking. It is something that acts on atopics (people who have a predisposition to allergy) and somehow makes them react allergically to pollen.

To put the matter another way, it somehow stops them learning to tolerate pollen. The immune system, as explained in Chapter Three, has to sort out the difference between harmful invaders and harmless ones, so that it can react effectively and promptly against disease-causing microbes, but not mount any damaging reactions against harmless items coming into the body, such as food molecules and pollen grains. The process of learning to shrug off harmless items is called **tolerance induction**, and it occurs when we first encounter a new allergen, usually as babies or young children.

It is difficult to investigate tolerance induction in human atopics directly, so we have to rely on studies with rats and mice. These show that an antigen which is inhaled *automatically* induces tolerance, in the sense of preventing production of the allergy antibody IgE (see p31). The action is specific: it applies only to the particular antigen that has been inhaled. It works by means of T suppressor cells (see p38), which can block the production of a particular type of antibody in response to a particular antigen. The T suppressor cells are like roving superintendents of the immune system, which patrol the body ensuring that other cells do not produce IgE to particular antigens, in this case pollen antigens.

That is what happens with antigens inhaled by adult mice and rats, and it is fair to assume that something similar happens in healthy adult humans encountering a new inhaled allergen as well (although there are other ways in which the allergic response is suppressed, see pp38–9). However, the system is not yet established in newborn mice and rats, which cannot produce the T suppressor cells. During the first weeks or so of life they can be sensitized by inhaled allergens. They do not start producing high levels of IgE immediately because they cannot produce much IgE at this stage – but the scene is set. Once they become old enough to produce IgE abundantly, the lack of T suppressor cells to the inhaled antigen becomes evident, and they can produce IgE to that antigen (although, they do not get any symptoms in the nose itself).

Even in adult rats and mice, and young ones past the vulnerable newborn state, certain things can interfere with the induction of tolerance, including the gas nitrogen dioxide. If animals inhale fairly high concentrations of this gas, it irritates the nose and airways. If they then inhale an antigen that they have never been exposed to before, they do not become tolerant as they normally would. (Again, there are no symptoms in the nose of the rodent, but a blood test shows them producing IgE to the antigen.)

How far can we apply these discoveries to human beings? That is a difficult question to answer, but studies of children with allergies, and the conditions they were born into, show some interesting associations. For example, the presence of a cat or dog in the house for the first year of life seems to make allergy to these animals later on in life more likely. Being born just before the pollen season may make hayfever as a child or teenager a little more likely. The general impression is that there is a period of particular vulnerability for the newborn child which lasts for three months or more. This could correspond, in some respects, to the brief period of vulnerability in the newborn mouse or rat, since human babies develop at a far slower pace.

However, looking back in time, it is clear that 300 years ago, babies (even atopic babies) did not react in the same way. They breathed pollen in their first few months, yet did not develop hayfever later. Something must have changed.

This could be something in our diet or way of life which influences the immune system and makes for a longer or more severe period of vulnerability in the young baby. Alternatively, it could be something in the air which irritates the airways, and thus directly interferes with tolerance induction by airborne substances when they are first encountered. This irritant could affect babies or children breathing in a potential allergen for the first time, but it might also affect adults in certain circumstances – immigrants from lands with different vegetation, for example. (It is known that immigrants sometimes develop hayfever; if they do so it is within two or three years of arriving in their new country.)

Whether airborne irritants such as nitrogen dioxide really can prevent tolerance induction in humans, as they do in mice and rats, is unknown at present. Scientists generally assume that they can, but there is no proof, and extrapolating from animals to humans is always risky. (Whether irritants can *break down* tolerance which has already been induced is an even trickier issue, but one which is relevant to those who develop hayfever late in life, see p43.)

The information about tolerance induction is useful in compiling our list of suspects. It is clear that we are probably looking for something that is able to affect atopic babies very early in life, when they will first be exposed to certain airborne allergens.

SUSPECT NUMBER THREE: AIR POLLUTION

As far as many journalists are concerned, this suspect has already been interrogated, charged, tried in a court of law and found guilty. 'Hayfever: the pollution sickness' was one memorable headline from 1992. To anyone who knows all the evidence in the case, however, it is clear that this verdict is premature. There are too many facts that do not fit:

- Hayfever began, not among the urban poor, living in the shadow of the Industrial Revolution and breathing the foul air of its foundries and factories, but among the upper classes. It then spread among the middle classes, and eventually reached the working class almost a century after it had begun.

- The incidence of hayfever is still rising in Britain, yet since the mid-1960s the air has been far cleaner than it was in the 1930s, '40s and '50s, thanks to the Clean Air Act, introduced to combat 'pea-souper' fogs.

- Hayfever does not naturally affect animals, with a few, rare exceptions. Our dogs, cats, cows and sheep share the same polluted air that we do, so why has hayfever not affected them?

- Hayfever is *four times* more common among eldest children and only children than it is among the youngest in a family, a huge difference which the 'pollution theory' cannot apparently explain.

That is the major evidence against. The historical evidence in favour lies in the link between hayfever and towns, a conspicuous link early on, but one which is gradually disappearing during the twentieth century. Some researchers believe that the spread of road traffic can explain this particular pattern: air pollution, originally a monopoly of urban areas, has now spread to the countryside as well with the growth in the number of cars and lorries.

This is an attractive theory, but to accept it involves classing *all* forms of pollution as one, and assuming that smoke from factory chimneys has the same effect on the nose as car-exhaust fumes. (Similarly, we may no longer experience the 'pea-souper' smogs of the 1950s, but there are some pollutants, such as ozone, that are more abundant in the air today.) Careful study of this subject makes it clear that 'air pollution' is not just one suspect, but a group of individual suspects. To lump them all together and call them 'pollution' simply leads to muddled thinking. The different types of pollutant must be considered separately.

Motor vehicle exhausts

The best evidence on exhaust fumes comes from Japan. Researchers have studied the incidence of hayfever to Japanese red cedar, comparing people from different areas. Those with the highest incidence of hayfever were living along busy roads lined with these trees. They were three times more likely to be affected than people living near forests of red cedar but well away from traffic pollution. Those breathing plenty of traffic fumes and only a little pollen came somewhere in between.

Japanese scientists looking for the cause of this phenomenon have made detailed studies of diesel particulates, tiny sooty particles that come from the exhaust pipes of lorries and diesel cars. When a bus or lorry spews out black exhaust fumes as it starts up, these particles are momentarily visible, but for the most part they are too small and too dispersed in the air for us to see. Nevertheless they are there, and an urban commuter could inhale as much as 500 millionths of a gram of diesel particles every day. According to the Japanese researchers, just one millionth of a gram can boost IgE production to 100 times its normal level, when placed in the nose of a mouse along with an antigen that has not been encountered before. The evidence suggests that diesel particles interfere with tolerance induction.

So far, so good – we seem to have a promising suspect. But what is frequently overlooked when people report these results is that the diesel particulates are basically small particles of carbon: soot. Any carbon particle has the same effect in inducing IgE, and there are carbon particles in the smoke from a wood fire, a coal fire, an oil lamp and a candle – forms of heating and lighting that humans have been using for thousands of years. If you have ever sat by a peat fire when it is still getting going, or a hearth burning slightly damp logs, *then* you have experienced pollution. The polluting capacity of wood-burning stoves has been well documented in the USA.

Of course, in the past, smoke from fires and stoves was mainly a feature of the cold winter months, whereas diesel particulates are plentifully inhaled in the summer, along with pollen. This may be an important difference, since it is the way the pollen allergens are absorbed on to the carbon particles that

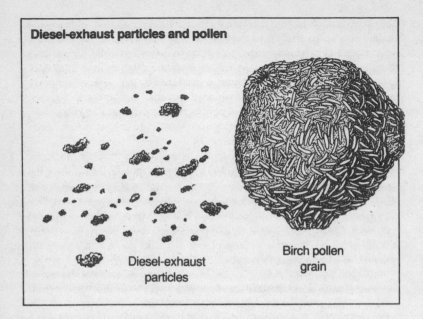

Diesel-exhaust particles and pollen

Diesel-exhaust
particles

Birch pollen
grain

seems to promote the allergic reaction. In the earlier stages of the Industrial Revolution, before the advent of diesel, the smoke from factories and steam trains would have injected carbon particles into the summer air, but probably in a more localized fashion than the ubiquitous cars and lorries of today.

To return briefly to Glasgow in the 1930s, where this chapter began, transport into the city from outlying villages and towns was by means of a steam train. On reaching the city, this railway ran through a tunnel under the suburbs. During their passage through this long tunnel the trains produced a horrendous build-up of smoke particles in the air, which were breathed by all the passengers. Smoke and 'pea-souper' smogs in the city centre were also plentiful. Yet, by Dr Morrison Smith's account, hayfever was virtually unheard-of. Once again, a piece of the jigsaw puzzle refuses to slot into place.

Could other constituents of modern exhaust fumes be playing a part, perhaps augmenting the effect of carbon particles from diesel engines? Nitrogen dioxide is known to interfere with tolerance induction in rats and mice (see p57) and it is one of the gases found in car-exhaust fumes. However, the link is not that straightforward because the levels used in the experiments described above were about *a thousand times* higher than those on a polluted city street. Nevertheless, nitrogen dioxide may still be relevant here.

Laboratory tests show that this gas, if it becomes concentrated in the air we breathe, acts as an irritant to the human nose and airways. Although the levels needed to produce symptoms are up to *a hundred times* higher than those found on city streets, a very different picture emerges from studies of nitrogen dioxide in the home. Here it is produced by gas cookers in poorly ventilated conditions, and old-fashioned paraffin or kerosene heaters. Children exposed to these sources of pollution are known to suffer more chest diseases, even though the levels of nitrogen dioxide are only moderate, often *less* than those on a polluted city street.

Presumably year-round exposure to moderate levels of nitrogen dioxide is more damaging to the airways than higher exposure for a few hours during a laboratory test. It is believed that the irritation to the airways is what makes nitrogen dioxide interfere with tolerance induction, so the levels created by traffic could indeed be a factor. When added to carbon particles, and inhaled along with a baby's first dose of pollen, they could well act to make hayfever more likely.

Another notorious gas produced by traffic should be mentioned here. Ozone is mainly formed in the summer months, and it too causes irritation of the nose and airways. It can easily build up to levels that affect those with asthma, making attacks more likely. During a photochemical smog (see p319), the levels reached will affect the breathing of healthy people too. Recent studies have shown that ozone also makes hayfever symptoms a little worse, producing more sneezing and itching of the nose. However, there is no evidence that ozone can interfere with tolerance induction in animals or humans. Making hayfever worse is one thing – starting it off in the first place is another.

Other forms of air pollution

Unfortunately, evidence about other forms of pollution is much less satisfactory. Apart from soot particles (see above) the only pollutants that have been studied in relation to allergy are sulphur dioxide and sulphuric acid.

Sulphur dioxide is a gas produced by coal fires, power stations burning coal, smelters and some factories. It was a major ingredient of the 'pea-souper' fogs of former days, and a lethal ingredient for those with bronchitis, the elderly or the very young. Sulphur dioxide is acidic and can severely irritate the airways, producing inflammation. In asthmatics it can provoke an asthma attack (see p70). Thanks to anti-pollution measures, sulphur dioxide is far less of a problem in cities today.

Studies of the effect of sulphur dioxide on tolerance induction in animals (see above) show that it may prevent tolerance from developing, even at quite low concentrations, such as those that could still be encountered in a polluted industrial area today.

Tiny droplets of sulphuric acid in the air are another form of pollution which affects the airways. No one has looked at the effect of this on tolerance induction, but it could well be similar to the effect of sulphur dioxide.

There are many other types of modern pollutant, and few have been studied for their effect on allergy.

CAN WE REACH A VERDICT ON POLLUTION?
Unfortunately, the answer to this question is 'not really'. There are clearly some aspects of the hayfever epidemic that it totally fails to explain (see p58). But if we accept that there are likely to be several causes rather than a *single* cause for this epidemic, pollution could at least be deemed 'guilty until proved innocent'. It seems likely that traffic pollution is playing a part in the present increase in numbers, and that smoke and sulphur dioxide may have been part of the problem in the recent past. But if smoke and sulphur dioxide can have this effect, why did it take so long for hayfever to touch the factory workers and poor city dwellers of the nineteenth century? This type of pollution was a widespread feature of industrial areas in the early nineteenth century, and even in the eighteenth century. In London, where nuggets of coal from seams under the sea were regularly washed up on the shores of the Thames, people had been burning this fuel to warm their houses for centuries. One writer of the seventeenth century recorded a 'hellish and dismall cloud of sea-coal' over the capital, while King James complained that St Paul's cathedral was being corroded by the smog. Sea coal can still be found today, and produces an unpleasant acidic smoke full of sulphur dioxide. If such smoke promoted hayfever, why did it not do so in the seventeenth and eighteenth centuries?

In some people, hayfever comes on suddenly in their thirties or forties. This is considered unusual, but there are hints that it is becoming more common nowadays. A careful scientific study is needed to check if this is really so. If it is, then pollutants from traffic would seem to be a prime suspect for breaking down the tolerance to pollen.

Having dealt with pollution, there are a few remaining suspects to be interrogated.

SUSPECT NUMBER FOUR: A DECLINE IN INFECTIONS
Certain infections have declined in the past 200 years, a decline that began long before vaccination was widespread, and which was largely due to better hygiene and sanitation. A few researchers think that this change could explain the association between small families and hayfever, since children with many brothers and sisters tend to catch more coughs and colds than only children. The suggestion is that infections educate the immune system

to behave in certain ways, and that, for those people with an atopic predisposition (see p39), encountering fewer infections results in an ill-educated immune system which overreacts to harmless antigens.

It has to be said that most scientists reject this idea. For one thing, virus infections (which include colds and flu) have been observed to trigger off asthma in some children, and the conventional view is that they make allergy *more* likely, not less. The opposing side argues that perhaps this is just a short-term effect, and in the long term infections protect against allergy.

The attractive aspect of this theory is that it might explain two other outstanding problems: why hayfever began among the upper classes and slowly worked its way down to the lower classes, and why it so rarely affects animals. The jury is still out on this one and will probably remain so for a long time.

SUSPECT NUMBER FIVE: 'MODERN LIVING'

No real culprit has been pinpointed here, but it is tempting to look for some aspect of modern living that was first enjoyed only by the very wealthy, but then gradually spread to the middle classes, and is now available to all sectors of our egalitarian society. If that luxury item was something which could irritate the nose, or subtly influence the immune system of a young child, it might qualify as a suspect.

A more varied and abundant diet is one possibility – perhaps it could affect the immune system in some way? No one has yet investigated this. Bottle-feeding has been suggested, but it does not seem to have much influence on hayfever, despite its effects in promoting food allergy (see p250). Something in paper or printing ink – an obvious culprit given the long-standing link between hayfever and education – has never been looked into, as far as we know.

The potential suspects here are innumerable, and it may take a collaboration between immunologists and social historians to come up with a useful shortlist of items worthy of further investigation.

SUSPECT NUMBER SIX: THE FINELY CHISELLED NASAL ORGAN

In 1887 Dr Edward Noakes of London concluded that hayfever was mainly due to a lack of space within the nose which compressed and irritated the membranes within. 'Perhaps this latter fact', wrote Dr Noakes, 'may explain the observation that the disease is most prevalent among the aristocratic classes, who are generally accredited with possession of that refined contour and delicate chiselling of the nasal organ, which necessarily diminishes the space for the internal structures, and compels some of these to lie in contact with each other.'

After a century on remand, we believe that this particular suspect should be released without trial.

AN UNFINISHED STORY

Unlike a detective story, there is no neat ending to this particular tale. We still cannot say what sparked off the hayfever epidemic, or made it steadily increase during the nineteenth century. We may have some answers to the question of why it is still increasing today, but several mysteries remain.

The temptation to place all the blame on pollution should be resisted, because it may prevent us from finding an important factor that lies behind hayfever – a factor that could allow us to combat the disease more effectively. The argument for controlling and reducing pollutants can be made on many grounds – the serious risks to asthmatics, the presence of carcinogens in exhaust fumes, the effects of some pollutants (notably ozone) upon the breathing of healthy people, and the sheer unpleasantness of living with polluted air. We believe that the continuing hayfever epidemic *does* add to the case against traffic exhaust fumes, but it is a mistake to attribute hayfever solely to pollution.

Chapter Five

TREATING HAYFEVER AND POLLEN ASTHMA: SELF-HELP AND MEDICAL HELP

Far too many people with hayfever choose to suffer in silence – if you can describe volleys of explosive sneezes, and regular snorting into handkerchiefs as 'silence'. According to one survey, for every hundred people with hayfever, fewer than twenty-five are getting treatment that relieves their symptoms fully. No doctor, however optimistic, would suggest that all the hundred could be entirely freed from their symptoms, but it is certainly true that many more people could be helped, and that many could experience far greater relief by reassessing their current forms of treatment.

Reassessment requires knowledge of the disease, knowledge of all the treatments now available, a consideration of the individual's lifestyle and preferences, and some intelligent experimentation. Unless family doctors were to devote themselves full-time to hayfever, abandoning interest in all other diseases, they would be hard-pushed to do this for everyone who needed such help. Consequently, there is a real role for patients to play here – in reassessing their own treatment and calling on their doctor for professional help when it is needed.

Do not expect a panacea – a single treatment that clears up your hayfever unaided. For the lucky few there *will* be a treatment that produces such magical effects, but for most the battle against allergy is one that has to be fought on several fronts at once.

The two primary forms of treatment – medicinal drugs and pollen avoidance – are dealt with in detail in Chapters Seven and Eight respectively. In brief, as far as drugs are concerned, there have been several major innovations in the past few years, including drugs with far fewer side-effects. One of the newer drugs may help you, even if you have, in the past, experienced unpleasant reactions to drug treatments.

Pollen avoidance can range from a few simple measures (such as wearing sunglasses or protective glasses and keeping windows closed at certain times of day) to high-tech 'pollen-proofing' of your home and car, combined with protection of your nose and eyes when out of doors. These measures are particularly useful to people with severe hayfever who are not helped very much by drugs, or who have strong objections to taking them.

Desensitization is another option for such patients, and this is fully described in Chapter Nine. The orthodox method, hyposensitization, is explained, along with two relatively new alternative treatments.

Finally, Chapter Ten deals with other treatments, mostly unconventional ones, such as dietary supplements, inhalations, homoeopathy, hypnosis, herbal remedies and acupuncture. Some of these may work, while others are probably a waste of money.

By reading each of these chapters in turn, you will have a clear idea of what you *could* do to tackle your hayfever symptoms. You can then choose from the various options available, selecting those that suit your home and lifestyle, your financial situation, your preferences for drug or non-drug treatments, and the severity of your symptoms. Be prepared to try different approaches and different combinations until you find one that suits you. Everyone is different.

As a very first step, however, you do need to be sure that you are actually suffering from hayfever. Chapter Six looks at how hayfever should be diagnosed. It suggests how you can diagnose yourself, and when a doctor should be called on to confirm the diagnosis.

If you are allergic to other airborne allergens, not just pollen, you may have a more complex task in dealing with your allergens. Chapter Twelve describes these airborne allergens, and the avoidance measures needed for each of them, in detail. The clearest sign of multiple allergies is if your symptoms continue at times of the year when no plants are in flower. Even though the symptoms may be very mild at these times, and seem scarcely worth noticing compared to what you go through in the pollen season, the other allergens are *definitely* worth investigating. It may be that the year-round effects of other allergens are making the nose unduly sensitive to pollen when it arrives. By dealing with the other allergens, therefore, you could make your hayfever much less severe. The most common allergens involved are those produced by house-dust mites, moulds or pets – and the good news is that control or avoidance of these allergens is much easier than pollen avoidance.

Allergens encountered at work that can produce rhinitis are also dealt with in Chapter Twelve, and this section looks in some detail at **sick building syndrome**. Finally, Chapter Thirteen deals with non-allergic forms of rhinitis, such as **vasomotor rhinitis**, and deals with sensitivity to food, which can produce a variety of symptoms, including rhinitis. The last part of the chapter explains how to carry out an elimination diet to diagnose such food problems.

Occasionally people with hayfever are allergic to another airborne substance, but never suspect that they are because they have symptoms only during the pollen season. What happens is that the response to the secondary allergen (such as the house dust mite or cat allergen) remains under control when the nose is in good health. But when spring or summer arrives, and the nose becomes inflamed by the reaction to pollen, it also becomes 'primed' to react to the other allergen. The basic mechanism underlying 'priming' is described on p41. To put it simply, once the nose becomes disrupted by its annual quarrel with pollen, it is over-sensitive and easily upset by other allergens. You should suspect this if any of the following apply to you:

- your hayfever is just as severe indoors with the windows closed (either at home or at work) as it is outdoors

- you seem to sneeze or blow your nose a lot when close to a cat, dog or other pet (but bear in mind that pets coming in from outside can carry pollen in their fur)

- you sneeze a lot first thing in the morning (most often a sign of house-dust mite allergy, or, less frequently, feather allergy)

- you are affected far more in some houses/buildings than in others, even though windows are closed in both

- you sneeze or blow your nose a lot when close to sources of mould spores such as compost heaps, dead leaves or rotten wood (see pp194–5 for a full list)

If you are reacting to other allergens during the pollen season, it is highly likely that they are aggravating your hayfever symptoms. Chapter Twelve will help you to identify the culprit, and give specific advice for avoiding that allergen.

IS IT ESSENTIAL TO SEE A DOCTOR?
It is traditional, in self-help books such as this, to 'play safe' and advise everyone to visit their doctor before trying to treat themselves or change their current treatment. However, a great many people with hayfever already treat themselves, and many have never consulted a doctor about the

problem. In most cases, this is probably quite satisfactory. Given the large numbers of people who now have hayfever, it would surely be an unnecessary burden on family doctors to have to see yet more hayfever patients, unless those patients have a specific need for professional help.

Self-treatment, based on pollen avoidance and medicinal drugs, should work well for all straightforward cases of hayfever. There are now several drugs that can be bought without a doctor's prescription: all those marked with an asterisk (*) in Chapter Seven. Only if these fail, or cause side-effects, should you need to consult your doctor about trying other drugs. Pollen avoidance is thoroughly covered in Chapter Eight, and it is unlikely that your doctor will be able to offer any additional advice, unless he or she is particularly interested in hayfever and has specialized knowledge of the local plants and climate.

The situations in which you should definitely go to see your doctor are as follows:

- if you suffer from asthma, either during the pollen season or at other times of year. Check the next section for asthma symptoms; these can be quite mild, and you could suffer from asthma without having recognized the fact

- if your rhinitis persists for most of the year, or well beyond the flowering season for plants, and you cannot identify a year-round allergen that might be causing the problem

- if your 'hayfever' has come on suddenly and is very severe

- if your 'hayfever' has come on following an accident that involved injury to the head, particularly to the face or nose

- if your mucus or saliva tastes salty; make a point of mentioning this to the doctor

- if you are suffering pain in the nose or face, or have earache; make a point of mentioning this to the doctor

- if you are suffering from nosebleeds

- if non-prescription drugs have failed to help you much and you are still suffering hayfever symptoms, despite pollen avoidance measures

- if you are not sure which pollen causes your hayfever and feel that you need to know (see p76). Your doctor can give you a skin-prick test (see p78)

- if your nose becomes completely blocked

- If your rhinitis is so severe that you have lost your sense of smell, cannot sleep properly, cannot work or study, or feel generally unwell

- if you would like desensitization treatment

On *very* rare occasions, cancerous growths in the nose have been mistaken for an allergic condition because they have produced symptoms that were almost exactly the same. If you have visited your doctor repeatedly and none of the medicines prescribed has had any effect, do go back again. The most likely explanation is that your allergy is highly resistant to treatment, but there is a remote chance of something more serious being wrong, and this should be investigated.

Another condition that can resemble allergic rhinitis is a leakage of the fluid that surrounds the brain (the **cerebrospinal fluid**) following injury to the face. The leakage may be intermittent, and it may not be apparent until some time after the accident. The tell-tale sign in this case is that the fluid is more salty than normal mucus from the nose, and that your taste buds detect this. Again, this is a rare condition.

COPING WITH POLLEN ASTHMA

Only a minority of patients with hayfever develop pollen asthma as well, but this can happen. The asthma tends to begin later in the pollen season than hayfever, and to continue for longer afterwards (see p23).

Some hayfever sufferers may experience asthma in response to other allergens, such as house dust mite, mould spores or skin particles from animals (see Chapter Twelve). This could simply be making the pollen asthma worse during the summer, or causing asthma attacks to continue into the winter months. Skin-prick tests (see p78) are valuable to pinpoint other allergies of this kind.

Most people think of asthmatics as suffering from severe attacks of wheezing and shortness of breath. This is indeed the case for many, but it can produce much milder symptoms instead. Feeling tight in the chest, having a persistent dry cough, or feeling short of breath when out in cold air are all possible signs of asthma. For some people, asthma only comes on when they exercise vigorously.

If you have any of these symptoms, you should see your doctor for advice. Drugs are usually prescribed for asthma, and the different kinds are dealt with on p88 and pp100–108.

If someone suffers from pollen asthma, heavy exposure to the allergenic pollen should be avoided in case it triggers a severe asthma attack. For example, a child with hayfever and pollen asthma, who is sensitive to grass, should be kept away from a lawn that is being mown, or a hay meadow being harvested.

It is a good idea to avoid heavily polluted areas if you suffer from asthma, as several pollutants can make attacks more likely. The three most heavily implicated are ozone, sulphur dioxide and acidic droplets (sulphuric acid) in the air. Ozone is most commonly found during the summer. Sulphur dioxide and sulphuric acid droplets are associated with domestic coal fires, industrial areas and fuel-burning power stations. Further details can be found in Appendix 7.

Sulphur dioxide is also used as a preservative in certain foods, and significant amounts may be given off when eating these. Sometimes this is sufficient to bring on an asthmatic attack. If you know that sulphur dioxide affects you badly, you should avoid all foods containing it, or approach them cautiously to see if they affect you. The foods concerned are listed in Appendix 8. If you have never reacted badly to any of these foods, there is no need to avoid them.

For anyone with severe asthma, cross-reactions are a potential hazard that should be borne in mind. Sometimes allergens in pollen cross-react with those in a food, and while most of these reactions to food are mild, they can be vigorous and produce anaphylactic shock (see p139). This is especially dangerous for an asthmatic. Cross-reactions are described more fully in Chapter Eleven.

Another hazard, but one that is easily avoided, is aspirin. Some asthmatics know that they are sensitive to aspirin (see p225), but others can take aspirin with no apparent ill-effects for many years, then suddenly develop a sensitivity to it. A bad reaction to aspirin can be life-threatening, so it is probably best avoided by all asthmatics. These are the aspirin and aspirin-like drugs:

aloxiprin (sold as: Palaprin, Palaprin Forte)
aspirin (Anadin, Angettes, Aspav, Aspro-Clear, Caprin, Claradin,
    Disprin, Doloxene Co., Equagesic, Hypon, Laborprin, Migravess,
    Nu-Seals, Paynocil, Platet, Robaxisal Forte, Solmin; there may be

other preparations available containing aspirin, so always read the packet
carefully)
benorylate (Benoral)
choline magnesium trisalicylate (Trilisate)
diflunisal (Dolobid)
salsalate (Disalcid)

Another group of drugs are chemically similar to aspirin and carry the same
risk. They are collectively known as non-steroidal anti-inflammatory drugs or
NSAIDS. The most commonly used drugs are:

ibuprofen (sold as: Nurofen, Apsifen, Brufen, Codafen Continus,
   Ebufac, Fenbid Spansule, Ibulere, Ibugel, Junifen, Lidifen, Motrin,
   Paxofen and Proflex)
felbinac (Traxam gel)
fenbufen (Lederfen)
fenoprofen (Fenopron, Progesic)
flurbiprofen (Frobe, Ocufen)
ketoprofen (Alrheumat, Orudis, Oruvail)
naproxen (Laraflex, Napratec, Naprosyn, Nycopren, Pranoxen,
   Synflex)
tiaprofenic acid (Surgam)

Most of these are prescribed drugs, used for rheumatoid arthritis, but some,
such as Nurofen, are available without prescription, as headache remedies
and general painkillers. Nurofen should not be taken by asthmatics. In the
case of prescribed drugs, discuss with your doctor whether these are safe for
you to take.

There are many ways in which asthmatics can help themselves. Knowing
how to use inhalers properly, and understanding when to use the drugs, are
two essential steps towards coping with asthma. If you feel unsure about
these points, do go to see your doctor again – you will not be wasting his or
her time. Self-help groups (see pp316–7) can also be very useful. In Britain
the National Asthma Campaign runs a phone line, charged at local call rates,
offering expert advice.

Using a **peak-flow meter** can also be very valuable. Your doctor should be
able to provide you with this piece of equipment and show you how to use it.
The meter measures how fast you can expel air from your lungs when
breathing out as hard as possible. This gives a good idea of how much
narrowing there is in your bronchi. Doctors use peak-flow meters in the

surgery to diagnose asthma, especially where the only symptoms are a cough, or tightness in the chest. At home the peak-flow meter should be used daily and the meter reading recorded. This regular reading helps to show whether your asthma is improving or not in response to drug treatments. It can also identify a deterioration in your condition before the effects become noticeable.

Asthma attacks can be frightening, but if one does occur it is important to stay calm. The emotions play a crucial role in asthma, and anxiety will make the tightening of the airways far worse. (Sometimes attacks are actually triggered off by tension and anxiety alone, although there is almost always an underlying cause for the asthmatic condition, usually an allergic one.) For a

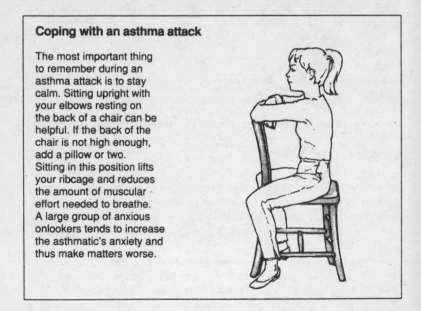

Coping with an asthma attack

The most important thing to remember during an asthma attack is to stay calm. Sitting upright with your elbows resting on the back of a chair can be helpful. If the back of the chair is not high enough, add a pillow or two. Sitting in this position lifts your ribcage and reduces the amount of muscular effort needed to breathe. A large group of anxious onlookers tends to increase the asthmatic's anxiety and thus make matters worse.

child, in particular, panicky adults are likely to make matters a great deal worse, whereas a soothing and reassuring person can actually alleviate the attack. For this reason, it is vital not to be over-protective with asthmatic children, and not to make them unduly fearful of their disease. They need to have as much freedom as possible, combined with a realistic understanding of the risks and their own limitations. This rhyme, written by an asthmatic boy with an asthmatic brother, sums up the ideal outlook for a child:

> Brothers are we,
> Both strong as sailors,
> But we never go nowhere,
> Without our inhalers.

Make sure that asthmatic children get enough exercise, by taking them to an indoor swimming pool, for example, where the amount of pollen in the air will be very low. Holidays by breezy coasts or high in the mountains are also beneficial, since pollen counts are usually low in these places, (mountains are also inhospitable to dust-mites, if these are an additional allergen). In Britain, the National Asthma Campaign organizes excellent activities and holidays for children and teenagers with severe asthma (see p317).

Chapter Six

DIAGNOSING HAYFEVER AND IDENTIFYING THE POLLEN CONCERNED

'If the waiting room is alive with the sound of sneezing, then I *know* it must be June,' observes a doctor with a busy practice in the London suburbs. Hayfever follows the seasons of the year more closely than any other disease, and for this reason the timing of the symptoms plays a major part in arriving at a diagnosis.

In many parts of the world the hayfever season is so clearly defined that patients can be diagnosed on this alone; if they have the right symptoms, and have them at the right time of year, then hayfever will be considered overwhelmingly likely and no further tests will be carried out. Tests are regarded as a waste of time and money – resources that are increasingly precious in health care.

This approach works when there are just two or three major pollen allergens whose times of release do not overlap too much. The cooler regions of the world are more likely to fall into this category because their vegetation is less varied and the growing season for plants is strictly limited. With only a few warm months available for growing, plants confine flowering to a brief interlude only, although pollen production may be prolific during that time to compensate.

In the Scandinavian countries, for example, birch pollen and grass pollens are the two major allergens. The birch season runs from late April through May, then stops fairly sharply. (Although research shows that people with birch-pollen hayfever often react to other plants as well, it is mainly birch pollen that is causing their symptoms.) The grass season begins in late May and runs through June and July. Most people with seasonal rhinitis suffer in one or both of these seasons. A third, and much smaller, group of patients does not start sneezing until July or August – they are sensitive to mugwort.

With only three principal allergens, each having a clear-cut season, skin-prick tests (see p78) are not used for the majority of patients. The sharply seasonal nature of the symptoms answers two questions at once: it shows that patients have hayfever rather than some other form of rhinitis, *and* it pinpoints the pollen primarily responsible. These are the two major aspects of diagnosis.

This diagnosis-by-season approach tends to be far less useful in warm, moist areas such as northeastern Australia. Here there is highly varied vegetation, including both native and introduced plants, and some very long pollination seasons. In much of north Queensland, for example, growing conditions are good all year round, and there is grass pollen in the air during every month of the year. Someone with year-round symptoms might be sensitive to grass pollen, or to mould spores or house-dust mite, or to some combination of these items. Other pollens might also play a part. The patient could, alternatively, have a non-allergic form of rhinitis (see Chapter Thirteen). In such a situation, skin-prick tests or other forms of medical diagnosis are vitally important.

In other warm regions with plentiful rainfall, such as Florida, California, or the Mediterranean countries, pollination seasons can again be very long, with a great deal of overlap between different plants. Pellitory-of-the-wall, for example, pollinates energetically from February to July around the Mediterranean, pauses for a brief rest in August, then flowers for yet another two months from September to November. During this time, a great many other allergenic pollens come and go in the air, and are abundant enough to cause hayfever. Given such circumstances, pollen seasons are too confused to be of much help in diagnosis.

The situation in Britain, and throughout northern Europe, falls somewhere between these two extremes, although it is closer to the Scandinavian example. Here grass pollen is the major offender and, as the doctor quoted earlier observes, the grass pollen season arrives with a bang in June. Since many different grasses cross-react (see p153), and most patients are allergic to the pollen of several species, a diagnosis of 'grass sensitive' is sufficiently accurate for almost all purposes.

Diagnosis by season becomes slightly less accurate for other pollens in Britain and northern Europe. There is a 'tree pollen' season in March, April and May, when sensitive people may react to the pollens of birch, alder, hazel, oak, ash, poplar or plane. Several of these species cross-react (see p154), particularly birch, alder and hazel, which belong to the same plant family, so it is reasonable enough to use 'tree pollens' as a diagnostic category. However, this may disguise some crucial differences between patients. (Unfortunately, skin-prick testing is usually done with 'mixed tree pollens', so it is no more accurate.)

A minority of patients in Britain and northern Europe have hayfever in August and September, usually in response to nettle, plantain, dock or mugwort pollen. While these are often lumped together as 'weed pollens', there is far less justification for this than there is with the trees: in general, there are no cross-reactions between weed pollens, except where the plants are closely related, and none of these are (see pp157–9). Someone with symptoms at this time of year could, alternatively, be reacting to mould spores. Diagnosis by skin-prick tests (see p78) would be worthwhile for anyone with late summer or autumn symptoms. Sometimes commercial extracts known as 'mixed weed and shrub pollens' are used for this. While they may differentiate a pollen allergy from a mould allergy, that is all they can do. Extracts of individual pollens are available to doctors (see p318) and should really be used for a meaningful result.

In the temperate regions of Canada and the northern USA the major allergen for most areas is ragweed, which pollinates from August to October. However, there are other allergenic weeds pollinating at this time, and skin-prick tests are helpful in pinpointing the culprit pollen. There is also a fairly well-defined grass season, usually from May to July. Those with hayfever symptoms in spring may be reacting to one of a range of different tree pollens. As in northern Europe, a rough diagnosis can be made on the basis of the season when symptoms occur. Moving southwards through the USA, the pollen seasons become longer, the allergenic plants more varied, and diagnosis by season increasingly difficult.

Appendix 1 lists the major allergenic pollens in different regions of the world, together with their pollination seasons. By noting when your symptoms occur, and studying the list for the region where you live, you may well be able to identify your problem pollen. Check with the illustration on pp112–13 (or with a local plant or tree field guide) to see if the likely culprit actually grows in the area where you live. If it grows densely in the surrounding area, then you can fairly assume that it is the problem. However, its apparent absence is not proof of its innocence. Pollen can travel for many miles on the warm airstreams of spring and summer, so even if the plant is not growing around your home area, it could still be affecting you. Check what plants grow in the surrounding countryside, or the areas from which the prevailing winds blow.

IS IT ESSENTIAL TO IDENTIFY THE POLLEN CAUSING HAYFEVER?

If it is not obvious which pollen causes your hayfever, you may be wondering whether it is crucial to identify your 'problem pollen', and whether you should therefore pay a visit to your doctor.

For those people who can control their hayfever symptoms well enough using antihistamines or other medicinal drugs, the answer to this is probably no. For those who do well with general avoidance measures, such as keeping windows closed when they have hayfever, the answer may also be no.

Identifying the pollen only becomes important if your symptoms are really troublesome and you want to try taking more specific avoidance measures – then you do need to know which plants cause your symptoms. Occasionally, the plant is growing in a very limited area indeed, and can actually be eliminated. For example, one patient with hayfever and pollen asthma discovered, through skin-prick tests, that the cause of the trouble was cypress pollen. Since she lived in a rural area of Australia, and the row of trees lining the driveway to her house were the only cypresses for miles around, eliminating cypress pollen from her life was a simple task.

The other situation in which it may be vital to identify your problem pollen is if you intend to travel abroad. The culprit pollen may be far more common at your destination than in the area where you currently live, resulting in a severe hayfever reaction that could spoil your trip. For example, someone with hayfever to 'tree pollen' might travel to Sweden during May (when birch pollen counts can reach 3,000 grains per cubic metre of air) and discover, to their cost, that the previously unidentified 'tree' causing their problems was birch.

DIAGNOSTIC TESTS FROM THE DOCTOR

The tests a doctor can offer you show whether your body *could* mount an allergic reaction to a particular pollen, not whether it actually does so. They are rather like the test used for the brakes of an elderly car: if this shows that the brakes are not all that good any more, it suggests that the car might become involved in an accident. The brake test does not predict absolutely that the car will have an accident tomorrow, because other factors are involved, besides the condition of the brakes.

The two medical tests most commonly used for hayfever both involve introducing a small amount of a specific pollen allergen – grass pollen, for example – into the skin and then seeing what reaction this provokes. If there is a reaction, this shows that the allergy antibody IgE (see p31) is present in the skin, and that it is an IgE which is specific for grass pollen allergens. That is as far as the test goes. It does not show that the person tested has hayfever to grass.

The interpretation of the test is based on previous medical research and runs as follows: if there is IgE to grass pollen allergens in the skin, then there are probably identical IgE antibodies in the nose, and if these are present in the nose they could produce grass-pollen hayfever. However, this is by no means certain. As explained in Chapter Three, the body has a great many different ways of regulating allergy, and even though it has produced IgE against grass pollen, it could well have seen the error of its ways and instigated a control mechanism to keep that IgE in check.

Skin tests, then, are only a clue to the nature of your rhinitis. They should always be looked at in the light of other evidence, such as the time of year when you suffer symptoms and the local types of vegetation. In this way, they can be used to confirm a suspicion about particular pollen allergens.

Alternatively, if someone has rhinitis all year round, a skin test can be used to suggest likely allergens, such as house-dust mite or cat allergen. These suspects must then be investigated in other ways – usually by trying to eliminate or avoid them and seeing if there is any improvement in the symptoms.

The skin-prick test

The test is usually carried out on the lower part of the arm, using the soft, hairless skin on the inner surface. Sometimes the skin on the back is tested instead. An extract of the allergen is used, with a single drop being placed on the skin. A pointed instrument known as a lancet is then used to lift the skin under the drop, puncturing it slightly so that some of the allergen extract enters the skin. This process is repeated for each of the allergens to be tested, usually ten or more, and sometimes up to thirty. Surplus extract is dabbed off, and the skin is left to react for between ten and twenty minutes. At the end of this time, the area of skin around each prick test is examined for signs of inflammation – this reveals whether the skin contains IgE antibody specific for that allergen. If there is any reaction, the size of the bump around the test site gives a rough idea of how strong that reaction is.

Antihistamine drugs (see p89), which can be bought without prescription, will interfere with skin-prick tests by inhibiting the reactions to allergen. If you are taking antihistamines and require skin-prick tests, you must stop taking the drugs at least two days before the test, and much longer for *astemizole* (Hismanal, Pollon-eze). Since the tests are quick and easy, they will probably be carried out at a first appointment, so it is worth stopping antihistamines before you see the doctor for the first time – assuming that you can manage without them. Always inform the doctor that you have been, or are taking, antihistamines.

After the skin-prick test, you may suffer a delayed reaction at one or more of the test sites. This can come on many hours later and can produce a large bump that is painful or itchy. It is just one example of the late-phase reaction (see p41). Should you experience such a reaction, it is nothing to worry about, and it will clear spontaneously within a day or so.

Intradermal testing

In many countries, including Britain and the USA, skin-prick testing (described above) is used almost exclusively, and intradermal testing is rarely practised. In some other parts of the world, however, intradermal testing is still the norm.

This test involves using a larger amount of allergen (but a weaker concentration) than the skin-prick test, and injecting it a little more deeply into the skin. As more allergen is used, there is a very small risk of **anaphylactic shock**, a major allergic reaction involving the whole body, which can be fatal if not treated promptly (see p139). If you suffer from asthma (whether to pollen or to some other allergen), make sure the doctor knows this before intradermal testing is carried out – the dangers of anaphylaxis are higher for anyone with asthma.

Blood tests

These are tests for the amount of IgE (the allergy antibody) in the blood. Usually the test is for a particular type of IgE, such as IgE to grass-pollen antigens. There are two versions of this test, whose technical names are the radioallergosorbent test (RAST for short) and the enzyme-linked immunosorbent assay (ELISA for short).

Such a test is far more expensive and troublesome than a skin-prick test, and yet it does not tell the doctor very much more. One occasion when it might be used is for a patient with a severe skin disorder that prevents a skin-prick test or intradermal test being carried out. It can also be valuable for patients taking antihistamines who are unable to stop taking them even for a few days for skin testing. Finally, there are patients who might be given a RAST rather than a skin test because they have suffered anaphylactic shock in the past and are regarded as a high-risk case by the doctor. This is probably overcautious, as anaphylactic reactions to skin-prick tests are virtually unknown, but given the severity and danger of anaphylactic shock, caution is probably wise.

The total amount of IgE in the blood (rather than particular types of IgE) can also be measured. This is rarely done for adults as it does not generally tell the doctor anything useful. However, it may be a valuable test for newborn babies who are considered at risk of allergy (see p246).

Intranasal provocation tests

In Chapter Four, the pioneering studies of Charles Harrison Blackley were described. This nineteenth-century doctor, as you may remember, was a hayfever sufferer himself, and the first to identify the true cause of hayfever. He did so by saving pollen during the summer, then inhaling it in mid-winter

The skin-prick test

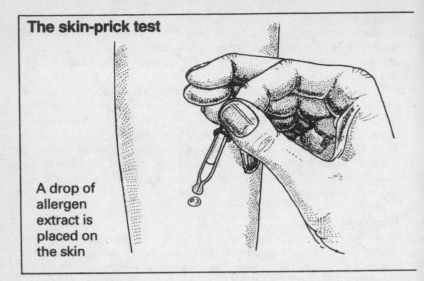

A drop of
allergen
extract is
placed on
the skin

to see what happened. He sneezed, and the rest is history. This seems to be the best, simplest and most direct test for hayfever, so why is it not used by doctors today? The answer is that a test of this type has sometimes been used in the past; it is known as a **nasal provocation test**. But it has fallen from favour because it is difficult to 'standardize', that is, to ensure that all patients are given the same dose of pollen allergen, and to measure their reaction in an accurate and scientific way. There is also some risk of provoking a severe reaction in the nose or, worse, an asthma attack.

However, if you are sufficiently curious about the cause of your hayfever and have not managed to identify the pollen responsible by the usual routes, then you could follow in Blackley's footsteps. Collect a few different pollens for comparison. Be very cautious about how much pollen you inhale – begin with the tiniest of pinches, spread it out on your hand and sniff very gently. *(Do not try this method at all if you have ever had an asthma attack.)* If there is no reaction, try a larger sniff. You may need to repeat this daily for a few days to get a reaction.

For a truly scientific approach, you should label the containers on the base, and not look at the label until you have carried out all the tests. In other words, test each pollen without knowing what it is at the time. This avoids the result being biased by your expectations. Test one pollen each day, without looking at the label either before or afterwards. Slip the container into an envelope that you have labelled with the day, and any symptoms you experienced.

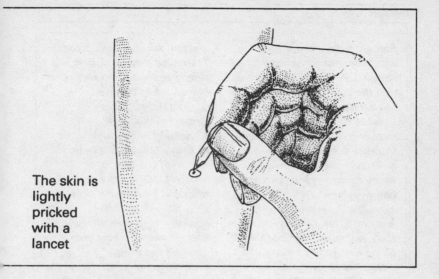

The skin is lightly pricked with a lancet

Repeat this until you have tested all the pollens, then open the envelopes to see which plants provoked your symptoms.

LIMITATIONS OF SKIN TESTING

Standard forms of testing available from the doctor have certain limitations. One which has already been mentioned is the chance of a **false positive** – a positive skin test (or blood test) to a pollen or other allergen that does not actually cause symptoms. It occurs fairly frequently, especially with house-dust mite allergen.

The opposite can also occur – the skin test can be negative even though the person *does* have symptoms in response to that allergen. This **false negative** reaction is most unusual, however. It only occurs when there is IgE for a particular pollen in the lining of the nose, but none in the skin. An allergist will usually look into such discrepancies using a nasal provocation test, although this too has its problems, described earlier.

Compared to the skin-prick test, the intradermal test has a greater chance of a false positive reaction and a lesser chance of a false negative.

One major shortcoming of *all* tests is that they can only find what they look for – and they mostly look for reactions to common allergens. If you are allergic to anything out of the ordinary, it is unlikely that the allergen concerned will be included in the set of extracts that the doctor has available. Some allergists will make up their own extracts to test likely suspects.

BARBARA

Barbara's day always began with a bout of exhausting sneezes. Wherever she lived it was the same. She had moved from New York to Israel to Britain, but the sneezing always followed her. During the rest of the day she suffered from a constant runny nose. Several doctors had wondered if she might be allergic to house-dust mite, and had given her skin-prick tests, but none were positive. Some had gone further and tested her blood for IgE antibodies (see p79) to dust mite, but again there was nothing. Finally, an allergist decided to test her nose directly. She carried out the test several times, sometimes puffing dust into Barbara's nose, sometimes an inert powder. Barbara was never told which it was, so her reaction was not prejudiced. The house dust produced severe sneezing and watery mucus, while the inert powder did not. Clearly, Barbara was allergic to something in house dust, probably house-dust mite. Although she was quite severely allergic, the skin tests and blood tests did not show this. Such **false negative** tests (see p81) can happen with medical tests because the allergy antibodies (IgE) may be present in the nose but not in the skin or bloodstream. Although this is relatively unusual, doctors should always bear in mind that it can happen. Reducing the mite population in her house (see pp175–92) produced a remarkable improvement in Barbara's health.

Occasionally, patients have strong suspicions about a particular pollen, only to be told that it cannot possibly be a cause of hayfever. This may happen with garden flowers (which are pollinated by insects), and with pine trees, both of which have gone down in medical lore as *never* causing hayfever. It is true that these two groups are not often implicated in hayfever, but there are plenty of exceptions among both insect-pollinated plants (see pp4–8) and conifers (see p6).

If it has proved impossible to identify your allergen, and the doctor or allergist is baffled, you may be able to get help from more specialist sources. There are pollen advice units in some countries, including Britain (see p316), that can help with information on the rarer pollens. Inhaled particles from insects are sometimes at the root of allergic mysteries, and there is a special research unit that can advise your doctor or consultant on allergenic insects (see p318). More information about insect allergies is given in Chapter Twelve (see pp212–13).

UNSUSPECTED ALLERGENS?

Until the late 1970s, tests for cockroach allergy were rarely carried out in the United States. Then allergists began testing for this particular sensitivity and found that it was remarkably common. Up to 30 per cent of people with allergies are sensitive to the faeces and skin particles of cockroaches. In some inner city areas in the southern states, where the warm climate suits cockroaches perfectly, they are the commonest cause of allergy.

Looking at a range of houses and using sensitive techniques to detect cockroach allergens, researchers found evidence of them in most samples of house dust. Even houses with no sign of cockroach infestation could show cockroach allergens in their dust, suggesting that if cockroaches are common in an area they may pay flying visits to every house on the street.

When the researchers looked at commercial extracts of house dust used for skin testing, they found that some contained cockroach allergens, while others did not. Thus a person with cockroach allergy might seem to be sensitive to house dust on the basis of one test, but if tested with house dust extract produced by a different company the test would be negative.

Cockroach allergy is also reported from India and other tropical countries, but no one knows how prevalent it is in Britain. Despite the cool climate, cockroaches are far more common than most people would like to think. A survey by the pest control firm Rentokil found cases of cockroach infestation in almost every region of Britain.

Until doctors begin including cockroach allergens in skin-prick testing, we will not know the extent of this problem. One intriguing aspect of this is that, in cool climates, cockroach numbers fall in winter and rise in the warm summer months. The amount of cockroach allergen in the air follows suit. Thus, someone with a runny nose or asthma due to cockroach particles might suffer symptoms only during summer, or might get much worse then. At present, such people would undoubtedly be diagnosed as having hayfever. If a skin-prick test were carried out, it could show no reactions to any of the allergens included, or it could show positive reactions to some allergens, including pollens. This might indicate that the patient is allergic to pollens as well as to cockroach allergen, or the pollen reaction could be a false positive (see p81). Either way, the patient would probably be diagnosed as having hayfever, when, in fact, this has little or nothing to do with the symptoms. The error should be obvious to the patient, because there will be far more symptoms indoors than outdoors. (This is unlikely to happen with hayfever unless you have a source of pollen indoors, see p115, or you live in a tower block, see p111.) It is up to the patient to impress this fact on the doctor, and to ask for a further set of tests.

Other insect allergies may also be more widespread than is commonly thought. Researchers in Japan decided to test this idea using skin-prick tests, and found a remarkable number of people who were allergic to insects such as silkworms and caddis flies. These are insects that generate a lot of airborne particles at certain times of year, and again they could produce seasonal symptoms that resemble hayfever (see p219).

Could there be pollens that are a widespread cause of hayfever but are not usually included in skin tests? Probably not, but there may be some exceptions. Scientists trapping pollen at the University of Cordoba in southern Spain found very large amounts of cypress pollen in the air during the winter months. They asked local doctors about cypress allergy and were told that it was unknown – but since no one tested for it, this was hardly surprising. Eventually, the doctors were persuaded to include cypress-pollen extract in their skin tests, and it turned out that cypress hayfever was quite common in the Cordoba region. Because the trees pollinate in winter, patients with this problem had always been diagnosed as having a prolonged cold, and therefore treated with entirely inappropriate medicines.

In the British Isles a weed known as pellitory-of-the-wall grows across the southern counties, the Midlands, Wales and Ireland. It was introduced from the Mediterranean region many centuries ago and tradition has it that medieval monks brought the plant to Britain, since it is frequently found around the ruins of monasteries. Pellitory-of-the-wall has never been regarded as a cause of allergy in the British Isles, yet it is a notorious hayfever plant in southern Europe. Doctors in Southampton decided to include pellitory-of-the-wall pollen in their skin-prick tests for a while, and discovered that quite a few patients gave positive reactions to the pollen. Whether this pollen actually causes any symptoms is unknown, but it probably does in some of these patients. Since pellitory can begin flowering in June, this type of hayfever could be mistaken for grass-pollen hayfever.

Chapter Seven

MEDICINAL DRUGS

Attitudes towards drugs present one of the most curious paradoxes of the modern age. On the one hand, there are a surprising number of people in our society who celebrate Saturday evening by sniffing an anonymous white powder, or swallowing an unlabelled white tablet, the powder or tablet being of unknown composition, and bought from a dubious character with absolutely no qualifications in pharmacy. Many more people regularly inhale another drug, supplied in a packet that is clearly labelled '. . . CAUSES LUNG CANCER'. At the other extreme, large numbers of people are terrified of taking any tablets, even those whose ingredients are known and carefully standardized, produced by reputable pharmaceutical companies, tested extensively for safety, and approved by the government.

In between these two extreme groups, the rest of the population hovers uncertainly, not sure whether medicinal drugs are a blessing or an insidious threat to its health. One of the problems lies in the word 'drug' itself, which includes everything from cough medicine to crack in one great tar-spreading brush stroke. The well-publicized scandals involving medicinal drugs, notably those about Thalidomide and Opren, have kept the fears going, and for many people the sense of mistrust is extended indiscriminately to all medicines.

In the case of allergy, particularly hayfever, we believe that this is unfortunate and deprives many people of the most useful help they can obtain. Drugs are not the *only* form of help, as the next two chapters will make clear, but they are not an option to be dismissed lightly, especially if your symptoms interfere with your life to any degree. The spring and summer are the best times of year – times to be enjoyed rather than endured.

Compared to the risk of driving down a motorway for an hour, the risk of taking an antihistamine is, for most people, very low indeed. Driving a car is dangerous, however good a driver you may be, but few of us give up driving because of the risks. Regularly spending an evening in a room full of cigarette smoke is slightly dangerous, but who would give up socializing to avoid this remote risk of lung cancer? In other words, we take some risks all the time, unconsciously weighing them up against our pleasure or convenience, and deciding that it is 'worth the risk'. Enjoying the sunny summer months is a pleasure one should not forgo unnecessarily.

This chapter is intended to inform you fully about the drawbacks, side-effects and risks of the drugs available for hayfever, other forms of rhinitis, and asthma. It does not minimize them but presents them in full. It explains, as far as possible, how the drugs work, and why they may cause side-effects. With this information you know what the 'cons' are. Discovering the 'pros' is up to you – you would have to try the drugs and see how much they help you. Once you know both the 'pros' and the 'cons', you can make a balanced and rational decision about taking drugs.

For anyone who is already taking medicines, this chapter can be of use in two ways. First, it can help to identify alternative drugs that may control the symptoms of hayfever or pollen more effectively, or simply cause fewer side-effects. Second, the chapter explains how to get more out of the drugs by using them more effectively. Many people with hayfever do not get the full benefits of the medicines they take because they start them too late in the season.

If you are already taking a medicine and do not know exactly what type of drug it is, you can use Appendix 5 to find out. There, and in the text that follows, the generic names of drugs (names that are used worldwide) are shown in italic, e.g. *chlorpheniramine*, while the trade names or brand names used in Britain are shown with a capital letter, e.g. Piriton. With non-prescription drugs, the generic name of the drug used is always given on the packet, although you may have to look hard for it. There are sometimes two drugs in a medicine, so be sure both to check in Appendix 5 and to read the information on each.

The information given here is intended as a guide only. If you buy non-prescription medicines, and feel you need further information, ask to speak to the pharmacist at the shop where you buy them. The pharmacist can advise you on the safety of the medicine, and whether you should consult your doctor before taking it. With prescription drugs, be sure to tell the doctor about anything that may be relevant to the choice of drug, such as other non-prescription drugs you are taking, or high alcohol consumption.

MAST-CELL STABILIZERS

There are only two well-established drugs in this category at present: *sodium cromoglycate* (also called *cromolyn sodium*) and *nedocromil sodium*. These are relatively new drugs that will probably become far more widely used in the future. They are very safe drugs, with fewer risks or side-effects than any of the other anti-allergy medicines.

A new drug, *lodoxamide* (Alomide), is believed to have a similar effect to the established mast-cell stabilizers.

How they work

These drugs are thought to tackle the allergic reaction at an early point by making mast cells more stable, that is, less likely to discharge their granules (see p32). However, there is some question about exactly how they work. Whatever their effect, they need to reach the mast cell before the allergen does.

Minor side-effects

Sneezing, stinging and smarting are fairly common reactions, but they are not a cause for concern as long as they pass quickly – which they usually do. With inhalers and nebulizers containing these drugs, there can be a transient cough as a result of throat irritation. Rinsing the mouth out with water, after inhaling the drug, will reduce these side-effects.

On rare occasions, when used as a nose spray or as an asthma treatment, these drugs have actually brought on an attack of asthmatic wheezing. If this happens, consult your doctor.

Even more rarely, there can be a true allergic reaction to the drug, in which case it must be discontinued immediately. *Nedocromil sodium* is the stronger of the two drugs, and can cause a transient headache or nausea when taken by mouth. You should see your doctor if you have these side-effects, or if you suffer a rash.

Precautions and interactions

Sodium cromoglycate is considered safe for use by anyone, even pregnant women and breastfeeding mothers. *Nedocromil sodium* should not be taken during pregnancy.

Usefulness

Suitable for symptoms in the eye or nose, and for asthma. These drugs do not work for everyone, but when they do work they are very effective. Since they are so safe and free of side-effects, they are worth trying.

Mast-cell stabilizers are particularly useful for young children if the doctor is reluctant to prescribe corticosteroid nose drops.

In the case of eye drops, those containing mast-cell stabilizers are considered much safer than corticosteroid drops.

How taken
Eye drops for conjunctivitis. These contain *sodium cromoglycate* (Opticrom) or *lodoxamide* (Alomide).

Nasal spray or drops for hayfever. These contain *sodium cromoglycate* (Rynacrom spray*) sometimes combined with a sympathomimetic, see p96 (Resiston One drops*).

Aerosols, nebulizers or spinhalers for asthma. These contain *sodium cromoglycate* (Intal, Cromolyn, Cromogen), or *nedocromil sodium* (Tilade).

Maximizing the benefits
With mast-cell stabilizers it is important to take them before encountering your problem pollen. If they get to the mast cell before the allergen, they are far more effective in stalling the allergic reaction. An asthma attack that has already begun cannot be relieved with this drug. However, some patients with hayfever do find that they are helped by these drugs, even after the symptoms have begun.

The benefits gradually build up, particularly with asthma and perennial (year-round) rhinitis. It can take up to six weeks of regular dosage for the anti-asthma effect to be established. With eye and nose symptoms due to pollen, the good effects are seen much more quickly, usually within a few days. But it is important that you use the drug regularly, and at the correct intervals, to gain the full benefit. Some doctors recommend starting the drug two or three weeks before the pollen season to ensure maximum effectiveness. The nose drops need to be used at least four times a day, so if you lead a hectic life and are not much good at remembering such things, this may not be the best drug for you.

With nose drops, a nose that is already profoundly blocked may be impermeable to the drops. In such cases, drops or spray containing an unblocking agent called a **sympathomimetic** (see p96) can be useful, in the short term, for opening up the nose to the mast-cell stabilizer, but they should not be taken for too long (see p97).

Some good effects will persist for several days after the treatment is stopped, but if you have asthma, or if the pollen season is still in progress, you should not discontinue the drug suddenly without consulting your doctor.

* No prescription required.

ANITA

Anita's hayfever began quite late in life, when she was twenty. She was prescribed antihistamines by her doctor, but found that they made her extremely dull and drowsy. She worked as a radio producer, and as her job required a high degree of concentration, taking these drugs was simply not feasible. Anita resigned herself to tolerating the hayfever symptoms. Six years later she was still suffering from hayfever when a friend showed her the tablets she took, a new form of antihistamine that did not produce drowsiness. These tablets could be bought without prescription and Anita was amazed to find that they reduced her hayfever to almost nothing without causing sleepiness. 'It was only through chance that I found out about this new drug,' Anita remarks. 'I'm glad I didn't go on just putting up with my hayfever year after year.'

ANTIHISTAMINES

These are the drugs most widely used for hayfever. There are several kinds that can be bought without a prescription because they are considered very safe.

How they work

Antihistamines work by interfering with the activities of histamine. This is a mediator (chemical messenger) released by mast cells (see p31), the cells that cause the allergic reaction. Although mast cells release several different mediators, histamine is probably the most powerful of them all. (Drugs to block other mediators, such as leukotrienes – see p32 – may well come on to the market within the next few years.)

When histamine is released into the bloodstream by mast cells, it affects the blood vessels themselves and certain muscles, known as smooth muscles. These smooth muscles are the ones over which we have no voluntary control, such as those in the bronchi, the digestive system and the bladder. Histamine makes these muscles contract, and the effect is particularly noticeable in the bronchi, where muscle contraction causes narrowing of the airways – an asthma attack. The effect of histamine on the blood vessels is to make them more leaky, so that immune cells can escape into the surrounding tissue –

part of the process of inflammation (see p34). Histamine also has several other actions that promote inflammation.

Histamine exerts its effects by binding to **receptors** on its target cells – cells lining the blood vessels, for example. When histamine binds, the receptor molecule passes a message on to the cell itself – it is rather like a doorbell that can be rung only by one specific messenger, histamine. Antihistamines work by being a little bit like histamine – similar enough to bind to the receptor, but not similar enough to make the receptor 'ring the bell' of the cell.

Like many of the chemical messengers in the body, histamine has a number of different jobs. It is released by various other cells in the body, not just mast cells, but in these cases histamine simply acts as a local messenger substance, carrying instructions to cells in the immediate vicinity only.

To allow messenger substances to have multiple jobs in the body, there is usually more than one type of receptor for each messenger. Cells in the brain, for example, may have a different kind of receptor from cells in the heart, so that the messenger can have different effects on each. In the case of histamine, three types of receptor are known, called H1, H2 and H3. It is the H1 receptors that are involved in the inflammation response, and which antihistamines block. The proper pharmaceutical name for antihistamines is 'histamine H1-receptor antagonists'. They do not bind to the second type of receptor for histamine, the H2 receptor, which is found in the lining of the stomach.

Minor side-effects

There is a range of antihistamines on the market, some of which have been in use for decades, while others are relatively new. A full list of those taken in tablet or liquid form is given below. Antihistamines in drops and sprays are listed on pp94–5, under 'How Taken'.

Older antihistamines:

(Several of these older antihistamines are also available combined with a sympathomimetic – see p98)

azatadine (Optimine*)
brompheniramine (only available combined with sympathomimetic, see p100)
chlorpheniramine (Piriton*)
clemastine (Tavegil*, Aller-eze*)

* No prescription required.

cyproheptadine (Periactin*)
dimethindene (Fenostil Retard*)
diphenylpyraline (Histryl Spansule)
hydroxyzine (Atarax)
mebhydrolin (Fabahistin)
mequitazine (Primalan)
oxatomide (Tinset)
phenindamine (Thephorin*)
pheniramine (Daneral*)
promethazine (Phenergan*)
trimeprazine (Vallergan)
triprolidine (Pro-Actidil*)

new antihistamines:
acrivastine (Semprex)
astemizole (Hismanal*, Pollon-eze*)
cetirizine (Zirtek)
loratadine (Clarityn)
terfenadine (Triludan*, Seldane*, Boots Antihistamine Tablets*)

The older types have quite a few side-effects, notably drowsiness. There can also be dizziness, nervousness, tremors, stomach upsets, dry mouth, blurred vision and, occasionally, impotence. In children, they sometimes have the opposite effect to drowsiness, making the child hyperactive. They have these effects because part of the histamine molecule is quite similar, chemically speaking, to some other messenger substances, including **adrenaline**, **serotonin** and **acetylcholine**. All these substances are involved in passing messages between nerve cells. Because of the chemical similarities, antihistamines can bind to some of the receptors for these nerve-cell messengers, partially blocking their action. Drowsiness results from antihistamines blocking the action of adrenaline, while the dry mouth and stomach upsets are a result of its blocking acetylcholine.

Anything affecting the nervous system has very noticeable effects, even if the degree of interference is actually quite small and causes no serious damage. This is generally the case with antihistamines, and the side-effects are usually nothing to worry about – they should certainly not put you off trying a different antihistamine. Having said this, *a minority of people do need to be careful about taking antihistamines*, because of pre-existing medical problems: these are listed on pp92–3, under 'Precautions and interactions'.

As everyone's body chemistry is different, these symptoms will be experienced to different degrees. Some people can even take the old-type antihistamines with no side-effects at all. Others find that the side-effects vanish if they persist in taking the antihistamines. The disappearance of the side-effects is due to an adjustment of the receptor-messenger interactions that were involved, and it is most unlikely that any damaging long-term effects are occurring. At the end of the pollen season, when antihistamines are no longer being taken, the system will shift back to its original equilibrium.

Although the side-effects of antihistamines can be distressing, they are not indicative of any major damage being done to the body. The only two side-effects to be a major cause for concern with most antihistamines are a skin rash, and hyperactivity in children. If either of these occur, stop taking the drug and consult your doctor. (With *terfenadine* there are some additional side-effects that are a cause for concern – see p93.)

Indirect harm is the greatest danger with antihistamines, because drowsiness is risky if you are driving a car or working close to machinery. It is important to check the effects of antihistamines before getting behind the wheel. This is less of a problem with the newer antihistamines (see below), but even with these you should proceed cautiously at first. Note that alcohol and other sedatives will make any such side-effects far worse.

The newer antihistamines have been available for several years now, and have far fewer side-effects. This is because they have more difficulty in crossing the barrier that exists between the bloodstream and the brain, so fewer antihistamine molecules reach the brain. They should not cause any drowsiness at all, although a few people do still find that they have this effect. They are variously referred to as 'second-generation antihistamines', or 'non-sedating antihistamines' (NSAs).

If you have tried one of these newer antihistamines and still suffered side-effects, it is well worth trying another one. They are different chemically, and there may be one that is just right for you. If you have found that they make you sleepy when combined with alcohol, try *cetirizine* or *loratadine*, which do not have this effect.

Precautions and interactions

There are a few situations in which antihistamines *might* be genuinely harmful. You should discuss the matter with a pharmacist or doctor if any of the following apply:

- you are pregnant or breastfeeding (see p108). For *astemizole* (Hismanal, Pollon-eze) you should definitely stop taking the drugs for several weeks *before* getting pregnant

- you have epilepsy, even *petit mal*, when the side-effects on the nervous system may be problematic

- you have liver or kidney problems, or urinary retention

- you have glaucoma

- you have prostate enlargement

- you are taking antidepressants, anti-anxiety drugs or sleeping tablets

- you have a thyroid disorder

- you have a heart condition or high blood pressure

- you have porphyria

- you have a stomach or duodenal ulcer

- you have Parkinson's disease

One of the most widely used antihistamines, *terfenadine* (Triludan or Seldane), has occasionally had side-effects on the heart. The same precautions apply as with other antihistamines (see above), but in addition you should not take *terfenadine* if:

- you are also taking *ketoconazole* (Nizoral), *fluconazole* (Diflucan) or related drugs. These are given as tablets, capsules or liquid and are prescribed for fungal infections, mainly vaginal thrush

- you are taking the antibiotic *erythromycin* (sold under a variety of trade names; ask the pharmacist if in doubt)

- you have any liver disease or damage, either now or in the past; liver damage can be due to infections, excessive consumption of alcohol, or other causes

- you have a heart arrhythmia

Stop taking terfenadine and consult your doctor if you experience any of the following: fainting, dizziness, palpitations or a skin rash. It should be emphasized here that the risks are very slight indeed, and that terfenadine has been in widespread use for ten years. You are most unlikely to suffer any ill-effects if you do not fall into any of the categories listed above.

Usefulness

Antihistamines are very effective in reducing most of the symptoms of hayfever, but they do not relieve a blocked nose. For this reason, they are often combined with a sympathomimetic (see p98). Corticosteroids, given as drops or spray, are useful for reducing nasal congestion, but not if the nose is absolutely blocked. In such cases, sympathomimetic drops or spray may be used first to open up the nose for the corticosteroid; alternatively, corticosteroid tablets may sometimes be used (see p105).

In the case of asthma, antihistamines are not particularly helpful. This is because asthma is a complex reaction in which other mediators, besides histamine, play a major role. The medicines used for asthma are described in the last two sections of this chapter.

Certain antihistamines have other actions as well and therefore deserve a special mention. *Ketotifen* (Zaditen) and *oxatomide* (Tinset) act as both antihistamines and mast-cell stabilizers (see p87). They have proved useful in preventing asthma attacks, but may have side-effects similar to those of the older antihistamines. *Terfenadine* (Triludan, Seldane) also stabilizes mast cells to some extent.

If antihistamines are taken regularly for many years, they may eventually become less effective. Switching to another form of treatment, such as corticosteroid nose drops or a mast-cell stabilizer, may be the best course of action in such circumstances.

How taken

Antihistamines are mainly taken by mouth, in tablet, capsule or liquid form. They are carried around the body in the bloodstream and reach the nose and eyes in this way. See pp90–1 for a list of the different ones available. Many can be bought without a prescription, but if none of these suit you, it might be worth asking your doctor about those available on prescription. (As far as cost is concerned, buying these drugs over the counter works out about the same as the prescription charge, and can be a little cheaper.)

Eye drops containing antihistamine are also available for anyone with conjunctivitis. A sympathomimetic (see p96) is included in these drops. The drops available at present all use the antihistamine *antazoline* (Otrivine-Antistin*, Vasocon-A). The presence of the sympathomimetic means that these drugs should not be used for too long, but a few weeks is probably safe.

---

* No prescription required.

Until recently, antihistamines have not been available in nose drops or sprays because they have various drawbacks in this form. One nasal spray is now available, containing *azelastine* (Rhinolast), but a prescription is needed for this. The number of antihistamines available in this form is likely to increase in the next few years. Current trends in drug use favour drops and sprays, which put the drug exactly where it is most needed. This more precise targeting of drugs means that the dosage can be much smaller, minimizing possible effects on other parts of the body.

New antihistamines are still being developed, and one, *levocabastine*, is intended for direct use in nose drops. This new drug looks very promising indeed – it is highly specific in its effects, and a very powerful blocker of histamine. Once it has undergone full safety trials, *levocabastine* drops and sprays should become available to hayfever sufferers.

Maximizing the benefits
A knowledge of how antihistamines work (see p89) can help in using them to best effect. To do their job, the antihistamine molecules must bind to the H1 receptors for histamine *before* histamine arrives. If histamine is already there and securely bound, the antihistamine cannot dislodge it. In time, the histamine will become detached from the receptor naturally, and antihistamine can then take its place, but by then the allergic reaction will already have begun, and the most the antihistamine can do is to prevent the next influx of histamine from making matters worse.

Once some histamine has been let loose and has bound its receptors, various changes take place which make the nose and eyes far more sensitive to pollen – the effect known as priming (see p41). Among other changes, more mast cells and basophils will gather in the nose, so more histamine can be released next time. This makes the task of the antihistamine far more difficult.

For these reasons, starting antihistamines a little *before* the hayfever season, and continuing them without a break, makes excellent sense. It can give far better results for the same dosage, and may even allow the dosage to be lower. If you do not have a personal record of when your hayfever symptoms began in the past, you can use Appendix 1 to work out when your problem pollen is likely to become airborne. Start taking the antihistamines a few days beforehand, or a week to be on the safe side. For summertime pollens, such as those of grasses, the season will begin up to three weeks earlier if the spring weather has been unusually warm, so adjust the time accordingly. Some pollen information services, such as those supplied on special telephone lines (see p127), include a prediction of when the grass pollen season will begin.

Of the two commonly used new antihistamines, *terfenadine* (Triludan, Seldane) acts much more quickly than *astemizole*, so it is the best choice if you have left treatment rather late. *Acrivastine* (Semprex) is even faster acting and is useful as a 'rescue' treatment, but you will need a prescription for this.

SYMPATHOMIMETICS IN NOSE DROPS, NOSE SPRAYS OR EYE DROPS

These drugs are for short-term use only. As long as this point is understood, they are very safe. They are widely available without prescription and, unfortunately, are often misused.

How they work

Sympathomimetics are drugs which mimic the effects of naturally produced adrenaline, the messenger molecule which produces the 'flight or fight' reaction. Adrenaline has various effects, but one is to make the small blood vessels (capillaries) contract. Thus it has an opposing effect to histamine.

By applying a drug that mimics adrenaline, the blood vessels in the nose can be persuaded to contract. This immediately reduces nasal congestion and makes it easier to breathe. If there is blockage of the sinuses (see p18) or the Eustachian tube (see p19), this will be relieved. When the drug is applied directly to the nose, only a very small dose is needed, and there should be little effect on the rest of the body.

Sympathomimetics are also included in some eye drops to reduce redness, swelling and pain.

Minor side-effects

As with most nose sprays, there may be some irritation at first. Stinging can also occur with eye drops and there may be some blurring of vision. Check that you are not affected by this before driving a car.

If significant amounts are absorbed from the nose into the bloodstream, effects will be noted similar to those of adrenaline: a faster or more noticeable heartbeat, irritability, insomnia and headache. Reduce the dose and these effects should disappear. These side-effects are harmless to most people, but may pose a risk to some because of other medical conditions (see below).

Precautions and interactions

For certain people, even a small amount of sympathomimetic reaching the bloodstream can pose some risk. Older people should use a lower dose, and young children should not be given these drugs at all. Discuss the use of these drugs with a pharmacist or doctor if any of the following apply:

• you have a heart condition

- you have high blood pressure

- you have epilepsy

- you have a thyroid disorder

- you are taking antidepressants (monoamine oxidase inhibitor type), or have taken them within the past two weeks

- you have glaucoma

- you are pregnant

The major risk with nose drops and sprays containing sympathomimetics, and one that affects *everybody* using them, is that the nose itself can become dependent on them. This usually occurs when the drops are used for more than two weeks, but it can happen more quickly, after just five days of continuous treatment. If you then stop using the drops, the nose goes 'cold turkey' and becomes completely blocked. The medical term for this is **rebound congestion**. Continuing with the drops will not solve the problem, as the nose will gradually become more blocked, and increasing the dosage will produce side-effects on the heart.

Once the drops are discontinued, the rebound congestion will slowly sort itself out, and the nose will return to normal, but the intervening period may be most uncomfortable.

It is vital with sympathomimetics to use the drops or spray as recommended on the package, and never to increase the amount, or to take an extra dose. If you find that your nose is becoming more congested, or the effects of each treatment do not last as long, then begin to phase them out. Even if the drops are working well, you should stop using them as soon as you can, preferably within a few days. Never continue for more than fourteen days.

If you experience any pain in the eye, palpitations or chest pain, stop using the drops immediately.

In the case of eye drops containing sympathomimetics, these can generally be continued safely for a few weeks, but ask your pharmacist's advice.

Usefulness
For instantaneous relief of a blocked nose, sympathomimetics applied directly to the problem are unrivalled, but it must be remembered that they are not treating the underlying condition. You could find them useful at the very height of the hayfever season, or at a time when a blocked nose is a

serious problem – when taking an exam or giving a speech, for example. They can also be useful occasionally if your blocked nose is preventing you from sleeping well.

The nose can also be unblocked in other ways, such as inhalations (see pp145–6), or with nasal drops containing salt water (see p146). Neither of these will give such dramatic relief as sympathomimetics.

One major use of sympathomimetic nose drops and sprays is in opening up a blocked nose for the delivery of other drugs, such as corticosteroids or mast-cell stabilizers. Use them only for three to five days.

One type of nose drop, Resiston One*, uses a very low dose of sympathomimetic combined with a mast-cell stabilizer (*sodium cromoglycate*). At this low dosage it is apparently safe to continue using the sympathomimetic for a prolonged period.

How taken
Nose drops and sprays. The main ones available are *oxymetazoline* (Afrazine Nasal Drops* or Spray*), *phenylephrine* (Fenox Nasal Drops* or Spray*) and *xylometazoline* (Otrivine Nasal Drops* or Spray*).
Eye drops or nose drops, combined with another drug, principally antihistamines (as in Otrivine-Antistin* and Vasocon-A eye drops) or mast-cell stabilizers (as in Resiston One* nose drops).

Maximizing the benefits
Since you cannot use them for long, save sympathomimetic nose drops for when they can be most useful – at the height of the pollen season, for example.

ANTIHISTAMINE AND SYMPATHOMIMETIC COMBINED IN TABLETS OR LIQUID
Another use for sympathomimetics is in a mixture with antihistamines, to be taken by mouth. All the mixtures contain the older type of antihistamines.

How they work
Antihistamines tackle the allergic reaction (see p89), while the sympathomimetic helps to unblock the nose and overcome the sedative effect of the antihistamine.

Ideally, the side-effects of the two drugs should cancel each other out: the 'speed-you-up' effect of the sympathomimetic should counteract the 'slow-you-down' of the antihistamine. At the same time, the sympathomimetic

* No prescription required.

relieves the one symptom that antihistamines have little effect on: nasal blockage.

Minor side-effects
The sort of side-effects occurring with sympathomimetic nose drops (see p96) can also occur when taking a mixture of antihistamine and sympathomimetic by mouth, but they are unusual. The drowsiness and other side-effects typical of antihistamines (see p91) are more likely.

Precautions and interactions
Those listed for antihistamines (see pp92–3) also apply here.

Some of the risks associated with sympathomimetic nose drops also apply here, and anyone with a heart condition, thyroid disorder or glaucoma should not take these tablets (see pp96–7 for the full list). It would be a good idea to talk to the pharmacist before taking one of these mixtures, as there are several other medical conditions which make them unsuitable.

The problem of rebound congestion (see p97) rarely occurs with these preparations, since the amount of sympathomimetic included is small, and it is not applied directly to the nose.

Usefulness
These mixtures were developed before the new antihistamines came on to the market, at a time when all antihistamines had a sedative effect on a high proportion of patients. To a large extent, these mixtures have been superseded by the new non-sedating antihistamines, but they may still be useful, particularly if your nose is badly blocked when you have hayfever.

How taken
The antihistamines used are mostly the same as the older antihistamines that can be taken alone (see pp90–91). The sympathomimetics used are often different from those found in nose drops and sprays, but have much the same effect. Although usually taken as tablets, liquid forms are also available.

Antihistamine/Sympathomimetic Mixtures

Brand name	antihistamine	sympathomimetic
Actifed*	triprolidine	pseudoephedrine
Aller-eze Plus*	clemastine	phenylpropanolamine
Contac 400*	chlorpheniramine	phenylpropanolamine
Dimotane Plus*	brompheniramine	pseudoephedrine

Brand name	antihistamine	sympathomimetic
Dimotapp*	brompheniramine	phenylephrine + phenylpropanolamine
Dristan Decongestant*	chlorpheniramine	phenylephrine
Eskornade Spansules*	diphenylpyraline	phenylpropanolamine
Galpseud Plus*	chlorpheniramine	pseudoephedrine
Haymine*	chlorpheniramine	ephedrine
Sudafed Plus*	triprolidine	pseudoephedrine
Triominic Tablets*	pheniramine	phenylpropanolamine

Maximizing the benefits

As for antihistamines (see p95).

CORTICOSTEROIDS

These are valuable drugs that need to be used with care, since too much can damage the body. However, when applied directly to the nose, in drops or a spray, there is very little risk involved, and the effect is superior to any other drug available for hayfever. Corticosteroids for use in hayfever and asthma are only available on prescription.

How they work

These drugs mimic the action of one of the body's own hormones, **hydrocortisone** (also called **cortisol**). Hydrocortisone has a variety of effects. It controls the amount of sodium and potassium that the kidney allows to pass into the urine, and releases glucose into the blood. It also moves protein out of the muscles and bones, and influences the way fat is deposited. Finally, it suppresses inflammation, but only at doses far higher than those normally found in the body. This last effect makes corticosteroids useful in treating allergies.

In using corticosteroids to treat allegic reactions, the trick is to persuade the drug to damp down inflammation, without carrying out any of its other actions. This has been achieved, to a large extent, by modifying hydrocortisone slightly. This chemical tinkering has produced *prednisolone, beclomethasone* and *budesonide*, which suppress inflammation but have very little effect on the excretion of salt by the kidneys, or other bodily functions.

When corticosteroid drugs are taken by mouth or injected, they simply act on the outcome of allergic reactions, damping down the inflammation. But when corticosteroids are applied directly to the nose, they also stabilize mast cells and thus reduce histamine release. This double action makes corticosteroid nose drops a very useful form of treatment.

---

* No prescription required.

JOHN

For John, hayfever came on suddenly and without warning when he was thirty-three years old. Initially he thought he had caught a cold, but when the violent sneezing and runny nose persisted for eight weeks this seemed unlikely. There was also an intense itching in his eyes and a congested feeling in the nose 'that made ordinary existence almost impossible'. His doctor suggested buying over-the-counter remedies, but John found that all antihistamines gave him a dried-out sensation in the nose, and a 'spacey' feeling. He decided he was more willing to endure the symptoms of hayfever than the side-effects of the antihistamines. The next year, however, his symptoms were worse, and the doctor prescribed a nasal spray containing a corticosteroid. At the very first try he found that the spray gave him an immediate and intense headache. When John reappeared in the surgery, it was clear to the doctor that this was a patient who was unusually sensitive to drugs. But he wondered if corticosteroid drops, which do not penetrate the sinuses as readily as a nasal spray, might be the answer. He therefore prescribed nasal drops, which turned out to solve the problem. They control John's hayfever very thoroughly and cause no side-effects. As John's case shows, it is always worth persisting with drugs until a suitable one is found. Sometimes the same drug will affect a patient differently, depending on the way in which it is 'delivered' – spray or drops, in this instance. The gas used in aerosol sprays can be an irritant for some people.

Minor side-effects

There can be some stinging, burning, irritation or sneezing when given as nose drops or sprays, and some forms affect the senses of smell and taste. Over-use of nose drops and sprays can produce drying out of the nose, crusting and nosebleeds. Some people suffer other side-effects with the sprays (such as headaches) but do well on nose drops. There are also differences between the various corticosteroids, and one may irritate your nose while another does not, so be prepared to try different types. Using salt-water drops in the nose (see p146), in between the doses of corticosteroid, may reduce the irritant effect of the drug.

The drug itself is only part of the story here – the way in which it is delivered can also affect the nose. Some preparations are water-based (aqueous) sprays, which are generally less irritating than aerosol forms using freon gas as a propellant.

Other side-effects include infections, which are a more serious matter, and are therefore considered in the next section.

In general, corticosteroids have few obvious side-effects, but can be dangerous if misused – the exact opposite of antihistamines, which tend to produce minor side-effects quite often, but are actually very safe.

Precautions and interactions

The first thing that needs to be said here is that corticosteroids are quite different from the anabolic steroids that periodically scandalize the sporting world. Nor have they anything to do with steroid hormones involved in sex and reproduction, such as testosterone, oestrogen and progesterone. (The last two are used in contraceptive pills and hormone replacement therapy, and both are quite distinct from corticosteroid drugs.) Rest assured, then, that taking corticosteroids will not turn you into the Incredible Hulk, allow you to win the Olympics, put hairs on your chest or stop you getting pregnant. Great confusion has been spread on this topic because people use the word 'steroid' indiscriminately for a variety of quite distinct substances.

What corticosteroids *can* do is to make infections more likely, particularly fungal infections such as thrush (*Candida*). In suppressing inflammation, they hamper a valuable part of the body's fight against disease.

However, the use of corticosteroids for hayfever or perennial rhinitis does not seem to be associated with a great increase in the risk of disease, as the dosage used is generally low. *Candida* infections in the nose are very rare. Consequently, the drops are safe as long as there is no infection in the nose to begin with: *corticosteroids should never be used when an infection is already present*. (There are medicines that combine corticosteroids with an antibiotic, and these can be prescribed in such circumstances.)

If you are using corticosteroid nose drops for year-round rhinitis, your doctor should see you every six months and examine the membranes inside the nose to ensure that no damage is occurring.

There is a small risk of infections in the eye with corticosteroid eye drops, and care should be taken not to expose the eye to infections. Avoid, for example, rubbing the eyes with unwashed fingers, using grubby towels on your face, or applying make-up that has been open for some time. The herpes simplex virus, which causes cold sores and genital sores, is particularly dangerous to the eyes, and great care should be taken not to expose them to this infection.

Corticosteroid eye drops should not be used by those with glaucoma. If anyone in your family has ever suffered from glaucoma, you should mention this to the doctor.

With inhaled corticosteroids, used for asthma, there is sometimes a problem with recurrent thrush infections in the throat. These can be combated by rinsing the mouth out with warm water after each inhalation. If infections do develop, they can be controlled with anti-fungal lozenges.

A more insidious problem arises if corticosteroids are taken over a long period of time, or at a high dosage, because the glands that produce hydrocortisone for the body feel somewhat redundant and tend to reduce their own production levels. Stopping the drug leaves the body with insufficient corticosteroids, which can lead to collapse in the worst cases. This means that corticosteroids taken as tablets should *never* be stopped abruptly if they have been taken for more than a few weeks. The glands must be given time to recover their natural level of activity, by gradually reducing the dosage. Even after as little as two weeks, corticosteroids should be withdrawn gradually, by halving the dose each day, to avoid a flare-up of the original symptoms.

Someone taking corticosteroids by mouth should carry a card as a warning to hospital staff in the event of an accident; they need to know that the natural production of hydrocortisone may be suppressed. Your doctor should give you such a card when prescribing the drug, or the pharmacist who fills the prescription can supply one. Make sure your card is always in your purse or wallet where it can be easily found.

Corticosteroids are sometimes given as a 'depot injection' (see below), which slowly releases the drug into the bloodstream over the following weeks. The dose declines naturally, so the problem of suddenly stopping the drug does not occur. However, it is still important for medical staff to know about the treatment in the event of an accident, so you should be given a card by your doctor and carry it *at all times*.

Another problem with the injection method is that there can be some wasting of the muscle at the site of the injection. This, however, is a temporary effect.

If you have been receiving a corticosteroid injection for hayfever every year for some time (it is the only form of therapy given as a single injection), then you may like to discuss the continuation of this treatment with your doctor. Perhaps, given the hazards involved, this approach should be reconsidered, especially if there are newer forms of treatment which you have never tried, such as non-sedating antihistamines or corticosteroid nose drops. In any event, you could be growing out of your hayfever now, making the injection unnecessary.

The problem of suppressing the body's own hydrocortisone production only arises when corticosteroids are taken by mouth or injected. There is no cause for concern with eye drops, or nasal drops and sprays, because the amount reaching the bloodstream is so small. The only exceptions to this rule occur with very young children, where any sort of corticosteroid preparation, even nose and eye drops, should be used cautiously. Significant amounts can be absorbed into the bloodstream and can affect the child's development. Make sure that the child is seen regularly by your doctor.

Usefulness

Corticosteroids are very useful for suppressing inflammation in the eyes, nose and bronchi. They often work for hayfever when all other drugs have proved ineffective.

Recent research shows that corticosteroid nose drops, used for hayfever, can also help to reduce asthmatic symptoms occurring in the pollen season, probably by interfering with the reflex reaction between the nose and the bronchi (see p21).

With inhalers used for asthma, and eye drops for conjunctivitis, it is a good idea to try out mast-cell stabilizers before corticosteroids are prescribed. They may do the job just as well, and are safer than corticosteroids.

How taken

Nose drops and sprays for hayfever and year-round rhinitis. Only a very small dose of corticosteroid is used. Although some enters the bloodstream, it is broken down promptly by the liver, before it can have any effect on the rest of the body. The drugs used include *beclomethasone* (Beconase), *betamethasone* (Betnesol, Vista-Methasone), *budesonide* (Rhinocort), *fluticasone* (Flixonase), *flunisolide* (Syntaris) and *dexamethasone* (Dexa-Rhinaspray, also includes other ingredients).

Eye drops for conjunctivitis caused by pollen. The drugs used include *betamethasone* (Betnesol, Vista-Methasone), *clobetasone* (Eumovate), *fluorometholone* (FML), *dexamethasone* (Maxidex), *prednisolone* (Minims, Pred Forte, Predsol).

Where there is a possibility of infection, nose and eye drops are available that contain an antibiotic as well as a corticosteroid; ask your doctor about these.

Inhalers and other devices for asthma. Very little of the drug enters the bloodstream when delivered in this way as the dose is small. Knowing how to use the devices properly is absolutely essential – ask the doctor to show you again if you are not sure. The drugs used are *beclomethasone* (Becotide, Becloforte, Becodisks, Aerobec Autohaler) and *budesonide* (Pulmicort).

Tablets, for dealing with a severe attack of asthma, or controlling troublesome hayfever symptoms during examinations. Sometimes this is the only effective treatment, but it has certain risks (see p103). Most doctors are cautious about prescribing such treatments. The tablets should be continued for a minimum of three weeks, and then slowly withdrawn. In the case of asthma, if they are stopped before three weeks, the asthma can flare up again shortly afterwards.

'Slow-release' injection into the buttock for controlling severe hayfever. A single injection at the beginning of the hayfever season leaves a reserve of corticosteroid in the muscle. This slowly leaks out into the bloodstream and continues combating inflammation for several weeks or months. As with corticosteroid tablets, this is a treatment with some risks attached, so it should not be used unless other methods have failed. (A similar form of treatment, in which corticosteroid is injected into the nose, should no longer be used as it carries a danger of blindness.)

Maximizing the benefits

Corticosteroid injections are given before the hayfever season begins. With nose and eye drops, it is also useful to start the treatment before the pollen becomes airborne, preferably about a week before. However, starting early is not as vital with corticosteroids as it is with mast-cell stabilizers or antihistamines. If symptoms do appear, begin using the drops or spray as soon as possible to avoid 'priming' (see p41).

With nose drops and sprays, it is important to learn how to use them correctly; ask your doctor's advice. If your nose is very blocked, the drops may be unable to reach their target. A sympathomimetic can be useful, in the short term, for opening up the nose to the corticosteroid drops, but it should not be taken for too long (see p97).

The maximum benefits from nose drops may not be felt until you have been using them for a week or two.

Corticosteroids are usually just one half of the battle against asthma: they help to reduce the inflammation in the bronchi, while bronchodilators (see p106) are used to open up the bronchi when an asthma attack does occur. The corticosteroids are treating the underlying inflammation and therefore need to be taken regularly, whereas the bronchodilators are used only when needed. A mast-cell stabilizer (see p87) may be added to the armoury, to further reduce inflammation – as with a corticosteroid, this must be taken regularly. Should you find you need to use your bronchodilator frequently – more than four to six times a day, for example – this indicates that the underlying inflammation is not being treated properly, so you should see your doctor again.

BRONCHODILATORS

These are used for asthma, and are only available on prescription. Your doctor will discuss their use with you before prescribing them, so the notes given here are fairly brief.

All bronchodilators make the bronchial muscles relax, and are used to alleviate or prevent asthma attacks. There are four types.

ß2-adrenoceptor agonists

Antagonists are drugs such as antihistamines, which bind to receptors and block the effect of the natural messenger that normally binds to the receptor. *Agonists* have the opposite effect. They bind to receptors and stimulate the cell, in the same way that the natural messenger would – in other words, they mimic the effects of that natural messenger.

The ß2-adrenoceptor agonists mimic the effects of adrenaline on the bronchial muscles, making them relax. They do so by binding to the receptors for adrenaline. These are called ß2 adrenoceptors, hence the name of the drugs. They include *salbutamol* (Ventolin, Ventodisks, Volmax, Maxivent, Rimasal, Salbulin, Salbuvent, Asmaven, Aerolin-Auto), *terbutaline* (Bricanyl, Monovent), *fenoterol* (Berotec), *pirbuterol* (Exirel), *reproterol* (Bronchodil), *rimiterol* (Pulmadil) and *salmeterol* (Serevent). Sometimes such drugs are combined with corticosteroids (see p100), as in Ventide, which contains *salbutamol*.

Of all the bronchodilators, these drugs have the most specific effects on the bronchi. They are now preferred to *isoprenaline* (Medihaler-Iso) which has a less specific effect, and tends to combine with adrenaline receptors in the heart muscles as well as those in the bronchi, sometimes causing irregular heartbeat, flushing and headaches. *Isoprenaline* is combined with a sympathomimetic, *phenylephrine*, in Medihaler-Duo.

Isoetharine is another non-specific ß-agonist. It is combined with *phenylephrine*, a sympathomimetic in Bronchilator. *Orciprenaline* (Alupent) is a drug of the same type that is partially selective for bronchial muscles, and has similar side-effects.

Side-effects *can* also occur with the specific ß2-adrenoceptor agonists, such as *salbutamol*, although they are generally less of a problem. They include tremor, nervous tension, headache, flushing and dry mouth. Taking the drugs from an inhaler reduces the side-effects by targeting the drug on the bronchi; this allows a much lower dose to be used than if the drugs were taken by mouth.

The effects of these drugs lasts for up to six hours, and the timing of doses should be geared to the patient's needs. Learning how to operate the inhaler properly is very important, as the drug can be ineffective if the inhaler is misused. Disk inhalers (Ventodisks) are easier to operate than conventional inhalers.

Even if they are used at quite high doses over long periods of time, there seem to be no serious ill-effects with these drugs. On the other hand, they do not reduce the sensitivity of the bronchi, as *sodium cromoglycate* does (see p87), so once they are discontinued, their beneficial effects cease. A combination of the two drugs is sometimes used.

Xanthines

These are naturally occurring substances that are chemically similar to caffeine. They include *theophylline* (Biophylline, Labophylline, Lasma, Nuelin, Pecram, Pro-Vent, Sabidal, Slo-Phyllin, Theo-Dur, Uniphyllin Continus), *aminophylline* (Phyllocontin Continus) and *choline theophyllinate* (Choledyl). They make the bronchial muscles relax, but affect the heart muscles as well. The dose must be exactly right, as there is only a small difference between the dose that will relax the bronchi and one which will cause irregular heartbeat. Other possible side-effects include headache, nausea, stomach upsets, depression, aching limbs and insomnia. Smoking and drinking will affect the dose needed, as will viral infections or taking other drugs, so it is important that patients taking these drugs have close medical supervision. As long as the dose is correct, they are suitable for long-term use, since there are no serious side-effects.

These drugs are usually taken by mouth. They can also be given as suppositories, inserted before going to bed, for those who suffer from early-morning attacks of asthma. They make the bronchial muscles relax by working *inside* the cells, whereas the ß2 agonists work *outside* the cell. The two different types of drugs therefore have complementary effects, and using both can be helpful for some patients.

Theophylline is combined with a sympathomimetic, *ephedrine*, in Franol and Tedral.

Anti-cholinergics

The main drugs in this group are *ipratropium* (Atrovent) and *oxitropium* (Oxivent), which are taken by inhalation. Side-effects are rare, except at high doses. They include dry mouth, difficulty in passing urine and constipation. Other anti-cholinergics include *butethamate* and *atropine*. Anti-cholinergics help to reduce the amount of mucus present in the airways, as well as relaxing the muscles, so may be useful where asthma and bronchitis occur together.

Sympathomimetics (see below), such as *adrenaline* and *ephedrine*, are sometimes combined with anticholinergics in inhalers. *Atropine* is combined with *adrenaline* and a muscle relaxant in Brovon. *Butethamate* is combined with *ephedrine* in CAM, which is taken by mouth. *Ipratropium* is combined with the bronchodilator *fenoterol* (a ß2-adrenoceptor agonist) in Duovent.

Other bronchodilators

Sympathomimetics (see p96) were once the main drugs used for bronchodilation, but they are much less specific for the bronchial muscles than the drugs described above. They produce side-effects more easily than modern bronchodilators and are much less used now. They include *adrenaline*, *ephedrine* and *phenylephrine*. Typical side-effects include nervousness, anxiety, tremor, irregular heartbeat and dry mouth.

COPING WITH HAYFEVER OR ASTHMA WHEN PREGNANT

This is obviously something that you should discuss with your doctor. The management of asthma during pregnancy is particularly important, as the lack of oxygen during an asthma attack can increase the risk of the baby dying soon after birth, being born prematurely, or having a low weight at birth. These risks disappear if the asthma is managed well. Ask your doctor to refer you to a specialist if you are concerned that your asthma is not under good control.

Some of the drugs used for asthma are not considered safe during pregnancy, so your medication may have to be changed.

If you suffer from hayfever and normally take non-prescription medicines, ask a pharmacist or doctor about their safety during pregnancy. Be sure that your family doctor knows what you are taking, whether a prescription or non-prescription drug.

With antihistamines, you should be aware of a danger that can arise in the very early stages of pregnancy, when you may not even know that you are pregnant. Some antihistamines carry a risk of deforming the baby, so you should not conceive while taking them, *nor for several weeks afterwards*. Reliable contraceptive measures should be taken throughout this time. The main drug implicated is *astemizole* (Hismanal, Pollon-eze), but it is wise to treat all antihistamines with the same caution, unless your doctor advises you that a specific antihistamine is safe.

You should not take *astemizole* when breastfeeding. Consult your doctor about other medications at this time.

The safest drug to use during pregnancy and breastfeeding is *sodium cromglycate* (see p87), which can help with both hayfever and asthma.

Chapter Eight

Avoiding Pollen

Avoiding pollen is like trying to avoid the Invisible Man, only more difficult, since it can be everywhere at once. Fortunately, science can offer some help here. In the past few years, research scientists have been hot on the track of pollen, and they now know quite a bit about its movements.

While you cannot evade pollen completely, you can certainly reduce the number of pollen grains you inhale every day. Indeed, some substantial reductions are possible if you are prepared to make certain changes. This could make your hayfever symptoms much less troublesome.

This approach may be sufficient on its own for some people, but for many more it will need to be backed up by use of medicinal drugs (see Chapter Seven) or desensitization treatments (see Chapter Nine). It can be particularly useful for those whose hayfever is only partially controlled by drugs.

THE INVISIBLE ENEMY

Most wind-pollinated plants scatter their pollen in the morning, but this is not true of all. The majority of grass species, for example, release their pollen in the morning, but a few species wait until the afternoon, so there is some pollen entering the air all day.

Knowing when pollen release is likely to begin in the morning is quite helpful. Grass pollen release occurs from about 7.30 a.m. onwards on a warm summer morning, when the ground and the grasses are dry, but if there is dew the timing will change. Pollen has to be thoroughly dried out before the plant disperses it, so pollen release will be delayed on a dewy morning until most of the dew has evaporated. Rainfall the previous evening will have the same effect. Ragweed generally gets going much earlier than grasses, releasing its pollen between sunrise and 9 a.m., although certain weather conditions can delay release until as late as 2 p.m. No precise figures are available for other types of plant but one study found birch pollen to peak between noon and 6 p.m.

Plants respond to the weather, and are more likely to release their pollen during a dry, sunny spell. During cool, damp periods, pollen builds up in the flowers, so the next warm day is likely to see a bumper pollen count as all this stored pollen is liberated.

As the sun's rays warm the earth's surface, the air above it also warms up, and then begins to rise, carrying the pollen with it. On a still day the rising pollen accumulates high up in the atmosphere. When the sun sets, and the earth begins to cool, the pollen is no longer buoyed up by currents of rising air, and gradually it falls to earth again.

How long this takes will depend on a variety of factors. It is much slower in built-up areas than in the country, because city pavements and buildings take longer to cool. In the countryside, most of the pollen descends between 8 and 10 p.m., but in the heart of the city the peak can be at midnight, and some pollen may not finally touch down until 2 a.m. This is why hayfever sufferers may wake in the night with an attack of sneezing.

The picture presented so far is a very simple one, which can be altered greatly by different weather conditions. Strong winds during the day will tend to blow pollen away and the heavy evening pollen-fall does not then take place. Should there be rainfall during the day, this washes most of the pollen out of the air, bringing relief to hayfever sufferers.

Inversions can make a big difference to the way pollen accumulates in the air. An inversion occurs when the air at ground level is slightly cooler than the upper layers of the atmosphere. The ground air cannot rise in the normal way, and the layer of warmer air above acts like a lid on a saucepan. This 'lid' keeps in the ground air along with its pollen and any pollutants it may contain (see p319). Cool temperate climates most often experience inversions in winter, but they can occur in summer too. In warmer climates inversions frequently occur in summer, and they are notorious in cities such as Los Angeles or Mexico City, where they contribute to smogs (see p319). In mountainous regions, temperature inversions can occur in valleys, because cold air sinks down the mountainsides at night, and can accumulate in the bottom of an enclosed valley. The layer of warmer air that sits like a lid over the valley can make pollen counts higher or lower. If the main source of pollen production is in that valley, then the pollen count will build up under the inversion. On the other hand, if the main pollen source is outside the valley, the inversion will keep that pollen out. When inversions are not present, the strong winds in mountainous regions tend to blow pollen away, and it is often blown straight across mountain ranges, missing the valleys.

Knowing the timing of pollen movements makes it possible to reduce your exposure. Stay indoors and keep windows closed when pollen is falling in the evening. For city dwellers, windows should remain closed at bedtime. To air the house, open the windows very early in the morning (to avoid grass pollen) or in the mid-afternoon (to avoid pollens such as ragweed that are released at sunrise).

If you live or work in a tower block, you should be aware that the warm air rising during the day constantly lifts pollen upwards, so the amount of pollen in the air at ground level may be quite low, whereas there are relatively high levels in the air ten storeys up. Keeping the windows closed while at these levels is the only real solution, but if you can get down to street level you may be more comfortable.

Pollen comes into cities from the surrounding countryside, but it is also generated locally, on railway banks, commons and waste ground, by trees growing in parks and gardens, or those lining the streets. Lawns in parks are not usually a problem, as they are mown regularly and this prevents the grasses from flowering. The grass in garden lawns may be mown less often, so may produce some pollen. If grass is your problem pollen, you should avoid areas with unmown grass in the morning, when the pollen is being released. In the evening, it will fall indiscriminately over everyone and everything, so any outdoor excursion will expose you to pollen.

Try to get out and take some exercise at times when the pollen count is lower – late afternoon and early evening, or very early in the morning if you are grass sensitive. Exercise improves your general state of health and should not be abandoned during the pollen season. Indoor swimming baths are a good place for pollen-free exercise, or you could use a mask and/or protective eyewear (see pp117–26) which would enable you to run or cycle.

AVOIDING POLLEN AT HOME

Pollen grains are fairly large particles, compared to some of the other items that can cause allergy, and this is one of their key advantages. The larger the particle, the faster it settles from the air. In an average room, with completely still air, all the pollen grains will have settled in about four minutes (see p202). The time taken depends on the ceiling height as well as the particle size: if you live in a grand old mansion with ceilings 6 metres (20 ft) high, it will take eight minutes. Add another four minutes for every 3 metres (10 ft) of ceiling height.

This means that if you go into a room, shut the windows and doors, and sit fairly still, you should be breathing air that is virtually pollen-free within five minutes. It may take a little longer for your symptoms to subside but they should ease off within an hour. During a long spell of sunny weather, when

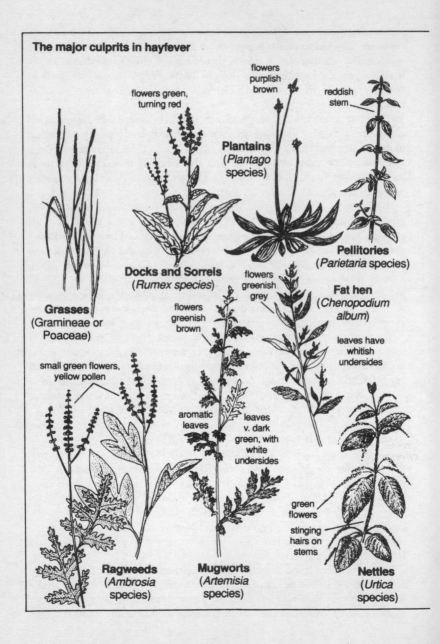

The major culprits in hayfever

flowers green, turning red

flowers purplish brown

reddish stem

Plantains
(*Plantago* species)

Pellitories
(*Parietaria* species)

Docks and Sorrels
(*Rumex species*)

flowers greenish grey

Fat hen
(*Chenopodium album*)

flowers greenish brown

leaves have whitish undersides

Grasses
(Gramineae or Poaceae)

small green flowers, yellow pollen

aromatic leaves

leaves v. dark green, with white undersides

green flowers

stinging hairs on stems

Ragweeds
(*Ambrosia* species)

Mugworts
(*Artemisia* species)

Nettles
(*Urtica* species)

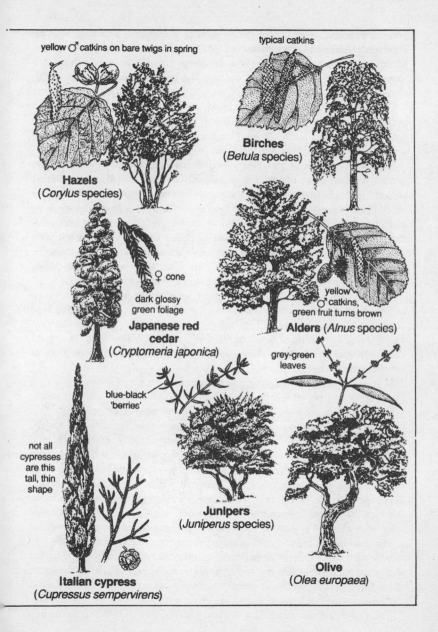

yellow ♂ catkins on bare twigs in spring

Hazels
(*Corylus* species)

typical catkins

Birches
(*Betula* species)

♀ cone

dark glossy
green foliage

**Japanese red
cedar**
(*Cryptomeria japonica*)

yellow
♂ catkins,
green fruit turns brown

Alders (*Alnus* species)

blue-black
'berries'

not all
cypresses
are this
tall, thin
shape

Junipers
(*Juniperus* species)

grey-green
leaves

Italian cypress
(*Cupressus sempervirens*)

Olive
(*Olea europaea*)

you are exposed to pollen for many days in succession, you may well be experiencing **late-phase reactions** (see p41) to the pollen of the previous day. In this case, your symptoms will not disappear entirely when you sit quietly indoors, but they should lessen because the nose and eyes are not being challenged by any new intake of pollen.

Even with doors and windows closed, there will, of course, still be some pollen coming in from outside, with the air that sneaks in around the edges of window frames and under doors. This may be so little that it does not bother you, but if it is a problem, you can deal with it in other ways (see below).

You may not want to spend very long sitting still, but once the pollen has settled, you *can* move around fairly normally without disturbing the settled pollen too much. Obviously, more vigorous and rapid movements will cause more disturbance than simply walking about. It may help to change your clothing on arriving home, putting on something you do not wear outdoors – that way you are not carrying a layer of pollen around with you on your clothes, to be disturbed whenever you move. Rinsing your hair may also be worthwhile, especially if it is thick or long. This will wash out the pollen grains, again reducing the amount you are breathing while indoors.

When in bed, we probably inhale quite a lot of pollen from our hair, and a nightly hair-rinse can reduce this. Another measure that is worth trying is to cover the bed and pillow with a bedspread or spare sheet during the day, then carefully roll it up at bedtime. This will prevent pollen from settling on the pillow and bed during the day and evening, and thus reduce the amount inhaled while asleep.

If you live with others, especially children, still air is probably a rare commodity, and pollen will be continually disturbed in the home. In this case you may want to use an air filter to reduce the airborne levels (see p119). This is not the only solution, however; you can also take steps to reduce the amount of pollen waiting to be disturbed. Regular vacuum cleaning will help (possibly with a filter fitted to the vacuum cleaner, see p119). Regular dusting using a wet cloth is also worthwhile; polished wood can be rubbed dry with another cloth to prevent marking. This will reduce the amount of pollen collected in the carpeting and on furniture, windowsills and other surfaces. Air currents created by movement in the room, doors opening and closing, or other disturbances will then churn up less pollen into the air you breathe.

Pets coming in from outside carry quite a lot of pollen on their fur, so people with hayfever may be better off keeping their distance from the family dog or cat for a while. Alternatively the pet could be excluded from the house during the pollen season. It should certainly be kept out of the patient's bedroom – this is a basic year-round precaution for anyone with allergies.

One rather obvious hazard for anyone with hayfever is bringing items into the house that produce the problem pollen. Hazel catkins and pussy willows might produce symptoms in some hayfever patients, for example, particularly hazel as there is often a cross-reaction from birch (see p154). In general, flower arrangements that only contain colourful flowers are unlikely to be a problem because these rarely cause hayfever (see p4). However, they may carry the pollens of other plants, such as grasses, on their leaves and petals. It is also possible that the scents of these flowers will be an irritant to the hayfeverish nose.

In the case of someone with ragweed sensitivity, there might be a cross-reaction (see p45) with other flowers in the daisy family (Compositae or Asteraceae) many of which are pretty garden flowers. Goldenrod is the worst offender, but any daisy, aster, dahlia, marigold, chrysanthemum, thistle or sunflower might cause problems. For more information on this see p157.

If, despite these basic measures, you still suffer from hayfever symptoms when at home with the windows closed, there are further steps you can take. It may be that a large amount of air is still coming into the house from outside – under doors, around windows, through catflaps or ventilation bricks. One obvious solution is to block off these entry holes, perhaps by installing better fitting windows and doors, or by simpler measures, such as plastic taped over the openings. However, this has some drawbacks for people with other allergies, besides hayfever. Someone who is allergic to cats or other pets, and still has those pets in the house, could be made much worse by a reduction in ventilation which can lead to a massive build-up of small allergenic particles in the air (see p208).

Blocking off draughts could well increase the moisture level in your house, and this will be a problem if you are allergic to either mould spores (see p193) or house-dust mite (see p172). As a short-term measure, reducing draughts is acceptable, but the ventilation must be increased again at the end of the pollen season. (The only other option is to use a dehumidifier, which takes moisture out of the air, see p306.)

Removing pollen grains from the indoor air, using an air filter or ionizer, is another option. With these devices it is important to make sure that what you are buying is up to the job – that is, powerful enough for the size of the room. Owing to the lack of restrictions or standards for air filters and ionizers in Britain, several devices are on sale that make vague and unfounded claims about filtering out pollen. Appendix 3 gives guidelines for choosing a filter or ionizer.

One firm produces a high-quality air filter that is also a powerful dehumidifier, capable of actually killing the house-dust mites in a room by making the air desert-dry for a few hours of the day when the room is not in use (see p189). This machine could be very useful if you are sensitive to mould spores or house-dust mite, as well as pollen, allowing you to keep the windows tightly closed without making the house damp, and actually killing many mites as well.

Air-conditioning systems are also of benefit to hayfever sufferers, particularly ducted systems that cover the entire house. As these take in only a small amount of air from the outside, less pollen enters the house, and much of that is removed during the cooling process anyway: cooling makes water condense from the air, and the tiny water droplets take pollen with them. The amount of pollen inside the house is small, and the coolness makes it far less of an ordeal to keep the windows closed. The moisture content of the air is controlled by the air conditioner, so there should be few problems with damp and mould.

Scientists in Wisconsin have studied the effects of air-conditioning systems on ragweed pollen and found that they remove about 95 per cent of the pollen. Adding a high-quality air-filtration unit to the intake on air conditioners reduced the pollen a little more – to about 2 per cent of outdoor levels. This further reduction in the pollen level was found to lessen night-time symptoms in ragweed-sensitive people a little, compared with air conditioning alone, but the researchers concluded that the extra benefits were small.

Unfortunately, there has been no comparable scientific research on air filters alone, which would be more relevant to countries such as Britain, where air conditioning is uncommon. However, it seems likely that air filters or ionizers will remove significant amounts of pollen from the air, and hayfever sufferers who have tried them frequently report good results. Several suppliers will allow you to try out a filter or ionizer in advance of buying it, either by hiring it out, or selling it on a money-back basis. This enables the purchaser to see whether a filter is of any assistance to them, and to choose from the different types available (see p298). If you do invest in a filter or ionizer, remember that it will only be effective when the windows are kept closed.

Free-standing air-conditioning devices that treat a single room only are also available. No one has checked to see how much pollen they remove from the air, but they probably take out some, and they make closed windows more bearable. Again, there are suppliers who will hire out these machines, so that you can see how much they help.

Teenagers represent a high proportion of hayfever sufferers, and it is often fairly easy to reduce the airborne pollen in a teenager's bedroom, by the methods already described, without affecting the activities of the rest of the household. This is worth the effort if the pollen season coincides with exams, as it gives the hayfever patient somewhere to study with a minimum of symptoms. One small additional measure that may help is to cover the desk and books with a sheet when not in use, and to roll it up carefully when studying begins. This will prevent a layer of pollen from accumulating on books and notepads, to be disturbed when the pages are turned.

REDUCING POLLEN EXPOSURE IN THE GARDEN

There is not a great deal that can be done here, and your neighbours' gardens will probably frustrate your efforts anyway, but you can avoid making your pollen exposure any worse.

Mowing a lawn can affect someone with allergy to grass pollen quite badly, even though the grass is not in flower. Tiny liquid droplets, containing similar allergens to those in the pollen, are thought to be at fault. The hayfever sufferer should not, therefore, cut the grass.

Cutting the lawn at frequent intervals will help to prevent it from flowering, although grasses will adapt to regular mowing and may flower when very short. Take a close look to see if flower heads are developing. Make sure the edges of the lawn are trimmed, and that grasses are cut down in the weedy corners of the garden.

Avoiding grass in the garden altogether is possible, and may be valuable for those who develop a rash when sitting on grass. Chamomile lawns or herb lawns are an alternative (but chamomile is not recommended for anyone who also has ragweed allergy, as the two plants are related and can cross-react). A good gardening book should tell you how to create such a lawn.

Certain plants should be avoided, such as ornamental grasses (e.g. pampas grass) and sedges if you are grass allergic, and goldenrod if you are sensitive to ragweed. If you are planning to plant trees, a skin-prick test may be advisable first, to find out whether any particular species could cause you problems. Birches are probably best avoided anyway. In warmer climates, hedges and windbreaks consisting of cypresses are quite often a source of hayfever problems. (Several plants seem to cause more problems in hot climates than cool ones, probably because the pollen becomes drier while on the plant, and is therefore dispersed more widely by the wind.)

If you have a large garden with large patches of ineradicable nettles, docks or other weeds, at least cut them down before they flower. Should you experience any symptoms while slashing or strimming the plants, these may be caused by droplets of plant juices in the air; get someone else to do the job for you next time.

PROTECTING YOUR EYES FROM POLLEN

Protecting the eyes from pollen is fairly easy. In fact, this is an area with considerable scope for self-help, and one that is often neglected by hayfever sufferers.

WHOLE GRAINS OR POLLEN PARTICLES?

A crucial question, in relation to any airborne allergen, is 'How big is it?' The size of the particle carrying the allergen makes an enormous difference to its becoming airborne and staying aloft long enough to be inhaled. Combating a very small allergen is an entirely different process from combating a large one. 'Very small' in this case means less than 4 microns (thousandths of a millimetre), while 'large' means 20 microns or more. The illustration on pp204–5 compares the sizes of major airborne allergens.

The size of the particle also influences the way in which it affects the human body. The size of pollen grains makes them highly likely to land in the eyes, which is why hayfever so often produces eye symptoms. Size also determines how deeply particles penetrate into the airways, an important factor in pollen asthma (see p203).

Most allergenic pollens fall in the range from 15 to 40 microns (thousandths of a millimetre). A full list of the different sizes is given in Appendix 2.

Life would be simpler if there were only intact pollen grains to cause hayfever.

Unfortunately, some plants also generate much smaller particles that contain pollen allergens (see p23). These are known for rye grass, ragweed, Japanese red cedar and Australian white cypress pine (*Callitris*). Whether they exist for other plants is uncertain, but it seems likely. The smallest of these particles may be a mere half micron across. Whether they are an important factor in hayfever will depend on how abundant they are in the air. At present this is not known, and more research is needed on this topic.

If these smaller particles are causing your symptoms, your efforts to avoid pollen allergens will be affected, but not to any major extent. There are four possible effects:

1. The particles take longer to settle than whole pollen grains. Particles of 2 microns take six hours to settle from an average room, compared with four minutes for most pollen grains. Thus, simply sitting still indoors, with the doors and windows closed, will not give you any prompt relief from hayfever. This makes air conditioning, or an air filter (see pp115–16) a more attractive option.

2. In theory, an air filter or dust mask that could remove whole pollen grains might not be effective against these smaller particles. In practice, this is unlikely, particularly with air filters. All good-quality air filters operate at very small particle sizes, usually down to a micron or less, because they are designed for a range of uses, not just for pollen removal. HEPA filters (see p298) must take out 99.97 per cent of particles at 0.3 of a micron to qualify as a HEPA filter. Electrostatic filters do not work on the basis of particle sizes anyway, and neither do ionizers.

With dust masks, pollen fragments will probably require a higher grade of mask. A Nuisance Dust mask (see p296) takes out particles of 5 microns and larger, and would therefore remove pollen grains easily but may not deal with pollen fragments. A mask that takes out respirable dust (anything sold in Britain that conforms to standard EN 149) would deal with both. Since masks are fairly cheap, you can test one to see if it works for you, and buy a better model if it does not.

3. Most good quality vacuum cleaners which use paper (rather than fabric) collecting bags, will retain the intact pollen grains that they pick up, but many smaller particles may escape and be given off as a fine spray into the air. If this is happening, you will be aware of hayfever symptoms when vacuuming (although this could also indicate an allergy to house-dust mite droppings, or something else in dust, see p172). In such cases, there are specialized vacuum cleaners on sale that can help considerably. For full information on these, and on filters that can be fitted to existing vacuum cleaners, see p308.

4. Fine particles become airborne more easily, and research with cat allergens shows that an air filter with a powerful fan can churn up settled particles, offsetting its cleaning action to some extent (see p208). If very small pollen particles are a problem for you, and you opt for an air filter, you may also need to reduce the quantity of settled particles in the home, by careful vacuuming and wet dusting (see p114).

SMALLER THAN SMALL?

While most hayfever involves pollen grains or pollen particles, some people are probably reacting to **volatile compounds** given off by plants. A volatile compound is any substance, solid or liquid, that readily turns into a vapour at normal temperatures. Alcohol is a good example. If you leave a glass of vodka or whisky out overnight, much of the alcohol will vaporize. Any scent depends on volatile compounds – it is because the molecules become airborne that they enter the nose and trigger off the sense of smell. Air fresheners consist of volatile compounds, and one can see solid air fresheners 'melting away' as the compounds become airborne.

Obviously, scented flowers give off volatile compounds, but so do the leaves and stems of many plants. Not all of these compounds have smells that the human nose can detect.

Why are these substances produced by plants? In some cases, they are compounds that insects dislike, and are released to deter them from eating the plants. Maize, on the other hand, gives off a volatile compound only when already attacked by aphids, and the scent attracts other insects that prey on aphids. No doubt, volatile substances play many other roles in plant life that we do not yet know about.

The question of whether volatile substances can affect hayfever sufferers is a difficult one, but there is some evidence that they can. It must be stressed, however, that it is probably only *some* plants having such effects, and only *some* patients being affected.

One plant that is known to produce volatile compounds in abundance is oil-seed rape, the yellow-flowered crop plant that has lately been accused of causing minor hayfever epidemics where it is grown. The volatiles from rape have an irritant effect on the nose that affects many people, not just those of an allergic disposition. It may be these that are responsible for the 'hayfever' outbreak, especially when it affects those with no previous history of allergy. Since the volatiles are acting as irritants, not allergens, this is not genuine hayfever. However, some people are genuinely allergic to oil-seed rape pollen.

Some people with allergies to tree pollen begin reacting very early in spring, before pollen is released. It has been suggested that tree buds release volatiles as they swell and open in the spring, and that this may be provoking symptoms.

In Sweden, volatiles coming from birch twigs in the spring are known to affect some people with birch hayfever. They also affect just as many people with no sign of hayfever or other allergies.

Only a minority of people with hayfever are likely to be affected by volatiles, and this is certainly not something to worry about. One possible sign of this problem is experiencing nasal irritation from the scent of flowers; your nose is clearly sensitive to the volatile substances making up the scent, and perhaps to other volatiles as well.

If you *are* sensitive to volatile compounds, how will this affect your efforts at pollen avoidance? Volatile compounds will not settle out of the air, although they will disperse very readily. They are unlikely to affect you at low concentrations, so you will probably find that, when outdoors you are affected by them only if close to the source. Whether they penetrate indoors, and what happens to them there, is unknown at present. Your nose will simply have to be the judge of that.

Since volatile substances are not particles, they will not be removed by air filters of the electrostatic or HEPA types (see p298), nor by dust masks. The only type of filter to take out these substances is one containing activated carbon (see p294). Such filters can be found in both air filters and masks, but care should be taken in using masks of this type (see p295).

Many people with eye symptoms from pollen already wear sunglasses in spring and summer, but this is only providing rather limited protection. Researchers in New Zealand and the United States have found that the protective effect of glasses can be much improved by adding shields at the top, bottom and sides of the frames. Simply adding shields to the top and sides of the frames can also be very helpful.

The cheapest way to achieve this is to make your own shields for an

CLIFF

Cliff was one of the most severe cases of hayfever that his specialist had ever seen. He was still in his teens, and the fact that the grass pollen season coincided with his final school exams was very worrying. Hyposensitization (see p134) had been tried without success.

Neutralization therapy (see p141) did not work either, and antihistamines were of little help. The specialist then tried cromoglycate *(see p87) and* corticosteroids *(see p100), but these only produced a minor improvement. Cases such as* this are rare, but when they do occur the only solution is to avoid pollen as far as possible. Cliff took to wearing sunglasses while walking outside, with a special filter mask over his nose too, at the height of the pollen season. His family kept the windows closed at home in the evenings, and bought an air filter to reduce the pollen level in his bedroom. Although Cliff still suffered with hayfever, he found the symptoms were bearable and no longer interfered with his work.

existing pair of glasses or sunglasses. Apart from low cost, the advantage of this is that you can extend the coverage right around the lens, giving thorough protection. Furthermore, the shape is personalized for your head, giving a very good fit.

The illustration opposite shows how to make these shields. Clear plastic sheeting can be bought in model and hobby shops, or in some shops supplying art materials. A thickness of 7.5 thou (thousandths of an inch) is the best, as it wraps around the frame easily.

Use glue or double-sided sticky tape to stick the plastic to the glasses frame. If using glue, check first that it does not dissolve the plastic of the frame, by testing a small inconspicuous area. Bostik All-Purpose Adhesive is probably suitable for most frames. Avoid 'superglues', because you want to be able to remove all traces of the glue at the end of the pollen season. Check that the glue you plan to use can be rubbed off or removed with a solvent, without damaging the frame. Should your glasses have plastic lenses, keep the glue away from these.

Cut a strip of plastic sheeting about 8 cm (3 inches) wide and 20 cm (8 inches) long. First, stick the plastic strip across the top of the frame (see illustration, stage 1). Once the plastic is stuck firmly to the top of the

Keeping pollen out of the eye

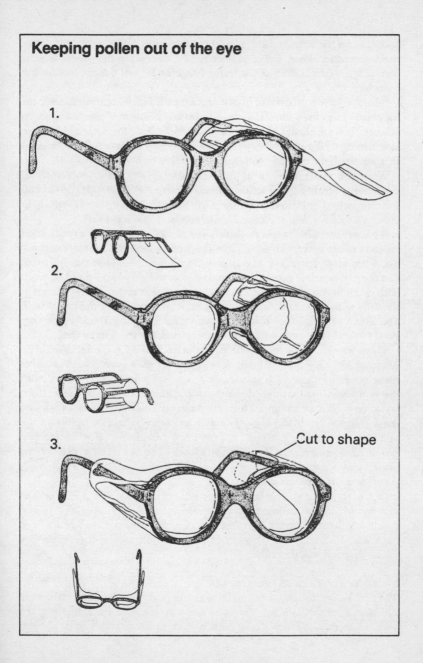

1.

2.

3.

Cut to shape

frame, wrap the strip around, mould it to the side of the frame with your hand, then stick down. Leave to stick firmly, then wrap the plastic around and stick it to the bottom of the frame (stage 2). Repeat this process for the other lens.

Once you have a cylinder of plastic around each lens you can cautiously cut the plastic away to fit your face (stage 3). Do this a little at a time, using sharp scissors. Try the glasses on after each cut, feel where the plastic rubs your face, and trim off a little more at that point. When you have achieved a good fit, smooth off the cut edge with an emery board or fine sandpaper.

When the weather is warm there should be very little problem with condensation (misting up) inside your customized spectacles. If you do find them fogging over occasionally, there are special cleaning fluids on sale in opticians that are 'anti-static' and make condensation less likely.

If you are prepared to spend a little more money, there is now a really good range of safety spectacles which are designed to look like ordinary glasses. There are several excellent and fashionable designs that look nothing at all like the plastic safety goggles sold in do-it-yourself shops and could be worn with no embarrassment whatever. Choose ones that give good protection at the sides of the lens, and a certain amount of protection over the top as well. The extent to which they shield the eye varies, but some models give very good top-and-sides coverage, and one extends below the lens as well.

These frames can be fitted with prescription lenses for spectacle wearers. Alternatively, they can be fitted with tinted sunglass-type lenses, or plain glass lenses, for those with good sight or contact lenses. Many people with eye symptoms find that they dislike strong light, and dark glasses give them welcome relief from the sun. There are occasions, however, when sunglasses make things difficult socially; you may want to keep them on indoors if the windows are open for example, but not taking sunglasses off when meeting people can seem impolite, especially in a work situation. Having both options available – a pair of protective glasses with tinted lenses and a pair with plain glass – is therefore useful.

Of course, plastic goggles sold for sports use or do-it-yourself protection can also be used against pollen. For a child who does not wear spectacles, plastic sports goggles may be the simplest and cheapest option. Combined with a bicycle and a trendy hat, they could be passed off as a fashion accessory rather than a medical necessity!

PROTECTING YOUR NOSE FROM POLLEN

The first person to use an umbrella was stoned by the outraged citizens of nineteenth-century London. Twenty years ago, someone running along the street in shorts and a vest would have been regarded as an oddball, whereas joggers are now commonplace. Ten years ago, cyclists wearing helmets were stared at and ridiculed. With so many people now suffering from hayfever, it will only take a few brave souls to start the ball rolling and make summertime dust masks seem entirely unremarkable. Already there are a few anti-pollution masks, aimed at city cyclists, that have been designed with looks as well as practicality in mind (see p296), and some are incorporated into attractive scarves to tie around the face Lone Ranger style.

Of course, there are other drawbacks to masks, besides loss of street credibility. They inevitably make it a little harder to breathe, and can become hot and uncomfortable in summer. However, if your hayfever is bad, and drugs have not helped much, the discomfort of a mask worn only when outdoors may be much less than hayfever, endured all day and night. Bear in mind that reducing your exposure substantially when outdoors can avoid the priming reaction (see p41) that will make you ultra-sensitive to pollen at other times, so the benefits could be substantial.

For some people, masks can prove useful as temporary protection from a particularly heavy load of their allergen – if they have to drive on a hot day, for example, or mow the lawn themselves. Some other instances in which masks can be valuable as a temporary protection, are listed in Appendix 3, where details of the different types of masks are also given.

A far less conspicuous way of protecting the nose is to insert a plug of foam rubber into each nostril. We know of only one hayfever sufferer who has tried this, but he reported excellent results, even when exposed to massive amounts of pollen, and says that the nose plugs cannot easily be seen when in place. The foam he uses is not the sort generally found in cushions or foam mattresses, where there are many small air bubbles within a solid mass of rubber. This does not let the air through, as the bubbles do not interconnect. The type of foam used is known as 'windowless' or 'reticulated' foam, and looks like a tangled net of fibres. The holes in the foam should be about 1 millimetre across. The nose plugs do not filter out all pollen entering the nose, but much of it gets stuck to the strands of the foam, so that the amount inhaled is reduced considerably.

Obviously, the foam needs to admit enough air to make breathing through the nose easy. If there is too much air resistance from the foam, you may begin breathing through the mouth, and this will mean that more pollen and pollen fragments penetrate the airways, perhaps triggering off pollen asthma. However, reticulated foam generally admits plenty of air.

Some hayfever sufferers report good effects from simply smearing petroleum jelly (Vaseline) on the skin just inside the nostrils. By making this surface sticky, it can detain some of the pollen that flows past on the incoming air, reducing the amount that reaches the delicate membranes beyond.

Farm workers with hayfever, who suffer serious symptoms when in contact with crops, can use a powered respirator helmet. The helmet itself is fairly light and comfortable to wear. The air filter, powered by a battery, is carried in the small of the back, attached to a belt that buckles round the waist. Air is taken in by this unit, filtered, then pumped up a flexible tube into the back of the helmet. Channels within the helmet carry it over the head and pump it out over the forehead. A plastic face shield extends down from the helmet, and the filtered air being pumped downwards keeps outside air from entering at the bottom of the face shield. Suppliers of this type of helmet are listed on p297. The high level of protection they offer may be valuable to anyone who cannot avoid contact with large amounts of their problem pollen or other allergen. Plant breeders, nurserymen, and laboratory technicians working with small animals (see p216) are among those who could benefit from such devices.

AVOIDING POLLEN WHEN DRIVING

There can be heavy concentrations of pollen in the air around country roads, and particularly on motorways. The movement of the traffic constantly stirs up pollen grains from the ground. In a long dry spell, when there has been no rain to wash the pollen away, a thick layer remains on the road and verges. Elsewhere, this does not easily become airborne again, but the considerable turbulence of air beside a motorway produces high airborne concentrations. Hayfever when driving is often a major problem, especially if you have eye symptoms and it affects your vision.

The simplest avoidance technique is to drive with the windows closed, and this is the standard advice given to hayfever sufferers. Needless to say, it can be sheer hell to be stuck in a hot little metal box on a sweltering summer's day, and most people yearn for another solution. Even with the windows closed there will still be some pollen intake, plus the pollen that was in the car to begin with.

The most sophisticated solution, if you can afford it, is a car with air conditioning, which will cool you off and cut down the pollen load considerably, since the air conditioner takes a great deal of pollen out, along with moisture droplets (see p116). There are also cars, such as the new Vauxhall Astra, which have special anti-pollen filters.

If a new car is beyond your means, there are various other solutions to the pollen in the car. For example, filters can be fitted over the air intake, or you could instal a car ionizer or air filter (see p303). These devices will reduce the quantity of pollutants inhaled, as well as protect you from pollen.

RICHARD

Richard first began to get hayfever when he was thirteen years old, and at forty he is still enduring the same symptoms, which last from early spring to midsummer, as he is sensitive to both tree pollens and grass pollens. His main problem is a very dry sore throat, a blocked nose and sore, itchy eyes. As a young man he tried antihistamines, but the forms then available made him extremely sleepy and he had to give them up, since his work as a travelling salesman required full concentration, especially when driving. Newer types of antihistamines have proved very effective for Richard and do not cause any drowsiness. He also uses eye drops that contain an antihistamine and a sympathomimetic (see p94). The medicines keep his symptoms under control and allow him to lead a relatively normal life, but Richard still finds his hayfever a nuisance and sometimes a social embarrassment. Five years ago he began driving a car with air conditioning and found to his surprise that he was substantially better. 'I actually enjoy being on the road during the summer now,' he says, 'as it is the only time when I am relatively comfortable.' For many people with hayfever, there is no single solution to their problems – they need to use several methods of coping with their illness, as Richard has done.

But you will still have the problem of heat to contend with, because the windows must be kept shut for them to be effective.

If you are a passenger in someone else's car, or simply hate the thought of closing the car windows, a pair of protective spectacles (see p124) may help. You could also consider wearing a dust mask to protect your nose (see p125).

MAKING USE OF POLLEN COUNTS
Not so long ago, pollen counts were for one type of pollen only (usually grass in Britain) and simply told you what yesterday's pollen count had been. The situation now is much better, and improving all the time. Several telephone lines currently offer pollen forecasts for the day ahead, and general outlooks

for the next three days. They also give pollen counts for a variety of allergenic species.

Not all the telephone services are the same. If the one you have been using does not offer pollen forecasts and outlooks, try another. The quality of information given in newspapers also varies considerably, and it is worth checking to see if another publication is giving more comprehensive details. In some countries, including Britain, good pollen forecasts are given by radio. Local stations may offer this service, as well as the national radio stations. Some early morning television programmes also give a pollen forecast for the day.

Pollen counts are always given in number of grains per cubic metre of air. The figures are usually averages for a twenty-four-hour period, which includes peak periods and low pollen periods. The actual pollen count at peak times will therefore be much higher. Sometimes pollen counts that relate to levels during the peak period are given, but this will usually be stated. Bear this in mind when comparing figures from different sources.

Some plant types provoke symptoms at quite low pollen counts, while others reach high counts before they set people sneezing. In Britain the count for grass might be about 150 grains per cubic metre at the height of the pollen season, whereas tree pollens can number 1,000 grains per cubic metre in the spring. Despite this, many more people are grass-sensitive than are tree-sensitive, suggesting that grass pollen is more highly allergenic.

There is only a limited value in pollen counts that relate to the previous day (retrospective counts). These cannot help you to avoid pollen, but they may help to explain a change in your symptoms. If you are uncertain whether you are allergic to pollen, or to some other allergen, then knowing how the pollen count changes, and seeing if this fits in with your symptoms, may be useful. However, if you are not entirely in step with the official pollen counts, this does not rule out sensitivity to the pollen in question. The changes in pollen levels in your immediate locality may be somewhat different from those elsewhere.

The pollen forecast is far more helpful in pollen avoidance, but it too has its limitations. The forecasts depend on computer models that predict pollen release based on the time of year, temperature of preceding days and weeks, predicted temperature, predicted rainfall and other variables. Some of the crucial facts and figures that lead to the pollen count prediction are obtained from weather forecasting, so if the weather forecasters are wrong, the pollen forecast will also be inaccurate. Similarly, the pollen outlook is as dependable as the weather outlook for the next three days.

Pollen count telephone lines usually open up in May in Britain, before the grass season has begun. If you are planning to take your medicinal drugs before the season starts – a good idea with antihistamines, mast-cell stabi-lizers or corticosteroids – the pollen count may be helpful in deciding when to begin. The telephone information should include a prediction of when grass pollen will first appear. (Once the grass season is underway, a predic-tion of when it will end is also given.) If the telephone line you are using does not do this, try another. The beginning of the tree-pollen season is far more difficult to predict, unfortunately, and there is no similar service for this yet.

Another use for the pollen forecast is in planning activities that involve high exposure to pollen, such as a trip to the countryside or to a park. The pollen forecast can help you avoid high-pollen days, but it will, of course, also help you avoid the best summer weather! If you are taking a long journey by car, and do not have anti-pollen devices or air conditioning in the vehicle (see p126), the pollen forecast can be very useful.

ESCAPING DURING THE POLLEN SEASON

If you are not too tied down by family or work commitments, and if your hayfever symptoms are severe, you may like to consider getting away from your home area at the height of the pollen season. Obviously, this is only practical if the season is relatively short.

A holiday in June or July is often recommended to those with severe grass-pollen allergy, and Appendix 1 can pinpoint parts of the world where there will be little grass pollen in the air. In general, moving slightly closer to the Equator will solve the problem because the grass will already have polli-nated in warmer climates. For those in northern Europe, the Mediterranean region offers a relatively inexpensive refuge.

It is not always necessary to leave the country to escape the pollen season. Coastal regions with an onshore breeze generally have low pollen counts because the wind pushes the pollen inland. In Britain, the west coast will be better than the east coast. Mountain and moorland regions have stronger winds and the grasses found there tend to pollinate less prolifically, so pollen counts may be lower. You cannot rely on mountain regions being better, however, and inversions in mountain valleys (see p110) can create pollen traps where the pollen count is very high. This is known to happen in the Swiss Alps, for example.

If you need help in identifying a retreat area with low pollen counts, some of the specialist agencies given on p316 may be able to help you.

HAYFEVER AND HOLIDAYS

Apart from coming down with dysentery or yellow fever, nothing can spoil a holiday as thoroughly as having severe hayfever. Many plants with allergenic pollen have a worldwide distribution – grasses in particular. Birches too are naturally widespread, occurring throughout the northern hemisphere, and are often planted in gardens in the southern hemisphere as well. Ragweed, once confined to North America, is now spreading across wasteland and farms in many parts of the world. The tree known as she-oak or 'Australian pine' is grown as a windbreak in warmer parts of the Americas and in the Caribbean, where the average Australian holiday-maker would hardly expect to find it. Cypresses are common worldwide, either as wild species or as garden shrubs and hedges.

Before booking a holiday, always check whether your problem pollen occurs at your destination, and find out when it is airborne there; the times of year will not necessarily be the same as those at home. Appendix 1 gives pollen seasons for the major allergens in all the most popular holiday destinations of the world. For pollen seasons in less visited areas, you will need to consult specialist information services, such as those listed on p316.

Another point to consider here are potential cross-reactions (see Chapter Eleven). For example, many people with cypress sensitivity show a reaction to Japanese red cedar, and vice versa. A holiday-maker with hayfever or asthma due to cypress pollen would be well advised to avoid Japan in the spring.

If you are going to a warm climate, where pollen seasons are often very long and not entirely predictable, it is a good idea to take a supply of your usual hayfever medicine with you anyway. This may prove useful in case of local quirks in pollen production or unexpected cross-reactions. The non-prescription antihistamines can be bought in many chemist shops, even in the depths of winter, so stocking up is no problem.

ELIMINATING THE POLLEN – COMMUNITY ACTION

Since the 1930s, a unique programme of community action has been under-way in the area around Montreal in Canada. At the instigation of a geography professor from the University of Montreal, people began an attempt to eradicate the two species of ragweed, native plants that were ubiquitous in fields, pastures and wasteland throughout the area. The programme has continued ever since, with poster campaigns, and organized ragweed-pulling by schoolchildren. There have been renewed efforts in the past decade, and research into different control methods has been carried out at Montreal's Botanic Garden. Researchers there have found that while hand weeding is the most effective method of reducing pollen production, it is also the most expensive if paid labour is used. Mowing, on the other hand, is fairly cheap, and if done with the mower blades set 2 cm (⅘ inch) from the ground it is highly effective, reducing pollen production by at least 88 per cent, and sometimes preventing it altogether. While ragweed has not been eliminated, the number of plants has certainly been reduced. Researchers have found that these efforts can cut the pollen count to about half the level it would otherwise reach, a significant achievement that brings relief to many hayfever sufferers.

Not all hayfever-causing plants are suitable candidates for this treatment. Grasses, for example, are vital to agriculture (although farmers might be induced to grow species with less prolific or less allergenic pollen). Birch trees and Japanese red cedar form vast and beautiful forests that few would wish to see eliminated. However, there may be some other weeds that are as unloved and as dispensable as ragweed, and they could be tackled with similar methods. This would only be worthwhile for those that are a major cause of hayfever among large numbers of people.

There is certainly a case for tackling ragweed – one of nature's most allergenic plants – in those parts of the world where it has become an unwelcome immigrant. These include parts of France (notably around Lyon), Hungary, Czechoslovakia, the regions that were formerly Yugoslavia, the eastern part of Austria, and parts of Russia, Switzerland and Japan. In general, ragweed seeds have arrived with grain imported from the USA. Hayfever in response to ragweed pollen is spreading in all these countries, and it seems clear that numbers will grow as the weed spreads, causing another hayfever epidemic. If the people of Montreal can make such an impression on ragweed on what is essentially its 'home ground', then areas where it is an invader should be able to achieve far more. The sooner this problem is tackled the better, for as any gardener knows, a weed problem simply grows worse with every passing year.

Britain is fortunate in not offering ragweed the right climatic conditions to become established. (The native ragwort, an untidy yellow-flowered weed, is an entirely different species, although it belongs to the same plant family.) Ragweed has been inadvertently introduced from the USA many times, but it has never gained a firm foothold. Ragweed flowers very late in the summer, and needs a long warm autumn to set seed. Only when there is an 'Indian summer' in Britain does ragweed set seed in significant amounts. Even then, the seed germinates very poorly in the normal springtime weather of Britain, so there are few years when new plants can establish themselves in any great number. Although ragweed can often be found on wasteland, especially near sea ports, and sometimes in gardens (it is believed to originate from birdseed in these cases), it rarely sets up thriving colonies. Its pollen sometimes turns up in noticeable amounts over London or East Anglia, yet there is no sign of the counts increasing from one year to another. When skin-prick tested with ragweed allergen, some hayfever patients give a positive result, but these are patients who react to many different pollens. Why they should react to

CROSSING THE LANGUAGE BARRIERS

Hayfever can be an embarrassing travelling companion. If, despite your plans and precautions, you are stricken by hayfever when abroad, you may feel the need to explain the explosive sneezing and red-rimmed eyes to the locals. You are more likely to get a hotel room if they know it's not infectious. (Explaining your problem will also be necessary if you have to buy drugs for your hayfever, but the best course is to purchase these at home and take them with you.) Since 'I have hayfever' does not feature in many phrase books, these are the words you need around the world:

Bulgarian:	*Stradam ot senna hrema.*
Danish:	*Jeg har hofeber.*
Dutch:	*Ik lijd aan hooikoorts.*
Farsi:	*Tabé yonjeh.*
Finnish:	*Minulla on heinanuha.*
Flemish:	*Ik heb hooikoorts.*
French:	*J'ai le rhume des foins* or *j'ai la fièvre des foins.*
German:	*Ich habe Heuschnupfen.*
Greek:	*Eecho anoixiatiki allerghia.*
Hungarian:	*Széna làzam van.*
Italian:	*Soffro di febbre da fieno.*
Japanese:	*Kafunshō desu.*
Norwegian:	*Jeg har hoy feber.*
Polish:	*Cierpię na katar sienny.*
Portuguese:	*Eu tenho asma dos fenos.*
Russian:	*U menya sennaya likhoradka.*
Spanish:	*Padezco de alergia al polen.*
Swahili:	There is no expression for hayfever in Swahili, and most people will not know of the disease. *Nina makamasi yaletwayo na mavumbi ya nyasi na majani* means 'I have catarrh brought on by the dust of grasses' which should be reasonably well understood. Pollen is *chanuva* in Swahili, but the word is not widely known..
Swedish:	*Jag har hosnuva.*

ragweed is not fully understood, but these may be false positives (see p81) or cross-reactions from people who are mildly sensitized to mugwort or golden-rod (see pp157–9), or the result of visiting the USA. There is no sign of ragweed hayfever at present. This could change if global warming becomes a reality, and if it produces warmer springs and summers, allowing ragweed to spread by seeding.

In some countries, particularly those with warmer climates, certain intro-duced trees (such as she-oaks or cypresses) are a major source of allergenic pollen. Where these trees are simply being planted as windbreaks, and another species would do just as well, it would seem sensible to discourage any further planting of the offending trees.

Chapter Nine

Desensitization Treatments for Hayfever

There is something very satisfying about tackling a problem at source – mending a broken pipe, for example, rather than just putting out a bucket to catch the drips. That may be why desensitization treatments for hayfever are so popular, since they apparently tackle the underlying problem, the malfunction in the immune system.

Desensitization treatments are far more expensive at least in the short term than most medicinal drugs, and are certainly more time-consuming for both the patient and the doctor. There is no guarantee of success, and the treatment must be repeated every year at the outset. Nevertheless, many people choose desensitization, because they like the idea of turning off the allergic reaction, rather than trying to damp it down with drugs.

For some people, desensitization may be the only viable treatment, since they have severe hayfever which is not helped by any of the drugs currently available. Other people use desensitization in conjunction with drugs, since they find that the combined effect is far better than using one treatment alone. In every case, some sort of pollen avoidance will also be valuable as well, reducing the allergen load so that the treatments have less to battle against.

The orthodox form of desensitization is sometimes known as **hyposensitization**. The prefix 'hypo-' means 'less', so the offer being made here is a limited one – sensitivity may be lessened, but perhaps not eradicated. For some people, however, there will be a fairly dramatic improvement. Another term for this treatment is **immunotherapy**.

Today there are two other forms of desensitization therapy, both of which are still hovering on the fringes of conventional medicine. One is known as **neutralization therapy**, the other as **enzyme-potentiated desensitization**. We will look at each of these three methods in turn.

HYPOSENSITIZATION: THE CONVENTIONAL TECHNIQUE

This treatment uses injections of pollen extract just underneath the skin. A series of injections are given, with each one employing a more concentrated allergen extract than the one before. For the first injection, an extremely dilute solution is used, containing only the most minute quantity of allergen. The dose is then increased gradually, which allows the body to learn to tolerate the allergen.

The treatment originated over eighty years ago, when hayfever itself was still something of a novelty. Dr Leonard Noon noted that hayfever was unheard-of in those with the greatest exposure to pollen: farmers and farm labourers. (This is no longer the case today.) This observation led Dr Noon to think that he might cure hayfever by exposing the patient to gradually increasing doses of pollen.

In Dr Noon's original version of the treatment, the patient was given between ten and twenty injections, usually at the rate of two a week. Similar treatment schedules are still used by some doctors today, although most draw the line at fifteen injections, and would not go up to twenty unless there were special difficulties. Alternatively, there are now some much shorter courses, where the pollen extract is combined with another substance which speeds up the process. These shorter courses use only three or four injections, given at weekly intervals, and while they can be helpful for some, the evidence available suggests that fewer patients benefit. Unpleasant side-effects, such as asthmatic attacks or anaphylactic shock (see box on p138) may also be more likely. Another approach is to use a large number of injections but to give them at daily intervals, known as **rush desensitization**. This too tends to bring on unpleasant reactions more readily. On the whole, the slow and laborious method, using ten, fifteen or even more injections, seems the most satisfactory.

This long re-education of the immune system has to be completed well before the pollen season arrives. An interval of at least a month is recommended between the last injection and the pollen onslaught. Some careful forward planning is therefore needed.

Time should be built in for possible set-backs. If an injection produces an allergic reaction (other than itching and redness at the injection site), it is clear that the treatment has progressed too quickly, so the allergist administers the same dose for the next injection, or even goes back to a lower one. Infections make people more reactive to the injections, so if a cold or flu strikes during the course, the concentration will be lowered, or kept the same, until it has passed. Set-backs such as these obviously lengthen the whole process.

It is vital that appointments are kept throughout the course of injections because missing a couple of weeks can wipe out all the benefits so far accrued. The treatment course may then have to start again, right from the beginning, and there will probably be insufficient time to complete it before the pollen season.

To allow for hitches in the schedule, a few extra weeks are added to the total time needed for the course. If things go smoothly, this means that the course finishes well before the pollen season. In such circumstances, the allergist usually gives a weekly maintenance dose, equal in concentration to the last dose injected, until one month before the pollen season.

Some allergists continue giving maintenance doses (but at a lower concentration) at monthly intervals throughout the pollen season. This seems to help sustain the good effects of the treatment. (At one time, hyposensitization courses were carried out *during* the pollen season, for those who had forgotten to start them in advance, but these have now been abandoned as they showed few good effects.)

To be sure of leaving enough time for the treatment, you should consult your doctor or allergist about hyposensitization well in advance. Make an appointment to discuss the treatment six months before the pollen season should begin.

If the hyposensitization treatment is carried out well, at least 80 per cent of those treated will probably benefit to some extent. While they may not lose all trace of hayfever, they will be far less reactive to pollen, and need smaller doses of drugs to keep their symptoms under control. The success rate seems to depend very much upon the technique used, and the care with which it is carried out. Don't be afraid to ask the doctor or allergist about their usual success rate before you decide on taking the treatment.

You may be able to judge in advance if hyposensitization is likely to help you. Observations by various doctors suggest that certain types of hayfever patients will not benefit from this treatment. They are the people whose symptoms do not come on immediately when they are exposed to the allergen, and who take a long time to recover when pollen clears from the air. Suppose, for example, that you are grass sensitive, but you know that walking through long grass in flower will not produce symptoms immediately – this is unusual for hayfever patients, and indicates a slower type of response. If a rainy day during the pollen season does not clear your symptoms, and it takes three days of rain to bring any relief, this too is a sign of unusually slow reactions. People in this group tend not to experience their worst hayfever symptoms when outdoors in the evening, but to wake up the following morning with a bad attack – a belated response to the previous evening's dose of pollen.

Anyone who recognizes this pattern of response in themselves is unlikely to do well on conventional hyposensitization, but may benefit from enzyme-potentiated desensitization or EPD (see p139). In general, those who have tried conventional hyposensitization without experiencing much improvement have a good chance of success with EPD: the two seem to have different effects on the immune system.

Conventional hyposensitization therapy is often continued for four to five years, and then stopped. About 60 per cent of patients who found the treatment helpful continue to show good effects without the annual course of injections. A great deal of research has been done into how hyposensitization works, and some answers obtained (see pp39–40).

Despite its advantages, hyposensitization is now very difficult to obtain in Britain due to a ruling by the Committee on Safety of Medicines in 1986. The Committee decided that hyposensitization should only be given where there was resuscitation equipment available (which rules out most local surgeries), and that patients should be kept there for two hours after the injection, in case of side-effects. This ruling turned an already lengthy process into a major ordeal, which few patients now go through.

The reason for this ruling was a spate of deaths due to hyposensitization. Between 1957 and 1986, twenty-six people died during their course of injections, with eleven of the deaths between 1980 and 1986, and five in the eighteen months just before the report. This alarming number of fatalities made the treatment seem far worse than the disease: whatever else hayfever may be, it is not life-threatening. Many of the deaths occurred as a result of anaphylactic shock (see box on p138) or a severe asthma attack. Some may have been due to errors in the way the hyposensitization was carried out, or a failure to give the right treatment when someone reacted badly, rather than to intrinsic problems of the hyposensitization method.

Hyposensitization is still freely available in all other countries, and many doctors now feel that the UK restrictions are unduly stringent. When carried out with proper care, the treatment rarely has adverse effects. The only patients who need to be kept under supervision for two hours are those with asthma. With other patients, any adverse reactions will appear within twenty to thirty minutes, and most can be dealt with promptly by an injection of adrenaline and antihistamine. Resuscitation equipment is rarely needed.

If you are having hyposensitization treatment, you can help to ensure your own safety. Enquire about the facilities for emergency care before you start the treatment. Once it begins, be sure to tell the doctor or nurse giving the injections:

- if you experienced any adverse reaction after the previous injection

- if you have an infection at present (this can alter your reaction to the treatment)

ANAPHYLACTIC SHOCK

One of the drawbacks of hyposensitization is the risk of **anaphylactic shock**, a massive allergic response affecting the whole body. Anaphylactic shock occurs when a large number of the body's mast cells (see pp31–5) discharge their mediators at once.

One effect of mast-cell mediators such as histamine is to make blood vessels wider and more leaky (see p34). This effect is beneficial during local infections, when it occurs in a restricted area of the body, but during anaphylactic shock it occurs *throughout* the body. With the same amount of blood coursing through a greatly enlarged set of channels, there is far less blood available to fill the vessels, and the blood pressure falls to a dangerously low level. Often, the patient's pulse becomes very weak.

Anyone suffering anaphylactic shock is seriously ill and needs immediate hospital treatment. There is a very real danger of death if treatment is delayed, especially if the person is asthmatic, since the bronchi also become severely narrowed during the attack.

Resuscitation equipment, of the kind available in hospitals, may be needed to deal with the attack. Adrenaline and antihistamine (sometimes with corticosteroids as well) are injected to counteract the effects of the massive histamine release. (Anyone at risk of anaphylactic shock can carry a syringe that is preloaded with adrenaline. These are made available to anyone with a strong reaction to bee or wasp stings, or to those with severe food allergy – see p162.)

During hyposensitization treatment, anaphylactic shock occurs if the patient's immune system has not 'kept up' with the gradually increasing concentrations of allergen. Instead of steadily becoming less sensitive to the allergen, the immune system suddenly takes a violent objection to the increasing dosage. Often there is a warning that this is about to happen – the preceding treatment session will produce some sort of adverse reaction, such as a very large local swelling, or a minor bodily reaction. The cautious allergist should always take note of such reactions, and reduce the next dose, or keep it the same.

- if you develop asthma, either during a course of injections, or between one year's treatment and the next; asthma may express itself as wheezing, tightness in the chest, shortness of breath (especially in cold air, or when exercising), or a persistent cough

Research is currently taking place on new and safer extracts for use in conventional hyposensitization. Various methods are being tried, all of which aim to change the allergen in some way, so that it activates the suppressive arm of the immune system (see p38) without being able to fire off mast cells. Chopping the allergen into small pieces, or attaching it to another chemical molecule, are just two of the methods that researchers in this field are trying out. If they succeed, a far safer method of hyposensitization may become available in the next few years.

LIMITATIONS OF HYPOSENSITIZATION

Needless to say, if you are being hyposensitized with extract of nettle pollen, when you are actually sensitive to mould spores, the treatment is not going to work. Accurate diagnosis is therefore essential. Before the treatment begins, you will be given a skin-prick test to confirm the diagnosis, but remember that the test can produce a false positive (see p81).

You can save yourself, and the doctor, a lot of time by not embarking on a series of injections with the wrong allergen. Read Chapters Six and Twelve, and consider whether the skin-prick test result agrees with the other facts, such as when and where you experience symptoms.

The other major limitation of the technique is that there are only a certain number of extracts available commercially, and if you happen to be allergic to yak sweat or passionflower pollen, you will be out of luck. Assuming your allergen has been identified, and can easily be collected, some allergists may be prepared to make the extracts themselves.

ENZYME-POTENTIATED DESENSITIZATION

This technique is practised fairly widely, and in Britain it may be possible to obtain treatment under the National Health Service, depending on where you live. Ask your doctor if you can be referred to a suitable allergist for this treatment. Otherwise you can be treated privately and your family doctor should be able to refer you to a suitable practitioner (see p318).

This desensitization method relies on the ability of an enzyme (see p12) to enhance the desensitizing effect of a pollen allergen. The enzyme in question is called β-glucuronidase. The enzyme is mixed with the pollen extract and then injected into the skin (an intradermal injection). Alternatively, the skin can be scratched and the pollen extract plus enzyme applied to the area in a small plastic cup. This latter method is safer for people with violent allergic reactions because the extract is not injected into the skin and should not therefore provoke an anaphylactic reaction (see p138). (It has never yet done so, despite years of use with some very sensitive patients.) This degree of caution is rarely needed in hayfever, but it might be appropriate for some people with pollen asthma who are at high risk of anaphylaxis, and it is also useful for people with immediate-onset food allergies: both conditions are regarded as too-dangerous for conventional hyposensitization to be used. The scratch method of enzyme-potentiated desensitization (EPD) is also suitable for children who are afraid of injections, and in the hands of an expert the method is safe for quite small children.

An unusual feature of EPD is that a standard mixture of pollen allergens is used, rather than individual pollen extracts, so each patient is treated with all the common allergenic pollens. However, a diagnostic skin-prick test is still used before the treatment, and where there are other sensitivities, such as house-dust mite or mould spores, the appropriate allergen extracts can be added to the pollen mixture.

The pollen mixture is produced in Britain, but it has been tried out by doctors in a variety of countries around the world and usually works well. The wordwide distribution of the common allergenic plants (such as grasses) plus the frequency of cross-reactions between many plants (see Chapter Eleven) seems to allow the mixed extract to work well in countries far from Britain, such as New Zealand and Italy. At present, the method has not been much used in the tropics or subtropics, and it may not give such good effects in these regions because of the presence of many different pollens.

Careful scientific testing of EPD has been carried out several times in both Britain and Italy, and these trials have shown that it works work well for grass, olive and pellitory pollen. Ideally, the method should be scientifically tested with other pollen allergies as well, but until this is done we must rely on the general observations of doctors using the method. These suggest that EPD is successful with many different pollen sensitivities.

Approximately 80 per cent of patients are helped by EPD, with about 40–65 per cent being a great deal better than before. When compared directly with conventional hyposensitization, using the same assessment methods, the two techniques produce equally good results, with EPD having far fewer adverse reactions and therefore being safer. It is also much less time-consuming, needing just one or two injections a year in most cases, compared to a series of ten to fifteen injections for hyposensitization.

Those who do not benefit at all from EPD are usually helped by conventional hyposensitization, and the reverse is also true. This suggests that the two techniques work by fundamentally different mechanisms.

The EPD treatment should be given before the hayfever season begins, preferably about three weeks before. Some patients benefit from having a second injection in the late autumn, which improves the response in the following year. The treatments will need to be repeated annually for three to five years, but after this period many patients find that they are free of hayfever.

Doctors are often suspicious of techniques that work by unknown means, and tend to reject both EPD and neutralization therapy (see below) for this reason. Yet the conventional technique, hyposensitization, was in use for many years before anyone understood how it worked. Even now, no one can say exactly how it works in each individual who benefits from it (see pp39–40).

NEUTRALIZATION TECHNIQUE

This is also known as intradermal neutralization therapy, or the Miller technique, after Dr Joseph Miller of Alabama, who spent many years developing it and investigating its applications. The treatment can be given in two ways – either using injections of allergen extracts under the skin, or giving the extracts in drops under the tongue, known as **sublingual drops**. With treatments for hayfever and other forms of rhinitis, sublingual drops are often used.

In both cases, the doctor must first discover which allergens are involved, by using a skin-prick test (see p78). Once the problem allergens have been identified, the next step is to establish the **neutralization dose**. This is the concentration of each allergen extract that is necessary to desensitize the individual patient to that allergen – different concentrations are required for different individuals.

To test for the correct dose, intradermal injections, which put pollen extracts into the skin, are used. These go deeper than the skin-prick tests, but are not especially painful. A tiny amount of the allergen extract is used.

If the concentration is too low to produce any significant reaction in the skin, the injection simply results in a small raised area, known as a wheal, which begins to go down soon afterwards. If the body does react, then the wheal grows slightly and takes on a characteristic appearance, becoming white, hard and raised, with a sharp edge. This is known as a positive wheal.

When a positive wheal is obtained, the dose is then reduced for the next injection, and repeatedly reduced, step by step, until a concentration is reached that fails to produce a positive wheal. The highest concentration of extract that fails to produce a positive wheal is the neutralizing dose. As well as producing desensitization, it can, for some patients, actually 'turn off' hayfever symptoms which have already begun.

Testing for the neutralizing dose can take one or two hours per allergen. Someone who is allergic to just a few pollens can have their neutralizing doses established in an afternoon, but for someone sensitive to several different allergens, a day or two of testing could be needed. Some practitioners speed up the process by using mixed pollen extracts and establishing a neutralizing dose for the mixture, but this does not give such good results as testing with individual pollen types.

Testing for the neutralizing dose is best done a month or two before the pollen season, but if necessary it can be carried out at any time of year.

Once the neutralizing dose has been established, it can be self-injected by the patient, or taken as drops, whenever needed. Most practitioners suggest a daily injection for the first week of the pollen season, then every other day for a few weeks. After that, the patient can experiment to find their own dosing regime – as often as necessary to keeps the symptoms under control. The drops are used two or three times a day at first, and then as often as needed.

· How neutralization therapy might work is not known. It is possible that, when the neutralizing dose is used, the pollen allergens are bound to skin cells inside the wheal for a long period of time, allowing them to exert a particular influence on the immune system. Perhaps they act by stimulating T suppressor cells (see p38), which could then damp down the immune response to pollen in the nose and eyes.

From a practical point of view, neutralization is less bothersome than conventional hyposensitization, in that the tests for the neutralization dose can probably be carried out in a single day, rather than involving repeated visits to a surgery. Compared to EPD, it is rather more time-consuming because of the testing process required. Furthermore, the neutralization point may change, so that the vaccine stops working as well. If this happens, you will need to go back for retesting. On the plus side, testing for the neutralization dose can be carried out during the pollen season, and therapy begun then, and while it may not be as effective as treatment begun earlier in the year, most patients will probably reap some benefits.

Neutralization is fairly widely available, and there is at least one centre in Britain which can offer it under the National Health Service. In practice, many patients will have to obtain treatment privately. Ensure that the practitioner uses a skin test to determine the neutralization dose. Once the neutralization dose has been determined, the drops (or injection vaccine) are relatively inexpensive. Most practitioners retest for the neutralizing dose every year.

Doctors experienced in this technique have found that it is important to neutralize for all the pollens (or other allergens) that give a positive skin test. If only one or two allergens are dealt with, even though these may be the major allergens for the patient, the results will be less satisfactory.

NEW FORMS OF DESENSITIZATION

Medical researchers continue to experiment with different approaches to desensitization. One new method, developed by researchers in Belgium, is to make a vaccine by extracting pollen-specific antibodies from the blood of hayfever sufferers and then combining them with pollen allergens. When allergen and antibody combine they form a complicated tangle that includes many molecules of each type. This is known as an **immune complex**. Having made their immune complexes, the researchers inject them into the skin of hayfever patients, and this appears to produce a beneficial desensitizing effect. In trials carried out so far there were no side-effects at all. If future trials are equally successful, this treatment may become available in the next few years.

Another new method tried by researchers is to give pollen or pollen extract by mouth, in capsules, with gradually increasing doses. The final dose reached is much larger than the amount of pollen that reaches the stomach by natural means (see p147). This method has proved successful in some trials, with a few patients suffering stomach upsets, but no serious reactions.

Many other new forms of desensitization are also being tried, but most of these are variations on one of the main methods described in this chapter.

Chapter Ten

OTHER TREATMENTS FOR HAYFEVER

Conventional medicine has some powerful weapons against hayfever, as described in Chapters Seven and Nine, but many people still turn to other forms of treatment. This chapter looks at all those which we have come across, and tries to assess whether they may help you or not.

You will, no doubt, meet people who have 'found the cure' for hayfever. There are two things to bear in mind when considering such claims. One is that most people grow out of hayfever as they get older, usually before the age of thirty. So the friend or colleague who claims that their hayfever cleared up as soon as they cut down on beer, stopped disco dancing, or started having a milky drink at bedtime is probably just reporting a coincidence. The second point to consider is the **placebo effect**, a phenomenon well known to medicine, whereby any new treatment will have some positive effect for most people. The placebo effect can operate with pills or capsules, with a visit to a helpful and reassuring doctor or therapist, a dietary supplement, a special diet, or a change in lifestyle. In all cases, belief that the treatment will work is the crucial element.

For example, in a trial of dust-proof mattress covers used for asthma (see p178), the **control group** of patients, who were given mattress covers that let through the dust mite allergen, showed a small improvement in their symptoms. This is why scientific trials always include a control group – a set of patients who are given a similar but ineffective treatment. The results observed in these patients can be deducted from the benefit seen with the real treatment, to take out the placebo effect from the real effect.

The placebo effect works for everyone, not just the gullible or dim-witted, and it seems to work by harnessing the body's own potential for self-healing. We all have far more control over our bodies than we are aware of, and a placebo (originally the name for ineffective sugar pills dispensed by baffled doctors) somehow taps into that inner power and makes it work in our favour.

Placebo effects are part of any medical treatment – they give a boost to the benefits available from medicinal drugs, for example, and to the good effects of desensitization. But with these conventional treatments, scientific trials have been carried out to verify that there is also a *real* effect from the treatment itself. With unconventional treatments, such as herbal pills, this is generally not the case: they have not been tested and compared with a control group, to see if they are any more effective than a placebo. Thus, the claim that such pills 'relieve hayfever symptoms' may be quite honestly made, yet the apparent benefits could be nothing more than a placebo effect.

If the placebo effect works, then why worry? This is a valid argument, but the placebo effect from a new 'drug' or other ineffective treatment only lasts a short while. Once the initial enthusiasm about the treatment wears off, the placebo effect ebbs away. Furthermore, the effect of a placebo will rarely match that of a genuinely effective drug or treatment. You may as well spend your money on something that really works.

Before leaving this subject, we should briefly mention **negative placebo effects**. These are seen, for example, when patients in the control group of a scientific trial – those taking a harmless placebo – report side-effects. Here it seems that some people *are* far more susceptible than others. Those who have had bad reactions to a drug in the past may suffer negative placebo effects from a new drug, particularly if they are worried about side-effects.

TREATMENTS TO UNBLOCK THE NOSE

A blocked nose can best be unblocked by means of corticosteroid nose drops (see p100), preceded if necessary by a brief treatment with sympathomimetic nose drops (see p96). For those who do not wish to use such drugs, there may be other ways of easing the congestion.

The traditional treatment used for colds – inhaling steam – can also be very effective in hayfever. Use a mixing bowl from the kitchen, pour in boiling water, put a towel over your head and shoulders, and sit face down over the bowl so that you are inhaling the steam. The longer you continue with this, the more effective the treatment will be. You may need to replace the water as it cools down.

Menthol, eucalyptus and other aromatic substances with a decongestant action are sometimes added to the hot water to improve its effects. They can be bought from any chemist, often in capsules (e.g. Karvol) or in liquid form. You could try adding these, but stop using them if there seems to be any irritation to the nose.

A high-tech version of this inhalation treatment, a device known as a Virotherm, is now available from some chemists' shops. It supplies a continuous stream of warm moist air, heated to exactly 43°C (109°F). The manufacturers recommend inhaling this air for twenty or thirty minutes. This device has been tested with those suffering from the common cold, and showed beneficial effects in reducing symptoms. It was superior to an ordinary steam inhalation. Although the effects on hayfever symptoms have not yet been tested to the same standard, the Virotherm is said to be valuable to some hayfever sufferers. Unfortunately, the machine is rather expensive, over £40.

Salt-water nose drops can also be useful in relieving congestion a little and soothing the irritated membranes of the nose. Sterile salt-water (or 'saline') solution can be bought in sachets (Normasol) at any chemist. You can also buy a dropper bottle, the lid of which contains a dropper for placing the salt-water drops in the nose. Fill the bottle with the salt water and change it every few days. Use the drops as often as you feel you need them.

Nose drops containing vitamin C have also been tried out by doctors in Israel, who tested them against placebo drops. They noted that the secretions of the nose are normally very slightly acidic, but that during a bout of rhinitis they become very slightly alkaline. It therefore occurred to them to try reversing this effect using a mildly acidic solution of vitamin C. About three-quarters of the patients tested experienced some benefit from these drops. Unfortunately, the concentration of vitamin C used in these tests was not reported. If you would like to try this treatment, start with a very dilute solution – a quarter of a teaspoon of pure vitamin C powder in a pint of water. Should there be no beneficial effect, increase the amount of vitamin C used slightly – but if it stings, the solution is too concentrated. The water used should be boiled for at least ten minutes beforehand, to kill bacteria. Alternatively, buy purified water from a chemist. As with salt-water drops, buy a small dropper bottle to contain the solution you have prepared and refill with fresh solution every few days. The drops should be used three times a day. Stop using the drops if you have a cold or other infection in the nose.

DIETARY SUPPLEMENTS

One treatment worth trying is to take cod-liver oil (two teaspoons a day). This contains certain natural oils that affect the production and control of **prostaglandins**, chemical messengers produced by the body which have a subtle influence on the inflammation process.

By favouring the production of some prostaglandins over others, fish oils reduce the tendency to inflammation in the body, which is why they are often recommended for rheumatoid arthritis. Recent studies have shown that they are also valuable in asthma, and possibly in hayfever. Since it is an inexpensive treatment, it is worth a try. Never take too much cod-liver oil, as it is a rich source of vitamin A, which is toxic in excessive doses. The effect of cod-liver oil on the prostaglandins takes about three months to become fully established, so do not expect any immediate benefits. To maintain the effect you need to keep taking the oil.

Evening primrose oil is likewise used for rheumatoid arthritis and has also been suggested as a useful supplement in hayfever. No one has yet carried out any tests to see if it really is effective, but it could be useful, as it too has an effect on the prostaglandin balance in the body. It can be used in addition to cod-liver oil, and may augment the effects. Again, it takes about three months to build up its protective action.

High doses of vitamin C were once proposed as a treatment for hayfever, but medical trials have shown that they are not effective. Ginseng and cider vinegar have also been suggested, but there is no evidence for these either. Scientific trials with ginseng in healthy individuals have shown that it can have unpleasant side-effects when taken for a prolonged period, such as diarrhoea.

Eating honey in a honeycomb has also been suggested as a treatment, because it contains some pollen. There are no trials of this treatment but it does not seem likely to work. The pollen in honey will rarely be the sort of pollen that hayfever sufferers react to (see p4). We all swallow quite a bit of pollen during the spring and summer anyway, as it catches on the saliva in the mouth.

IONIZED AIR

Air ionizers work as cleaning devices, removing particles from the air (see p304). It has also been claimed, by some hayfever sufferers, that the stream of ions coming from the ionizer has a direct therapeutic effect. By facing the ionizer at close range, and so allowing the ions to flow over their face, they apparently experience relief from existing symptoms of hayfever, such as itchy eyes and a streaming nose. One German manufacturer has even produced a portable air ionizer to be worn around the neck, which emits ions over the face.

There is nothing known about ions to suggest how this might work, and most doctors and scientists are dismissive of such claims. To the best of our knowledge, no one has tested the direct effects of ions on hayfever symptoms. However, claims of substantial improvement in hayfever have been made repeatedly, and there is probably no harm in trying the effects of ionized air, if you feel inclined to do so. Shops that specialize in selling ionizers often have one running, so you can try it out in the shop itself – the effects are supposed to come on within a few minutes. Some of those who supply air filters and ionizers (see p302) will allow you to hire a device for a while to check if it is beneficial.

Some ionizers may produce a small amount of ozone (see p319) which you could inhale if at close range. Should you experience any coughing, or irritation of the nose or airways, then stop the treatment immediately.

HYPNOTHERAPY

A scientist in the USA has looked at the effect of hypnosis on relieving congestion of the nose in hayfever sufferers. He classified the patients studied into 'high hypnotizable' and 'low hypnotizable' subjects.

The 'high hypnotizable' set showed considerable benefit from hypnotherapy sessions aimed at reducing their congestion. However, they also did well on sympathomimetic drops (see p96) and on placebo drops. Compared with 'low hypnotizable' patients, they did much better on all three treatments, and still showed the benefits a month later, when they had fewer hayfever attacks and were using their medicinal drugs less often.

It seems that 'high hypnotizable' subjects are more susceptible to placebo effects, although other studies of placebos have not found this link.

The practical conclusion from all this is that if you respond to hypnosis you will respond equally well to any treatment that you believe in, so hypnotherapy is probably a rather expensive option. Self-hypnosis might be worth trying, if you are an enthusiast for totally natural cures. There are various tapes available that teach self-hypnosis – enquire in health food shops or 'alternative' bookshops.

HERBAL MEDICINES

There are herbal tablets sold in pharmacies that claim to alleviate hayfever. As far as we know, these have not been tested in a controlled trial. Their main ingredient is garlic.

Chinese herbal treatments are also available. While the good effects of Chinese herbal treatments for eczema have been demonstrated scientifically, no tests have been carried out on those offered for hayfever.

Before taking any herbal medicine, consider the possibility of allergic cross-reactions (see p167), particularly if you suffer symptoms in the mouth from certain foods. Although it must be very rare, some medicinal herbs may also be toxic to some people.

ACUPUNCTURE

This is a system of medicine that originated in China, and which involves stimulating specific sites on the body, known as the acupuncture points. Stimulation of these points is generally done very gently with needles, but

MADELEINE

Madeleine was very sensitive to several pollens, including silver birch, plane tree, various grasses, plantain and nettles. She suffered from asthma as well as hayfever, and because so many pollens affected her, she had to endure the symptoms from early spring right through to the autumn. Although she tried antihistamines, they did not help much, and as she disliked taking drugs anyway, she gave them up. After four years of 'summer misery'

Madeleine decided to try alternative treatments, and found that the most successful one for her was acupuncture. The treatment is carried out each spring, with two twenty-minute sessions. Sometimes these are enough to protect her from symptoms for the entire summer, but occasionally she needs a booster dose later. Most hayfever sufferers find that they need more treatment sessions than this, usually five or more.

there are many different versions of acupuncture treatment, some using harder pressure, some using needles that carry an electrical current, others using suction cups.

There is a traditional explanation for how acupuncture works, which most Western doctors find difficult to accept, as it bears no relation to what is known about human physiology. It would seem that acupuncture was developed on a trial-and-error basis, and a theoretical framework then constructed to explain how it worked. An alternative explanation, based on nerve reflexes between the skin and the internal organs, has now been proposed by Western practitioners of acupuncture and seems plausible. It looks as if acupuncture stimulates these reflexes, which can have beneficial effects.

Few would deny that acupuncture is an effective system of altering bodily responses – its dramatic effects in producing local deadening of the nerves, so that surgeons can operate on a fully conscious patient, are convincing evidence that this is a powerful form of treatment. Whether acupuncture effectively treats *all* the ailments for which it is offered is another matter. There have been only a few proper scientific trials, and as far as we know, none have been carried out for hayfever.

Since there are nervous reflexes that control the production of mucus, and the swelling of blood vessels in the nose (see p226), it is not implausible to suggest that acupuncture could help in reducing hayfever symptoms. During the 1980s, scientists in the USA also discovered tiny nerve cells that lie alongside mast cells (see p31) and which may influence their action. This unexpected discovery offers another route by which acupuncture could affect an allergic reaction such as hayfever – and affect it at a more fundamental level.

Acupuncture is said to work for hayfever, but five or six treatments are generally needed during the pollen season to maintain the good effects. Some patients are helped by just two treatments in the spring, but this is unusual. In terms of value for money, neutralization (see p141) or enzyme-potentiated desensitization (see p139) would cost about the same per year as a course of acupuncture treatments.

HOMOEOPATHY

Homoeopathy is a form of treatment first devised by a German doctor, Samuel Hahnemann, at the end of the eighteenth century. Hahnemann was appalled by the drastic effects of some of the remedies then used by doctors, such as blood-letting, emetics and cathartics: in this he was undoubtedly right. Hahnemann abandoned the medical techniques he had been taught and devised his own system based on the idea that 'like cures like'.

Homoeopathy uses substances – animal, vegetable or mineral – that produce the same symptoms as those it aims to treat. The substance used is called a similium. The similium is ground up in alcohol, and the extract is then diluted, one drop in 99 drops of alcohol. A single drop of that mixture is taken and diluted with another 99 drops of alcohol. This process is repeated many times, and each time the dilution is made the mixture is succussed. This means repeatedly hitting the container against 'a hard but elastic object, such as a leather-bound book' (to quote Hahnemann). The dilution process might be repeated as many as thirty times, producing a C30 potency. According to homoeopathic ideas, the power of the extract to treat the patient *increases* with each dilution, so that one diluted twenty times (a C20 potency) is *less* effective than one diluted thirty times.

Having made the C30 potency, this is then 'impregnated' into tablets made of lactose, the sugar found in milk. Homoeopaths take a bottle of 'blank' lactose tablets, add a few drops of the potentized solution, then shake the bottle. The drops of potentized solution only fall on a few of the tablets near the mouth of the bottle, and most of the tablets are untouched by them. Yet *all* the tablets in the bottle are said to acquire the same therapeutic power.

One of the reasons that scientists are so sceptical about homoeopathy is that they can calculate, approximately, the number of molecules of the active substance (the similium) in the first drop of extract used. They can then calculate how many there are in the first dilution, the second dilution, and so on. Quite early on in the process, there are only one or two molecules of the similium left. By the thirtieth dilution, there is unlikely to be even one molecule left. *The thirtieth potency contains none of the similium.*

Homoeopaths argue that, during succussion, the similium somehow imposes an 'informational structure' on the alcohol, and that this is what makes homoeopathic medicines active. But substances such as alcohol are extremely simple chemically, and very well understood by science (far better understood, for example, than the subtle workings of the human body). Chemists can state fairly confidently that there is nothing in the alcohol which can take on a 'structure', and certainly no way in which that structure could be passed on with successive dilutions, becoming more potent each time. Even if there were such a 'structure', how could it be communicated to lactose tablets at the bottom of the bottle, where no drop or splash of the C30 potency is felt? Such explanations seem to be invoking something akin to magic.

Despite all this, many people report good effects from homoeopathic medicines. There have also been proper scientific trials of homoeopathy, and some have shown that homoeopathic tablets have a greater effect than placebo tablets (see pp144–5). (None of these, incidentally, used the similium employed for the homoeopathic hayfever remedy widely sold in Britain.) However, other trials have found no effect. Where benefits have been seen, this could be due to chance (always a possibility, even in the best scientific trials) or due to some other unanticipated effect.

This may sound like special pleading, because we would probably take such positive results at face value if they concerned a conventional drug or a desensitization treatment. But the sort of logic being applied here is one that any sensible person uses. If someone tells you that they saw a dog in the garden yesterday, you will probably accept that they are telling the truth. If they say they saw a lion, you might be a little doubtful, and would want further evidence. If they say they saw a unicorn, you are going to be profoundly sceptical. The claims made by homoeopaths about succussion, potencies and 'informational structures' are definitely in the unicorn league.

Medical historians suggest that homoeopathy acquired a good reputation early on because doing nothing was infinitely better for patients than subjecting them to the horrors of conventional medical treatment at the time. Many recovered naturally, since the body has its own healing powers which simply need time to work. But because they were being treated by a homoeopath, their recovery was attributed to homoeopathy. We believe that this good reputation, passed down from generation to generation, and endorsed by the British monarchy, gives homoeopathy a 'super placebo effect', which continues to work wonders today.

Where the patient visits a homoeopath (rather than buying over-the-counter homoeopathic remedies), there is the additional benefit of a long consultation with a sympathetic therapist, which is helpful for almost any medical complaint, especially one where some psychological factors are involved. Homoeopaths ask a lot of questions about diet and lifestyle, and may often give useful advice. This, rather than the homoeopathic remedies, is probably the source of their success. In the case of hayfever, however, psychological factors are of minimal importance, so this holistic dimension of homoeopathy will not confer much benefit.

In conclusion, if you believe in homoeopathy, it will probably do you some good, but if you could transfer that belief to some aspect of conventional medicine, it would probably do you far more good.

Chapter Eleven

UNDERSTANDING CROSS-REACTIONS

None of us is perfect, and that goes for our antibodies as well. In theory, they should bind to just one type of antigen, but they can mistakenly bind to something that has a very similar chemical feature or epitope (see p11). In the fight against disease this can sometimes have advantages (see p46), but for anyone with hayfever, cross-reactions may multiply their problems by making them sensitive to other pollens, to foods, and even to cosmetics, insecticides, timber or wood pulp.

CROSS-REACTIONS BETWEEN POLLENS

In forming antibodies to pollens, we are true individualists – each of us makes the antibodies by our own unique (and entirely random) process (see p30). The antibody's binding site may fit the epitope like a tailor-made glove if you are lucky, but it might only fit it like a mitten – which would leave plenty of scope for that antibody to fit on to another, similarly shaped epitope. This is what causes a cross-reaction. Thus, two people who are sensitive to the same pollen do not necessarily show the same cross-reactions. Those with pollen-specific antibodies like tight-fitting gloves will probably have few cross-reactions, while those with the mitten-like antibodies may cross-react with several other pollens.

Bear this in mind when looking at the lists below. The fact that a cross-reaction is listed here simply means that it is *possible* and affects quite a few people. It does not mean that you will automatically suffer from it.

CROSS-REACTIONS BETWEEN GRASSES

Grasses belong to the family Poaceae (formerly called the Gramineae). Within that family there are many different species and these are not at all closely related. Despite this, there appears to be a great deal of similarity between grass pollen antigens.

All grass pollens seem to have the potential to cross-react. Thus someone from Britain with grass pollen allergy can react to sorghum pollen, although they have never been exposed to it in their life. There are more cross-reactions among grasses than in any other plant family.

Even with grasses, however, not everyone cross-reacts. A Danish study showed that three-quarters of grass-sensitive patients reacted to timothy grass, a major allergenic pollen, but the remaining quarter did not. Taking four common grasses (timothy, meadow fescue, false oat grass and couch grass) 95 per cent of grass-sensitive patients react to one or more of them, but that leaves 5 per cent of patients who are allergic to some other grass, and show no reaction to any of these four.

Reeds and sedges (Cyperaceae) sometimes cross-react with grasses, and so may rushes (Juncaceae) and reedmaces or cattails (Typhaceae).

CROSS-REACTIONS BETWEEN TREE POLLENS
The birch family

Birch, alder and hazel all belong to the same family, the Betulaceae. Birch produces the most allergenic pollen of the three, and many people are allergic to birch alone. However, quite a few people with birch hayfever show a cross-reaction to alder or hazel or both. Hazel and alder begin pollinating very early in the year, so those showing this cross-reaction may suffer symptoms up to two months before the birch pollen season begins. In Britain hazel bushes in sheltered gardens may even start to pollinate before Christmas, and might cause some symptoms.

Hornbeams are usually put in a separate family, the Carpinaceae, but they are closely allied to the Betulaceae. People who are sensitive to birch may also react to hornbeam pollen, but this type of hayfever has not been widely reported except in the USA.

Birches, oaks and beeches

A variety of cross-reactions occur between trees in the order Fagales (see box article). These include the oaks, beeches and chestnuts, the hornbeams, plus all members of the birch family – birches, alders and hazels.

These wide-ranging cross-reactions help to account for the usefulness of the diagnosis 'tree sensitive', used in Britain and Scandinavia (see p75).

Again, birch seems to be the prime offender. In Scandinavia, 90 per cent of people who react to springtime pollens are sensitive to birch pollen, and it seems likely that this is the pollen which began their hayfever, with reactions to other pollens developing subsequently.

There may also be cross-reactions between birch and the pollen of unrelated trees (see p159).

Willows and poplars
Willows, poplars and aspens all belong to the same family, the Salicaceae. Cross-reactions between different trees and shrubs in this family probably occur quite frequently. Sallows and osiers are also forms of willow.

Cypresses, junipers, thujas and 'cedars'
Cypresses and junipers belong to the family Cupressaceae, along with the trees known as thujas. There seem to be extensive cross-reactions between the pollens in this family. If you have a problem with cypress, always check the label before planting evergreen shrubs in the garden. Some cypresses and junipers have common names such as 'mountain cedar' so it may not be obvious from the common name that they are part of this family. Check the scientific name: if it begins *Cupressus*, *Chamaecyparis*, *Cupressocyparis*, *Juniperus*, *Thuja*, *Thujopsis* or *Fitzroya*, it is a member of this family.

There is a possibility of cross-reactions with some trees in the next group, the Taxodiaceae.

Redwoods, bald 'cypress' and Japanese red cedar
Japanese red cedar belongs to the same family as the sequoias and redwoods of North America, the Taxodiaceae. Swamp 'cypress' or bald 'cypress', *Taxodium distichum*, is also a member of this family. Cross-reactions between the different trees are possible but not yet shown.

Cross-reactions between Japanese red cedar and true cypresses have been found by several researchers, so it seems that this family has similar pollen allergens to the Cupressaceae (see above). Whether those with allergy to redwood or swamp 'cypress' pollen also cross-react with cypresses is unknown.

Olive, ash and privet
These three species belong to the same family, and there is some cross-reactivity between them. The only one whose pollen contains powerful allergens is olive, which is a frequent culprit in hayfever around the Mediterranean, and in parts of Australia and the USA. Those who are sensitized to olive may then react to ash, which is a heavy pollen-producer, and a very common tree in Britain, but rarely causes hayfever of its own accord, being only mildly allergenic. People who are sensitive to olive can also produce a reaction to privet. Privet is insect-pollinated, yet its pollen grain is small and quite large numbers become airborne.

RELATIONSHIPS OF LIVING THINGS

The more closely related two living things are, the more likely they are to have allergens that are chemically similar.

For the purposes of allergy studies, it is usually assumed that all members of a single species share the same antigens. A species is a group of animals or plants, all of which can potentially breed with each other. We are usually aware of species as creatures that we can recognize and put a name to, because they all look similar: a tiger, for example, or a giraffe, or a silver birch.

Groups of related species, such as silver birch, downy birch, yellow birch and paper birch, are grouped together in the same genus. When the scientific name of a plant or animal is given, the first word is always the name of the genus. In the case of birches, it is *Betula*. Silver birch is *Betula pendula*, downy birch is *Betula pubescens*, yellow birch is *Betula lutea*, while paper birch is *Betula papyrifera*.

For the most part, species in the same genus seem to share chemically similar allergens, so doctors describe someone as being allergic to 'ragweed', even though there are several different species of ragweed. The ragweeds are referred to collectively as '*Ambrosia* spp.' (spp. is shorthand for 'species'), *Ambrosia* being the name of the genus. The same goes for nettles (*Urtica* spp.), docks and sorrels (*Rumex* spp.), plantains (*Plantago* spp.), pellitories (*Parietaria* spp.) and mugworts (*Artemisia* spp.).

Related genera (the plural of genus) are grouped together in a family. At the family level, there may still be enough in common between the different species for them to cross-react, but they will not necessarily do so. Some families, such as the grass family, show extensive cross-reactions among the many different members, even between species that belong to distant branches of the family and are not closely related. In other families there may be few shared allergens: nettles and pellitories belong to the same family, for example, but cross-reactions have never been observed between them.

Related families are grouped together in an order, and while few cross-reactions occur at this level, there are some. The only well-known ones are within the order Fagales, a collection of trees that includes birches, alders, hazels, hornbeams, beeches and oaks.

There is an exception to most rules, and the domestic dog provides one here. Although this is a single species (yes, a Chihuahua *could* still mate with a Great Dane, given a stepladder), there are substantial differences between the allergens of some breeds. This has become apparent because a few people show an allergic response to *only one breed of dog* and not to others.

However, this highly selective response to dog breeds is rare. Most people who are allergic to dogs respond equally to all the different breeds.

CROSS-REACTIONS INVOLVING 'WEED' POLLENS
Ragweeds and their allies

Ragweeds belong to the daisy family, the Compositae (also called the Asteraceae). Cross-reactions with other members of this family do occur for some ragweed-sensitive patients. The most commonly reported cross-reactions involve:

Bur ragweed or false ragweed *(Franseria)*
Marsh-elder *(Iva)*
Burro-bush *(Hymenoclea)*
Cocklebur *(Xanthium)*
Groundsel bush or tree *(Baccharis)*
Mugwort, wormwoods, 'sage', sagebrush *(Artemisia)*
Feverfew *(Parthenium)*
Goldenrod *(Solidago)*
Boneset or thoroughwort *(Eupatorium)*
Sunflower (*Helianthus*)
Dandelion (*Taraxacum*)
Broom weed (*Xanthocephalum*)

Goldenrod illustrates the question of cross-reactivity perfectly. In Britain it is grown as a garden flower, a fact that amazes hayfever sufferers from the other side of the Atlantic. In the USA, goldenrod is regarded as a noxious weed, along with ragweed itself, since 30 per cent of ragweed-sensitive people are also allergic to goldenrod. Clearly, goldenrod only causes such problems (or only causes them on a grand scale) if ragweed pollen has set the stage for it to do so. The same is also true for dandelion pollen (see p5).

Many other members of the daisy family show cross-reactions with ragweed, but far less frequently than those listed above. They include several garden flowers such as asters, chrysanthemums, dahlias, various daisies, coneflowers (*Dracopsis* and *Rudbeckia*), marigolds, African daisies (*Arctotis*), and zinnias. Among wild flowers, thistles, knapweeds, brittle bush, chicory, rosinweed, sneezeweed, rabbit brush, coltsfoot and ironweed are all implicated occasionally.

Chamomile flowers, when used in teas and cosmetics, have caused cross-reactions for ragweed-sensitive people. The allergens concerned are found in the chamomile pollen, which in theory could cause hayfever, but this has never been reported. Perhaps there is too little of the pollen becoming airborne.

The daisy-like flowers of *Pyrethrum* can also show some cross-reactions with ragweed pollen. It is these flowers that are used to make pyrethroids, a type of insecticide and acaricide (mite-killer) that is often marketed as 'natural' and safe. In fact most pyrethroids used today are synthetic ones, made in a laboratory but based on the chemicals found in the flowers. Like their natural counterparts, they can cross-react with ragweed pollen. However this does not happen often, which is fortunate since pyrethroids are widely used in household sprays to kill house-dust mites. A few ragweed-sensitive patients react badly to pyrethroids, however. Another acaricide, benzyl benzoate, is available and anyone with a severe reaction to ragweed might be best advised to choose this, especially if they are asthmatic.

Mugwort

Mugwort and other members of the genus *Artemisia* (see p157) belong to the daisy family, along with ragweed. There are reports of cross-reactions between ragweed and mugwort, so people who have never been exposed to ragweed pollen but are sensitive to mugwort may show a positive skin-prick test to ragweed. They might also react badly to ragweed pollen on visiting North America or some other part of the world where ragweed is common. A skin-prick test for ragweed might be advisable before travelling, to see if this is likely. The trip can then be planned to avoid the ragweed season (see Appendix 1).

Cross-reactions between mugwort and other members of the daisy family have not been reported. It would seem that mugwort is not such a potent sensitizer as ragweed anyway, and has fewer shared antigens with others in its family.

Goosefoot and amaranth families

There are often cross-reactions between the plants in these two closely related families. The plants most often implicated are:

Fat hen, Lamb's quarters or Pigweed (*Chenopodium album*)
Mexican tea (*Chenopodium ambrosioides*)
Goosefoot (*Chenopodium berlandieri*)
'Russian thistle' (*Salsola pestifer* or *Salsola kali*)
Burning bush (*Kochia scoparia*)
Wingscale (*Atriplex canescens*)
Lenscale (*Atriplex lentiformis*)
Wedgescale (*Atriplex truncata*)
Common orache or orach (*Atriplex patula*)
Allscale (*Atriplex polycarpa*)
Saltbush and Annual saltbush (*Atriplex argentea* and *Atriplex wrightii*)
Sugar beet (*Beta vulgaris*)
Red glasswort (*Salicornia rubra*)
Winter fat (*Eurotia lanata*)
Smotherweed (*Bassia hyssopifolia*)
Greasewood (*Sarcobatus vermiculatus*)
Russian pigweed (*Axyris amaranthoides*)
American seepweed (*Suaeda americana*)
Palmer's amaranth (*Amaranthus palmeri*)
Redroot pigweed (*Amaranthus retroflexus*)
Spiny pigweed (*Amaranthus spinosa*)

Note that some of these plants are found only in Europe, others are found only in North America, while some are found in both.

CROSS-REACTIONS BETWEEN UNRELATED POLLENS

When cross-reactions occur between pollen and food, plant relationships are frequently irrelevant, as we shall see. This raises the possibility that there are also cross-reactions between pollens from unrelated plants. It is a topic that has not been studied a great deal as yet, except in the case of birch pollen.

The one well-documented case relates to birch pollen cross-reacting with apple pollen. The fact that birch pollen and apple fruit cross-react so often (see p164) inspired researchers to see if the same could occur with apple pollen, and it did.

Birch appears to show other cross-reactions of this kind, as with bog myrtle, a wild shrub that is in an entirely separate plant order. Over 80 per cent of those sensitive to birch pollen give a positive skin-prick test to bog myrtle.

Skin-prick tests of Swedes with birch-pollen hayfever reveal that they frequently react to pollen from a wide range of other plants, including many that are not close relatives, such as elder and horse-chestnut. Whether these are true cross-reactions remains to be proved. It could simply be that the allergic reaction to birch pollen makes the nose more easily sensitized to other pollens which are airborne at the same time of year.

Could the pollen of other plants, besides birch, produce cross-reactions to the pollen of unrelated plants? At present, this is a question that researchers have not even begun to look at.

CROSS-REACTIONS TO FOOD

Only a minority of hayfever patients are affected by cross-reactions to food, and if you are one of the select few you will probably know about this sensitivity already. It usually causes symptoms in the mouth only, generally itching or tingling. There can also be hayfever-like reactions in the eye and nose which usually pass quite quickly, along with the symptoms in the mouth.

More severe symptoms can occur, however, including a swelling of the tongue, lips and throat, an outbreak of itchy urticaria (nettle rash) all over the body, or an asthma attack. In the most serious cases, there can be a reaction affecting the whole body, known as **anaphylactic shock** (see p138). Such reactions can be life-threatening because the throat swells so much that the airways become blocked, or because there is a prolonged and severe attack of asthma, or through the effect of anaphylactic shock on the blood vessels which makes the blood pressure fall to very low levels.

If you do not suffer from cross-reactions to food at present there is *no point whatever* in worrying about them – the chances are they will never occur, and if they do, they will be mild and transient.

The only people who do need to be cautious, even though they have never reacted to food before, are those with asthma. As the case described on p166 makes clear, a cross-reaction can be very dangerous. If you are asthmatic and you begin to feel odd after eating a food (e.g. with tingling or itching in the mouth or lips) then stay close to a telephone for an hour at least, so that you can summon help if necessary. In most instances the symptoms will wear off, and nothing further will happen. In this case there is no cause for concern, but do avoid eating that food in future. Should any further symptoms appear (see box on p162), do not hesitate to seek medical help.

It must be emphasized that for the majority of hayfever sufferers, cross-reactions to food are very mild and affect the mouth only. Such reactions should be regarded as a warning, and the food avoided as much as possible, but there is no need for scrupulous avoidance in most cases. By 'scrupulous avoidance' we mean never consuming the food under any circumstances, which can involve considerable vigilance when eating away from home (see box on pp168–9).

The exceptions – those instances where the food should be avoided altogether – are as follows:

- if you have asthma (see above)

- if the food concerned is celery, since this is particularly likely to provoke a swelling in the throat that can lead to suffocation if not dealt with promptly

- if peanuts or any other type of nut is involved; these tend to provoke severe reactions

- if the symptoms you experience on eating the food have been getting progressively worse

- if you have ever experienced swelling of the tongue, lips or throat, difficulty in breathing, or urticaria (nettle rash) all over the body

- If you are taking the drugs known as ß-blockers (beta-blockers), used for a variety of heart conditions; these increase the risk of a severe anaphylactic reaction

- if you have ever collapsed after eating a food (anaphylactic shock); in no circumstances should you eat it again, or eat any food that has been in contact with it

Of all hayfever sufferers, those most often affected by allergies to foods are children. Quite often there is a sign of an impending reaction, because the child instantly dislikes the smell or taste of the food. Of course, children often react like this to new foods, so it is hard to judge when the child's objection should be taken seriously and when it should be ignored. In general, however, if a child with hayfever strongly dislikes a fruit or vegetable, you should not insist on it being eaten, nor try to present it in a disguised form.

TAKING CARE WITH FOOD ALLERGIES

Anyone who has had an allergic reaction to food in the past should be aware that a further exposure can sometimes precipitate a worse reaction. Even a relatively mild reaction, such as localized urticaria in response to a food, can be the foretaste of something much more serious, and it is vital that such warnings are heeded.

An initial test that can be done at home is to apply a small amount of the food to the face, making sure that none of it goes anywhere near the mouth. If this produces a rash, then the food should not be eaten.

For those who have had a severe anaphylactic reaction to food in the past, it may be advisable to carry a syringe containing emergency medication, in case the food is inadvertently eaten again. The syringe can be used only once, and contains adrenaline, which counteracts the effects of histamine and other mast-cell mediators, by causing the blood vessels to contract. It is still necessary to avoid the food, of course – the contents of the syringe will only be effective if a very small amount has been eaten.

An aerosol spray containing adrenaline (Medihaler-Epi) can be issued to those who have suffered severe swelling of the throat in the past, in case they unintentionally eat the food again. It may also be useful if you feel you could not cope with giving yourself an injection in an emergency. Your doctor should be able to prescribe either the injection or the spray.

Do not delay in using the syringe or spray if you begin to experience a severe reaction to food. In this situation a 'wait-and-see' attitude could be disastrous. The sooner you use the adrenaline, the more effective it will be, and you will avoid the possibility of lasting, irreversible damage to the body. Having used the syringe or spray, contact your doctor or go to a hospital quickly, because you will probably need further treatment. The adrenaline injection should be repeated every fifteen or twenty minutes until you are fully recovered. Tell the doctor if you have been taking corticosteroids, as these may suppress your body's normal ability to produce its own corticosteroids, which are needed in this crisis situation. Extra corticosteroids can be given to counteract this.

Not all anaphylactic reactions come on immediately. They can sometimes take an hour or even two hours to develop. There are usually some initial signs that things are amiss, such as itching or swelling in the mouth, nausea and stomach pains. If the food is affecting the throat, hoarseness or a 'lump in the throat' sensation may be the first signs. Should these be followed by more generalized feelings, such as itching all over, sneezing, runny nose, diarrhoea and weakness, a serious anaphylactic reaction may be developing. Other odd sensations that may accompany this stage are a feeling of warmth, and a peculiar sense of dread or apprehension. Incontinence, disorientation and abdominal pains may also be experienced.

If there are any signs such as these, **do not delay in getting medical help**. Go to an accident and emergency department if you can, and make sure you are seen quickly – don't sit quietly waiting your turn.

Anyone who has had a severe reaction in the past should consider wearing a medical-information bracelet with the relevant information on it. (You can find out how to obtain such a bracelet from your doctor or pharmacist.) If you were to eat your culprit food by mistake while away from home, and were found unconscious, it could save your life. Without it, you might not get the correct medical help.

THE LINKS BETWEEN POLLENS AND FOODS

Not all pollens are involved in cross-reactions with foods. The prime offender here is birch pollen, which causes a great variety of reactions with different fruits, nuts and vegetables. Mugwort, grasses and pellitories are also linked to some cross-reactions.

One or two of the cross-reactions make sense in terms of plant relationships, such as grass hayfever and wheat sensitivity, or pine pollen and pine nuts. But these are the exceptions, and most of the cross-reactions cannot be explained in this way. It seems that some fruits and vegetables just happen to have substances in them that are similar to pollen allergens. In the case of birch, which has been studied far more than the others, some of the shared allergens seem to be 'heirloom' molecules, like profilin (see p46), which were found in ancestral plants and have been retained by many different plant families.

These are the known cross-reactions, with the most commonly implicated foods listed first for each pollen:

Pollen	Food
Birch	Apple
	Carrot
	Cherry
	Pear
	Peach
	Plum
	Fennel
	Walnut
	Potato
	Spinach
	Wheat
	Buckwheat
	Peanut
	Honey
Mugwort	Celery
	Carrot
	Spices
	Melon
	Watermelon
	Apple
	Chamomile tea
Grass	Melon
	Tomato
	Watermelon
	Orange
	Swiss chard
	Wheat
Pellitory	Cherry
	Melon
Ragweed	Melon
	Chamomile tea
	Honey

	Bananas
	Sunflower seeds
Pine	Pine nuts
Hazel	Hazelnuts, filberts, cobnuts

There are a number of other fruits and vegetables that may cause symptoms in people with hayfever, but these are not strongly linked with any particular pollen.

The last example does not involve a pollen, but we will include it here for completeness. It is probably the strangest cross-reaction of all – between house-dust mite and kiwi fruit. This is a true cross-reaction due to an entirely coincidental similarity in the epitopes (see p11). Occasionally people with house-dust mite sensitivity react badly to kiwi fruit the very first time they eat it. There are reports of the same cross-reaction between dust mite and papaya fruit (paw-paw).

Sensitivity to foods can sometimes be so pronounced that they do not have to be eaten to produce symptoms. For example, some patients with birch pollen hayfever cannot even peel or scrub potatoes without reacting to them. One woman with grass pollen hayfever suffered asthma, red eyes and a streaming nose at the smell of boiling Swiss chard.

Very often the allergen in the food is destroyed by cooking, or even by storage, so it is worth some cautious experimentation with cooked, canned, or frozen and defrosted versions of the culprit food. Cooked apples are almost always tolerated by apple-sensitive people. You can always apply some of the food to your skin first, before eating it, to see if it produces a rash – this will warn if a severe reaction is likely.

Treatment of hayfever symptoms is rarely of any help in clearing up responses to food.

CROSS-REACTIONS TO OTHER ITEMS

A beautician who suffered from hayfever in late summer, brought on by ragweed pollen, found that she was developing a congested nose all year round, along with itchy hands which grew worse when she was at work. A resourceful allergist looked into the cosmetics she was using, and discovered that they contained chamomile. Switching to other brands of cosmetics cured the hands and the stuffiness in her nose, although her hayfever still came back every year as expected.

Chamomile is found in a great many different items, from shampoos and face creams to teas and herbal remedies. Fortunately, only a tiny minority of those with ragweed hayfever are sensitive to chamomile, but if you are you should read labels on cosmetics with care.

JACK

Jack was six years old and had suffered from hayfever since he was five. Skin-prick tests showed him to be sensitive to a wide variety of pollens, including ragweed and mugwort. The doctor gave Jack a course of injections with pollen extracts, a treatment known as hyposensitization (see p134). The treatment was successful and Jack continued with it for two years.

One spring evening, when Jack had just completed his second annual course of injections, he began to cough, and later became breathless and wheezy. His mother suffered from asthma herself, so she knew the signs, but she did not take Jack back to the doctor immediately. The night-time coughing and wheeziness continued, and one evening, when Jack could not sleep, his mother decided to give him a cup of chamomile tea, which she thought would be soothing.

Jack drank a few sips of the tea, but didn't like it and refused the rest. A few minutes later he began wheezing violently, and was clearly having difficulty in breathing. He began scratching himself hard, as he felt itchy all over, and complained of a terrible pain in his stomach. Soon afterwards, Jack was sick and he then became very pale,

Insecticides containing pyrethrum or synthetic pyrethroids can also cross-react with ragweed pollen (see p158).

Those sensitive to cypress pollen sometimes react to the wood of cypresses or other conifers. This type of cross-reaction may well occur with other pollens from coniferous trees. Wood pulp, used for making paper, is also reported as causing allergic reactions in some hayfever sufferers, perhaps as a result of a cross-reaction.

Just occasionally there can be allergens in the stuffing used for furniture. In former times, furniture-makers of the New World sometimes used 'Spanish moss' (*Tillandsia*) to stuff their settees and armchairs, and those sensitive to the pollen (found in the air in some southern states) may react to the furniture as well. (Similarly, old sofas stuffed with horsehair will almost certainly contain microscopic flakes of horse-skin as well, and this could provoke symptoms in someone who is highly allergic to horses.) Allergy to kapok, a soft plant fibre used for stuffing toys, is also known.

began sweating violently and collapsed. His terrified mother had by now telephoned for an ambulance. The doctors in the emergency department at the hospital were equally alarmed – Jack was clearly close to death. However, they were well versed in the treatment needed for such a case, and quickly injected the boy with adrenaline, antihistamine and corticosteroid. The colour began to return to his cheeks a few moments later, and within an hour and a half he had regained consciousness. Tests later showed that the IgE antibodies (see p31) he produced to ragweed and mugwort pollen could also react with an antigen in chamomile flowers – it is the flowers which are used to make chamomile tea.

Chamomile belongs to the same plant family as ragweed and mugwort, the daisy family (Compositae or Asteraceae). Shared antigens are quite common among related plants, although they rarely cause such a violent reaction to a food as they did in Jack's case. In fact, a cross-reaction to chamomile tea is remarkably unusual, considering how common ragweed allergy is. However, anyone who is ragweed sensitive would be wise to approach this herb tea with some caution.

HERBAL MEDICINES

Herbal medicines, naturopathic remedies and the like could well contain plant materials (e.g. feverfew) which cross-react with certain types of pollen. Before taking these, you should check that you are not likely to be sensitive to them. Find out the ingredients, if possible, and see whether any of these belong to the same plant genus or family as your problem pollen (you may need the help of a plant field guide). Reject any medicines that contain closely related plants. Proceed cautiously with others, testing some of the medicine on your face first. If this provokes no reaction, try a very small dose of the medicine at first, and gradually build up to the recommended dose.

EATING OUT WITH FOOD ALLERGY

If you have to avoid a food entirely, eating away from home can be problematic, particularly if the food is likely to turn up 'in disguise'. Apples can be used in sauces for meat, for example, or added to cakes and pastries. Concentrated apple juice is the sweetener in 'sugar-free' wholefood jam. Celery is usually obvious, but celery seed, sometimes used as a spice, can contain the same allergens. Carrots, which affect some people with mugwort hayfever, can appear in carrot cake or may be mashed (and therefore unrecognizable) in soups and stews. Fennel seed, which may share allergens with fennel itself, is sometimes used as a spice. Melon, a problem for some with mugwort or grass hayfever, is found in Aqua Libra and similar drinks.

Dinner invitations are something of a problem, and the best approach is to tell your host or hostess in advance what you cannot eat. Offer to bring your own food if this is more convenient. For buffets and parties, eat beforehand, or take something safe with you.

When eating in restaurants or cafés, enquire about the contents of prepared food, and watch out for unsuspected ingredients. Plain food, such as steak and a salad, where 'what you see is what you get' is much the safest option. All sorts of odd things can be found in casseroles, stews, pies, sauces, cakes and puddings. You could ask your waiter or waitress to check with the chef what ingredients have been used, but unless you are absolutely sure they will do so, it is better to speak to the chef yourself.

A particular word of warning about peanuts: cross-reactions between birch pollen and peanut are rare, but straightforward allergy to peanut is one of the most common food allergies. It kills a few people every year, due to the fact that peanuts are so widely used, often in unrecognizable forms. Peanut has turned up unannounced in sweets, cakes, biscuits, cookies, Chinese egg rolls and even (as peanut butter) in chilli con carne. If you are peanut-sensitive, watch out for nuts generally, as there is a new product being launched which looks like an almond or walnut, but is actually made from peanuts. The packets will have to declare their ingredients, of course, but the bowl of nuts on a bar or party table may not be quite what it seems. There are also pretzels available now with a peanut-paste filling which is quite unexpected and therefore dangerous. Satay dishes contain peanut, as do many traditional Thai recipes.

Never try to pick out the offending food from a dish that has already been prepared, and then eat what is left. There will be some unseen molecules of the food that have seeped into the mixture, and you may be sufficiently sensitive to react to them.

Anyone with a severe and potentially dangerous food allergy may be helped by enzyme-potentiated desensitization (see p139). This is a very safe technique, and while it will not allow you to eat the food freely, it may protect you from life-threatening reactions if you encounter the food accidentally. It can also be helpful for those who are affected by the smell of the food alone, as some unfortunate people are.

Chapter Twelve

WHAT'S IN THE AIR? ALLERGENS AND IRRITANTS OTHER THAN POLLEN

'You can't live on fresh air' is an old saying, but it is not entirely true. The air around us actually contains millions of tiny particles, both animal and vegetable, which would provide a good balanced diet, full of protein, vitamins and minerals – if only you could filter out enough of the particles.

Many of these airborne particles are only a few thousandths of a millimetre in diameter, but they can be seen, even without a microscope. Look at any landscape (or any landscape painting) and you will notice that the distant hills or trees are bluish in colour, more blurred and less colourful than items in the foreground. This is the result of particles in the air scattering light. Distant trees are viewed through a far thicker 'layer' of air than trees close to, and this changes their colour from green to blue. (On a damp misty day, when there are minute droplets of water in the air as well as the usual particles, the effect is even stronger.)

We are breathing a veritable zoo – there are particles from insects, spiders and mites, scales from the wings of butterflies, flakes of skin from people, dogs, cats and other animals, and tiny fragments of feathers. In addition to the 'animal', there is plenty of 'vegetable' – pollen grains, plant hairs and particles, volatile molecules (see p120) from plants, and the spores of fungi. Finally, there is also a fair amount of 'mineral' – particles of rock and soil dust. And, of course, there are bacteria and viruses.

Those are just the *natural* airborne particles. Small wonder that, in the course of evolution, we acquired noses, whose job is to filter out all this junk from the air destined for our lungs.

When human ancestors discovered fire, about 1.5 million years ago, a new kind of particle joined the natural ones in the air – man-made smoke. We have been adding new synthetic particles ever since, and at increasing speed in the past 200 years.

The nose that originally developed to cope with natural particles has proved fairly adept at handling the new synthetic particles as well. But among the hundreds of different particles that we now breathe, several can cause a bad reaction in the nose – reactions similar to hayfever, including sneezing, a runny nose or a blocked nose.

These reactions are covered by the general term **rhinitis**, meaning inflammation of the nose. (Sometimes, you may also hear doctors use the word **rhinopathy**, a broader term meaning something wrong with the nose that might or might not involve inflammation, or **rhinorrhea** which just means a runny nose.) Strictly speaking, rhinitis should only be used when there is genuine inflammation, that is, an immune response in the nose. In practice, the term is often used rather more loosely than this.

Those particles that cause rhinitis through an allergic process (see Chapter Three) are called **airborne allergens**. Those that cause rhinitis or rhinopathy in other ways are generally referred to as **airborne irritants** and are dealt with at the end of this chapter.

Of all the microscopic items that we inhale, only a very few can act as allergens. Even those that *can* act as allergens do not necessarily do so. Most people never react to any allergens, and even severely allergic individuals do not react to *all* potential allergens. This is an important point to remember, otherwise the thought of that airborne 'zoo', which sweeps into the nose with every intake of breath, may induce a feeling of panic!

The six major groups of airborne allergens (other than pollen) are:

- house-dust mite droppings

- mould spores

- fragments of animal skin

- proteins from the saliva or urine of animals

- fragments of feathers

- particles of insect bodies, or their droppings

Of these, most can cause either rhinitis, or asthma, or both. They do not cause symptoms in the eye as readily as pollen does, but eye symptoms certainly can occur. Symptoms are usually present all year round, but they can be seasonal in some people (see p218).

Other allergens may be encountered at work, such as wheat flour or wood dust in the air. These are dealt with on p216.

HOUSE DUST

House dust is the major source of airborne allergens, after pollen. Dust itself is largely a human product – flakes of dead skin that we shed unknowingly every day of our lives. Mixed in with the skin flakes are hairs, human and animal, and tiny threads from clothing and upholstery. Not a very appetizing mixture, you might think, but to some animals that dusty corner behind the sofa is a land flowing with milk and honey; those animals are house-dust mites, which feed mainly on skin particles. There are several different kinds, the most common being known as *Dermatophagoides*, or 'skin-eater'.

Skin is made of a protein called keratin, and to a microscopic creature such as the house-dust mite, a discarded human skin flake must be like a large, tough, dried-up piece of steak – chewy but very nutritious. Part of the difficult job of digesting these skin flakes has already been done, however. Like a piece of well-hung game, they are already colonized by microorganisms such as moulds, yeasts and bacteria long before the house-dust mite eats them.

If house-dust mites did not produce allergies, we would all get along with them quite happily. Quentin Crisp, the English eccentric and writer with a famous aversion to housework, once observed that 'after the first four years the dust doesn't get any worse' – no scientist has ever investigated Mr Crisp's observation, but perhaps, when four undusted years have passed, the house-dust mite population reaches a peak level, and the mites promptly devour all newly arriving dust. Unfortunately, if you are allergic to house-dust mite, you cannot take Mr Crisp's sanguine view. Dust and dust-eaters alike have to be kept to a minimum. There will be further details on how to achieve this later in the chapter.

One point to emphasize here is that many people with an allergy to house-dust mite are quite unaware of the source of the problem, because they may not feel any worse in a house that is apparently very dusty, nor much better in a house that is spick and span. This is because our main exposure to house-dust mite comes from mattresses, sofas, armchairs and other upholstery. However clean these might seem on the outside, they will contain our skin flakes within, and conditions there are ideal for the dust mite. There are often huge and thriving populations of mites, and whenever we roll over in bed, or flop into an armchair, a blast of air, rich with mite allergens, is expelled from within the mattress or upholstery. The older the mattress or armchair, the more mite allergens there will be.

Most allergens are proteins (see p12), and in the case of house-dust mite, the main allergen is a digestive enzyme (see p12) that the mite produces to break down the skin proteins. This enzyme, and other mite proteins, are found on the mite's droppings or 'faecal pellets'. Thus, the inhaled particle that affects the nose of the rhinitis sufferer is not the mite itself, but its droppings. These are much smaller than the mite, and crumble to produce even tinier particles (see p204) which can become airborne easily and stay airborne for a long time.

Some people, however, react to allergens found on the mite itself, while a certain number react to some other component of dust, not to the house-dust mite or its products. Some of these individuals react to moulds or mould spores in the dust (see p193). Others are allergic to sheep's wool, a difficult allergy to diagnose (see pp211–2). A few people react to a different mite, one which preys upon *Dermatophagoides* (without, unfortunately, reducing its numbers very much). It is also possible to be sensitive to cockroach particles in the dust (see p83) or to fragments of other insects, such as house flies or carpet beetles (see p213). A tiny minority of patients are allergic to human skin itself.

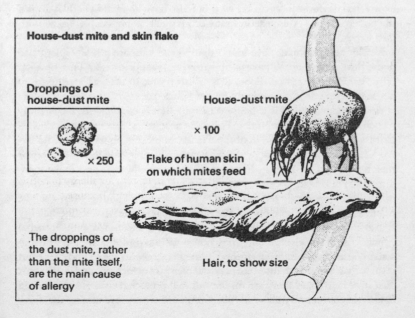

House-dust mite and skin flake

Droppings of house-dust mite

× 250

House-dust mite

× 100

Flake of human skin on which mites feed

Hair, to show size

The droppings of the dust mite, rather than the mite itself, are the main cause of allergy

Although dust mites mainly favour houses, substantial populations can also be found in cinema seats (the older the better), and fabric-covered car seats. The sort of dust encountered on building sites, or in factories, does not cause any problems. There are rarely many dust mites in offices either, as the harsh cleaning fluids used tend to see them off. However, recent reports have identified high dust mite levels in some offices, and linked them to outbreaks of 'sick building syndrome' (see p218). Hospitals generally have very few mites, which is a large part of the reason why asthmatic children recover when in hospital, dust mites being the major allergen in asthma.

Identifying house-dust mite allergy

An allergy to house-dust mite can produce rhinitis or asthma or both, and where it produces rhinitis in children, this is often accompanied by glue ear (see box article on p176). It can also cause eczema and, much more rarely, stomach cramps, vomiting or diarrhoea. Even nasal polyps (see p228) can be due to house-dust mite allergy.

It is possible for house-dust mite allergy to coexist with pollen allergy, resulting in year-round symptoms that get worse in the pollen season. Alternatively, someone may be allergic to both, but not sufficiently sensitive to house-dust mite for it to cause symptoms on its own. Such people will experience hayfever in the usual way, but also have a reaction to dust during the pollen season – this reaction may or may not be noticeably linked with dust exposure.

Researchers in Japan have found that people who are already allergic to house-dust mite tend to have a far stronger reaction if they then develop hayfever. For this reason alone, it is worth trying to prevent sensitivity to house-dust mite in children (see Chapter Fourteen).

How do you know if it is house-dust mite that is responsible, or partially responsible, for your symptoms? For some people, the reaction is so obvious that the diagnosis is not in doubt, particularly those who have to do house-work and are afflicted by symptoms when dusting, vacuum cleaning or making the bed, activities which stir up the mite allergens and make them airborne. For others, sneezing attacks that only come on in bed or first thing in the morning are a tell-tale sign – the allergens coming from the the mattress (see p172) are to blame. (Bear in mind, however, that feather allergy is also a possibility, since pillows and duvets are often stuffed with feathers.) People with house-dust allergy may notice their symptoms are far worse in some houses than others, even though the house seems clean and free from dust. A cosy home with fitted carpets and plenty of armchairs and cushions is dust-mite heaven, as there are millions of well-protected crannies where skin flakes can collect and mites can hide within upholstery and among the fibres of the carpet. Apart from wall-to-wall carpeting, another modern improvement has proved highly congenial to dust mites: tightly fitting windows and doors, intended to provide total draught-proofing. While this may save on heating bills, it increases the moisture in a house by sealing it in, so that fewer mites perish through desiccation now. In the draughtier conditions of unimproved, old-fashioned houses, the air is drier and many mites die a thirsty death, which helps to keep the numbers down. Moulds also grow more slowly, making the skin flakes less digestible for the mites.

Houses that are damp, such as those built near rivers or near the sea, usually have many more dust mites than those at higher altitudes. Symptoms are likely to be worse in such locations, but this could also indicate mould allergy (see p193) and you would need a skin-prick test to determine which was important.

There is another clue, but it is not a very reliable one. Seasonal variations in symptoms are possible, because damp weather favours the mites, and in some houses they tend to be more numerous during autumn and winter. (Note that moulds may give the same sort of seasonal pattern, however – see p218.) This clue is unreliable because, according to a study carried out in Germany, not all houses are affected by the outside climate. Some are so sealed off from the outside world that the dust mites are only affected by the house's internal conditions.

Finally, shampooing carpets stirs up the mites and their droppings, producing an unusually heavy load in the air for some time afterwards. This can provoke a severe attack of symptoms, especially in children playing on the newly cleaned carpet.

If you think that house-dust may be your problem, but are not sure, ask your doctor to carry out a skin-prick test (p78). You should be given tests for both house-dust mite and house dust. If both are negative, you can be fairly sure you are not allergic to dust mite or anything else in dust, but there is a remote possibility that the result is a false negative (see p81) and you really are sensitive to dust. In this case you will need a nasal provocation test (see p79).

A positive result should be interpreted carefully, as quite a few people give a false positive skin-prick test to house-dust mite – that is, the skin test is positive but they actually show no symptoms. Before you set about reducing house-dust mite allergen in your home, you should be sure the diagnosis is correct.

Dealing with house-dust mite
The measures needed for adults and older children are described here. Babies and toddlers need a slightly different approach, described on p188.

GLUE EAR

Rhinitis can lead to 'glue ear', particularly in children. This is especially likely when there is allergy to house-dust mite (see p173) but can also happen with other forms of rhinitis. Glue ear arises when there is so much build-up of mucus in the nose that it works its way up into the Eustachian tube (see p19) and blocks it off. (The proper medical name for this condition is **chronic secretory otitis media**. Not surprisingly, even doctors prefer to call it 'glue ear'.)

Once the Eustachian tube is blocked, air can no longer get into the middle ear, so pressure on either side of the eardrum cannot be equalized. This may cause pain and 'popping' in the ears. In time, the air that was already in the middle ear is gradually displaced by a thick, sticky liquid exuded by the ear. Part of the function of the healthy Eustachian tube is to let this treacly stuff drain away, but now there is nowhere for it to go. Eventually it fills the cavity, gumming up the three tiny bones that are a crucial part of the hearing apparatus. This impairs hearing and may produce an uncomfortable feeling in the ears.

A baby or toddler with glue ear may be too young to complain of earache or

The recommendations largely refer to cool climates. In hot and humid climates the mites will thrive even better, and ventilation will not help much in controlling them.

People vary greatly in their sensitivity to house-dust mite. Some remain well unless confronted with a massive amount of the allergen. In their case, the only thing causing problems may be an old armchair or mattress, one that has housed generation upon generation of dust mites and is now richly endowed with their allergens. Replacing this item may be all that is needed to put a stop to their symptoms, although it is also advisable to seal a new mattress (see pp177-8) so that the mites do not move back in. It is also possible, rather than replacing a mattress entirely, to use a treatment that kills the mites (see p179), and then to seal the mattress.

Other sufferers need more thorough measures that substantially reduce the house-dust mite population in the rooms they spend most time in – the bedroom and living room. Only the most sensitive individuals need to reduce the dust mite population to a bare minimum throughout the home. This 'popping' in the ears, but there are other signs that can alert you to the problem. Often children scratch at their ears, or shake their head repeatedly in an unusual way. Deafness is usually obvious, although it is sometimes mistaken for simple disobedience. Occasionally the first sign that anything is wrong is that a baby does not begin talking as soon as it should, because it cannot hear properly. (There can, of course, be many other reasons for delayed talking.)

Glue ear becomes a serious problem for some children, and sorting out the problem is vital as impaired hearing can interfere wih their mental development and success at school. If nasal drops do not relieve the symptoms, then the condition is usually treated by inserting small tubes, called grommets, into the eardrum. Where allergy to house-dust mite or some other airborne allergen is the underlying problem, treating the allergy can often avoid the need for grommets.

Children with recurrent glue ear and adenoids sometimes turn out to be suffering from an allergic problem, even though there is no obvious sign of allergic rhinitis. Some children suffer glue ear as a result of food intolerance (see p232).

involves quite a lot of effort, so the obvious thing to do is to start with minimal changes and gradually work your way up.

First you should deal with your mattress. The best thing is to replace your mattress with a new one, and to seal it immediately in a cover that acts as a barrier to dust-mite droppings, to skin flakes and to the mites themselves. The cover prevents dust mites from repopulating the new mattress: research has shown that they usually colonize new bedding within three months. The cheapest way to seal a mattress is with a cover made of plastic sheeting, either home-made or a ready-bought one. (The sort of cover used for small children who wet the bed will also protect against dust mites, as long as it has no holes anywhere, and the seams are reasonably airtight. You could make it more airtight by sealing the seams, or any holes, with packing tape.) This sort of smooth plastic cover can create a problem in that the bedding tends to slip off, but a few small strips of double-sided sticky tape can help to solve this.

In recent years these plastic covers have been superseded by a much

JUNE

At five o'clock every morning, June woke with a volley of sneezes. Once her husband decided to count them and the total was 53. During the summer, the sneezing and streaming nose were not as bad, so June was clearly not suffering from hayfever.

Her problems had begun two years earlier, when they had first moved to Britain from the south of France. The family had been forced to live in temporary accommodation for a while, and the flat they had taken was very damp. Although her symptoms had improved since moving into a house, they were still troublesome.

It seemed clear to June's doctor that an allergy to house-dust mite or mould spores was the most likely cause: both are favoured by damp conditions, and both are worse in autumn and winter. However, the fact that June's symptoms peaked when she had been in bed for a few hours pointed more strongly towards house-dust mite. Mites thrive in mattresses.

As it turned out, June was sensitive to both these allergens: the doctor used skin-prick tests (see p78) to discover this. Before prescribing any drugs, the doctor asked June to try simply reducing these allergens in her house. June bought a plastic mattress cover and improved the ventilation in the house to reduce any dampness. Later, she bought a dehumidifier for the bedroom. These measures improved her symptoms considerably and she decided against any further treatment.

improved product made of **microporous material**. Such material lets water vapour through while acting as an impenetrable barrier to mites and their allergens. (Water vapour is the gas produced by the **evaporation** of water; under warm conditions water can become water vapour, while in colder conditions water vapour becomes water again, the process known as **condensation**.) With the older, completely impermeable plastic covers, a drop in temperature could produce condensation on the inside of the cover, from water vapour leaving the mattress, and might result in mould growth. With the new microporous materials this will not occur. The material is not as slippery as ordinary plastic covers, so it has an additional advantage in that the sheets stay put. Similar covers are also sold for pillows, duvets and the box springs at the base of the bed. See p307 for a list of suppliers and a guide to prices.

In the past, those with house-dust mite allergy were often advised to choose a foam mattress rather than the traditional interior-sprung design, since foam – or so it was claimed – harbours fewer skin particles, and therefore fewer mites. Pillows filled with synthetic materials were also said to be better than feather pillows. Recent research has failed to confirm this, and it is now widely accepted that microporous mattress covers, pillow covers and, possibly, duvet covers, are much the best measure that can be taken against dust mites. With these covers on, it does not matter what the pillow or mattress is made of. Duvets that can be washed regularly (see p181) are also useful, instead of the duvet covers.

Another recommendation often made in the past was to vacuum clean the mattress regularly, but this is now considered far less valuable than sealing the mattress. There is also the possibility of increasing the level of mite allergen in the air while vacuum cleaning, unless you have a specialized type of vacuum cleaner or have equipped yours with a filter (see below).

If a new mattress is out of the question, there are ways of reducing the number of mites in an existing mattress, prior to sealing it in a plastic cover. One is to spray the mattress with an **acaricide**, a chemical that kills mites and ticks (see box article). Another is to treat the mattress with **liquid nitrogen**, which is very cold and freezes the mites to death. Suppliers and further details of both these treatments are given on pp309–10.

In both cases, the treatment needs to be followed by thorough vacuum cleaning, because killing the mites is only half the battle – you also need to remove their old droppings, and their tiny corpses since these can release allergens as they decompose. Once the vacuuming is done, you can seal the mattress into its new cover.

Why go to all this trouble, when the mattress is going to be enclosed in plastic or microporous material anyway? It might seem just as effective to cut out the mite-killing treatment and vacuuming, but this is not recommended by doctors who have studied mites in mattresses. If enclosed by a cover, the mites will be locked in with their food supply, and will continue to feed and breed. Allergens will build up inside the cover and if it then develops a small hole, the allergens will seep through and begin to cause trouble again. (There could also be some seepage around the seams of the cover, depending on how these are constructed, although most manufacturers do their best to prevent this.) Similarly, if the plastic cover has to be removed for any reason, the allergens will flood out. However, if you are aware of these drawbacks, and watch the cover carefully for holes, then this shortcut method could work

EIGHT LEGS OR SIX?

Mites are often referred to as insects, but in fact they are different creatures entirely. They are related to spiders, and the most obvious difference is in the number of legs: insects have six, spiders and mites have eight. These eight-legged creatures are called **arachnids**.

Mites, along with their close, and equally unloved relatives, the ticks, make up the zoological order called the Acari, a subdivision of the arachnids. The chemicals that kill mites and ticks are therefore called **acaricides**.

Note that an insecticide will not necessarily act as an acaricide, although some do, notably **permethrin** and those based on **pyrethroids**. Some acaricides, including **benzyl benzoate**, are specifically mite-killers and do not work against insects. For this reason, flea sprays, fly killer and other household insecticides will not necessarily affect house-dust mite, and it is better to buy a spray that is sold specifically for this purpose. For more details on these products, and suppliers, see p309.

just as well. If the cover has to be removed at some point, make sure the allergy sufferer is out of the room, and remains out of it for a whole day, during which time the room should be thoroughly vacuum cleaned and dusted.

At the same time as treating or replacing your mattress, you should deal with your pillows. Replacing them with new ones is a good idea, but as with new mattresses it is vital to put a plastic or microporous barrier over the new pillow, underneath the pillow case, to prevent recolonization by mites. Old pillows can be treated with liquid nitrogen first, but not with acaricides, as the amount inhaled will be too great.

Blankets and duvets should be replaced with new ones if at all possible, or washed. Some launderettes have machines large enough to wash a whole duvet. A wash temperature of at least 58°C is needed to kill the mites. Lower temperatures will wash out the droppings and their allergens, but leave many live mites to replenish the stocks. Dry cleaning will kill some mites and remove some of their allergens but is less satisfactory than washing at high temperatures. Duvets should be aired outside for a day after dry cleaning. If these measures are difficult because you have no other bedding available, simply putting a duvet into a tumble-drier and keeping it hot and dry for a couple of hours should kill off many of the mites, and may also **denature** (see p182) some of the allergens.

One of the advantages of buying a new duvet is that there are some special ones available (see p307) which separate into three layers. This allows them to be washed in an ordinary washing machine at home, one layer per wash. They are also suitable for laundering at 60°C.

Maintaining the low dust-mite levels

Once the changes to your mattress and bedding have been made, a little extra effort every week will help to keep the mite population down. The bedding should be shaken outside and hung in the sun at regular intervals – dust mites, like vampires, have an aversion to sunlight. If this is impossible, a long spin in a hot tumble-drier is valuable. Sheets, pillowcases and underblankets should be washed once a week at 58°C or higher. If there are problems in washing underblankets, you could just place them on a radiator once a week, making sure that they get good and hot for a while. This will kill the mites but not remove the allergen, so it is a measure that is only useful if they have been washed at least once.

Always make sure that beds are aired thoroughly before they are made, as the body produces moisture at night, which penetrates all the bedding. The duvet or blankets should be pulled back, and left for at least an hour before the bed is made. As an additional measure, an electric blanket can help to reduce the moisture in the bed, creating hot dry conditions that dust mites dislike. (This can be useful as a temporary measure, if you cannot afford mattress covers.)

Needless to say, while these activities are going on, the level of allergen in the air will rise dramatically. The allergy sufferer should not have to dust, vacuum clean, sweep floors or make beds if there is anyone else in the household who can do the work. Wear a mask (see p295) if this sort of housework is unavoidable.

The most important measure of all is to increase the ventilation in your bedroom, and in the rest of the house. As long as it is not raining outside, opening a window will reduce the amount of moisture in the air, making conditions far less congenial for mites (see p190). Airing the room at the same time as you air the bed makes excellent sense. Try to get a good blast of air through the whole house every day.

Tackling dampness in the house

Anyone living in a house that is clearly damp should take steps to combat this, as the mite problem is bound to be worse in such conditions. Many of the measures described for combating moulds on pp195–9 are relevant for

DENATURING THE ALLERGENS

An allergen can act as an allergen only as long as it keeps its particular chemical features – the ones that make it recognizable to allergy-producing antibodies (see p30). If those features are changed in some way, the allergen no longer binds to the antibody, and there is no allergic reaction.

Most allergens are proteins. Proteins can be **denatured** – have their shape changed – in various ways, and such changes often stop them from acting as allergens.

One way to denature a protein is to heat it to a high temperature. Heating to 75°C will denature the main dust-mite allergens, but some are not affected.

Another way to denature proteins is to treat them with certain chemicals. One that is widely sold is **tannic acid**. Tannic acid is assumed to be safe, since it is found in tea and red wine at concentrations only a little lower than those in the sprays. Thorough vacuuming is essential after use of the spray, and this is said to remove most of the tannic acid (which dries to a powder) anyway.

However, there have been no tests involving close contact with tannic acid for long periods of time and it is just possible that residues left in a carpet could act as an irritant to the skin of a baby or toddler playing there

dust mite as well. You should try to reduce the damp coming into the house, *and* the moisture being generated indoors. However, measures aimed solely at reducing condensation on walls and windows are not relevant to controlling house-dust mite.

Taking further steps

Reducing night-time exposure to dust-mite allergens is enough for many people. We spend an average of eight hours a day in bed, far longer than in any other single place, which makes the bed a happy hunting ground for the mite, since we shed a lot of skin while sleeping. Being in bed also gives us a prolonged exposure to the plentiful mite allergens found there. By reducing the allergen load experienced at night, many people reduce the sensitivity of their nose or bronchi, which makes them less likely to suffer symptoms at other times.

regularly, especially if that child has sensitive skin.

Tannic acid can be used on carpets, mattresses and all upholstery, and the formulations that are sold are said not to stain fabrics. Other allergens will also be denatured, so tannic acid could be helpful for those allergic to pets, if the pet is still in the house. (However, if the allergen exists as very small airborne particles, the tannic acid sprayed on to surfaces will have limited usefulness.) The treatment needs to be repeated every three to four months. Suppliers and approximate costs are given on p310.

Note that tannic acid is *not* an acaricide – it does not kill the mites. However, it destroys the reservoir of mite allergens. Although these build up again with new mite droppings, it apparently takes at least three months for the allergens to reach the sort of levels that generally cause symptoms.

If you are reluctant to use acaricides (see p309), and cannot afford liquid nitrogen treatment (see p310) or a powerful dehumidifier that will kill mites (see p306), then tannic acid may be a good option for carpets and furniture. Unlike bedding, this cannot be dealt with using microporous covers.

If symptoms are still experienced after dealing with the mattress and bedding, then you should turn your attentions to the rest of the bedroom, particularly the carpet, if there is one. Mites in a fitted carpet can rapidly re-colonize the bedding, and if there are enough of them, they could undermine your efforts at keeping the bedding mite-free.

The major problem with carpets is that dust mites cling to the fibres for dear life, using eight tiny suckers, one at the end of each leg. When a vacuum cleaner zooms overhead, a few of the mites may be caught unawares and sucked up into the mouth of the roaring monster, but most hang on to the fibres around them and live to fight another day. A research team found that, even if a carpet was vacuumed thoroughly three times in quick succession, 65 per cent of its mites still remained. Where vacuuming *is* effective is in removing the mites' droppings, but since each mite produces about twenty faecal pellets a day, the surviving mites soon replenish this source of allergen.

There are three things that can be done about this problem. One is to use an acaricide or liquid nitrogen treatment to kill the mites, before you follow up with vacuuming. The second is to banish fitted carpets and have rugs. The third is to use a dehumidifier to kill the mites (see p306).

If you choose the first option, the acaricide treatment needs to be repeated every six months at least. Some manufacturers recommend that it be done every two months, while others specify three-monthly or four-monthly intervals. Obviously you need to think about the safety aspect, particularly if there are small children playing on the carpets. Some experts believe there is very little risk from these sprays, while others are more cautious. If you decide on a spray, the allergy sufferer should stay out of the house while it is being carried out and for some hours afterwards (see p309). So should any children, whether they have allergies or not.

Liquid nitrogen has no safety risk, since it simply produces nitrogen gas, which is the major component of the air we breathe. Tests have shown that it does not damage carpets or upholstery in any way. As it is extremely cold, it has to be handled carefully, so these treatments are only carried out by trained personnel. They will treat a whole room at a time, or a whole house if you prefer. If the whole house is treated, you can assume that the dust-mite population has been eliminated, but you are not free of them for ever, unfortunately. Dust mites also live in clothing, particularly overcoats and old sweaters, so they will be reintroduced by people coming into the house. The liquid nitrogen treatment therefore needs repeating every six months.

With either of these treatments, thorough vacuuming afterwards is very important, otherwise the allergens will remain in the carpet. (After the treatment the dead mites are much more easily vacuumed up, as they can no longer cling to fibres.) You may need to invest in a new vacuum cleaner, one that retains all the dust mites and their droppings within its bag (see box article on p185), or at least add filters to your existing cleaner. Make sure every room is vacuumed fully, including areas behind the furniture and under the bed. In the case of liquid nitrogen treatments, thorough vacuuming is done for you as part of the service.

Carpets with a very deep pile are likely to prove resistant to acaricide treatment, because the spray will not penetrate right down into the carpet. With liquid nitrogen, you should ask the advice of the supplier about deep-pile carpets.

If you are choosing new carpets, those with short pile are preferable, and synthetic fabrics are best. The synthetic fabric has a slight electrostatic charge which helps to hold the mite droppings within the carpet, so that fewer become airborne. A more radical solution is to get rid of fitted carpets entirely, and for those with severe dust-mite this may be the only solution.

VACUUM CLEANERS

Most ordinary vacuum cleaners have tiny pores in the bag that are large enough to let the fragments of dust-mite droppings escape — so, as you vacuum up dust, many of the allergenic particles are spewed out again through the bag, leaving the vacuum cleaner via the exhaust. This can actually *increase* the amount of dust-mite allergen in the air.

Special vacuum cleaners, designed for those with dust-mite allergy, are now available (for suppliers and approximate prices see p308). These use better bags, which help retain the particles, backed up by a high-quality filter that cleans the exhaust gas before it leaves the machine. Their suction power is generally higher than an ordinary vacuum cleaner, so they pick up more dust. One model can be fitted with a dust-detection device to show that an area of carpet has been vacuumed fully and all dust removed.

If you suffer symptoms during or after vacuum cleaning (the particles could take several hours to settle from the air), one of these vacuum cleaners could be the answer. A new and cheaper alternative is to fit a pad of filter material to your existing vacuum cleaner (see p308). This will not give quite such good results, but may be sufficient for your needs.

Someone who suffers from dust-mite allergy should not change the bag on a vacuum cleaner, even on one of these specialized models, as the potential for spillage of dust, and high exposure to allergens, is always there. If this is absolutely unavoidable, wear a high-grade face mask (see p295).

The great advantage of rugs is that they can be hung up outside, beaten to remove dust, and then left in the sun. This purges dust mites far more effectively than any amount of vacuum cleaning. Try to give all the rugs this treatment once a week. If buying rugs, avoid those with foam backing or a thick pile.

The floor itself can be wooden boards, vinyl flooring, cork tiles or linoleum. Cork tiles are the warmest to the feet, and sealed cork tiles, with a thin coat of vinyl on them, are now available and easily kept clean. Whatever the surface, it should be vacuum cleaned regularly to remove dust mites from the crevices. On a bare floor, vacuum cleaning removes about 80 per cent of the mites.

Dust in the living room

If reducing your exposure to mite allergens in the bedroom has only helped a little, you should tackle the carpet and upholstery in the living room.

Armchairs and sofas should be vacuumed, especially the areas where the arms and head normally rest. This treatment, like the thorough vacuuming of the carpet, should be repeated weekly.

Those who are still suffering symptoms may need to treat the carpet with acaricide or liquid nitrogen (see p179) followed by thorough vacuuming. Again, this may not work well for deep-pile carpets. A very elderly sofa or armchair can also prove resistant to treatment sometimes. The living mites may be killed, but there are seemingly inexhaustible reserves of allergen within the upholstery, and each new treatment simply releases more of them. In this case, new furniture, or regular treatment with tannic acid (see p182), may be the only options.

Having taken care of the carpet and upholstery, you may need a general 'spring clean'. Needless to say, the person doing the cleaning becomes exposed to a higher level of dust while at work, so it is preferable if the allergy sufferer goes out for the day and someone else does the work. Paying someone to clean the house may be worthwhile, but make sure it is understood that the work needs to be done very thoroughly. If the cleaning has to be done by the allergic person, the mouth and nose can be protected with a dust mask (see p296 for the type of mask needed). Another useful tip is to use a damp cloth when dusting, to minimize the amount of dust going into the air, rinsing the cloth out in water at intervals. (To prevent staining of polished wood, rub all the moisture off immediately with a clean, dry cloth.) Even if someone else does the cleaning, damp dusting is a worthwhile measure. There are now special dusters for sale that retain the dust by an electrostatic charge, so that very little becomes airborne (see p309).

The dust from picture rails, architraves and door tops should all be included in this spring clean, and again, a damp cloth should be used. Long-handled feather dusters are obviously out, because they simply scatter the dust around in the air. A vacuum cleaner with dusting attachments can be useful, and the special models designed for allergy sufferers have these (see p308).

Relatively few people will need to go beyond these measures, but for the unfortunate sufferers who are ultrasensitive to dust mite, it may be necessary to treat all fabrics with acaricide or liquid nitrogen. Alternatively, remove as many fabrics as possible. This means doing without curtains where possible, or choosing thin, smooth materials. Textured materials, or those with a pile, such as velvet, can harbour dust. All curtains should be washed every month or two. Any fabric items in the bedroom should be removed unless really essential. Hang clothes elsewhere if possible, and remove soft toys, dressing gowns, armchairs and cushions. Overcoats and sweaters should be dry cleaned or washed, as these can contain many mites. There is a special test kit available, which will show you how well these control measures are working (see p310).

As a last resort, you could move to a new house! Old houses, particularly if they are damp, are absolutely infested with house-dust mites. A newly built house, or one that has been stripped and thoroughly refurbished, is largely free of mites, and it takes about five years for the numbers to reach their normal level. Timber treatment for woodworm is likely to kill dust mites as well, if it uses **permethrin** or **pyrethroids** (see p180).

Pros and cons of mite control

One of the drawbacks to controlling mites in the home, apart from the effort and expense involved, is that allergy sufferers may become preoccupied with the problem of house-dust mite, and may become 'prisoners in their own home', feeling unable to venture into other people's houses for fear of the hordes of mites lurking there. This fear is largely unfounded, because reducing your exposure at home will mean that your nose (and your bronchi if you have asthma) are not being constantly irritated by an allergic reaction. They are in far better condition generally, and not likely to be upset by a brief dose of dust in someone else's home. (Sleeping on an old and untreated mattress in someone else's house is a slightly different matter, however.)

Before you begin, consider the other options. If you simply have rhinitis, you could well use drugs to control the symptoms, or some form of desensitization. The information about anti-allergy drugs, given in Chapter Seven, and desensitization, in Chapter Nine, is as relevant to house-dust mite as it is to pollen. Understanding the other options fully can help you to decide on the best way of tackling your allergy. For those who have asthma, and are allergic to dust-mite droppings, some form of mite control is considered sensible.

Most people eventually find a mixture of treatments that is right for them. A sensible, balanced approach is to reduce dust exposure in bed by using mattress and pillow covers, and then to reduce exposure in other parts of the home as much as possible without excessive fuss. This minimizes the basic level of sensitization in the nose or bronchi, and drugs or desensitization can then be employed to control any remaining symptoms.

To some extent, the decision taken will be influenced by the severity of the symptoms. In this respect, asthma should always be taken more seriously than rhinitis, because the bronchi, once sensitized, can become increasingly reactive to both allergens and irritants, and sometimes to emotional stress. An asthma attack is alarming, especially for small children, and asthma can prevent children from getting enough exercise, or developing a healthy independence as they grow up. All in all, any cleaning measures in the home that can prevent a child's asthma from getting worse are probably worth taking. (Bear in mind that irritants such as tobacco smoke also need to be eliminated.)

Mite avoidance for babies and toddlers

For babies and small children, avoiding dust-mite allergens is basically a similar process, but with some changes in emphasis. An infant's mattress is probably sealed or coated with plastic anyway, to guard against bed-wetting, so the mattress is unlikely to be a major source of allergens. Pillows and bedding do need to be kept mite-free however, and microporous covers (see p178) are recommended. New bedding for a new baby is a good idea, unless you can thoroughly clean the old bedding before putting on the microporous covers. Any bedding that cannot be covered with allergen-proof covers, nor washed regularly at 60°C, should be avoided.

There should be much more emphasis on carpets – babies and toddlers spend a lot of time at floor level, after all, and are close enough to breathe the allergens that they stir up while playing or crawling about.

Some quite difficult choices need to be made here. If you abandon fitted carpets and opt for rugs (see pp185–6), the level of dust mite will be greatly reduced but your child will have fairly cold hard floors to crawl and toddle about on. Cork tiles are one solution to this, or old-fashioned linoleum, both of which are fairly warm to the touch. Looking on the positive side, children brought up on a carpet-less floor from birth will probably not know what they are missing, and develop into hardy little individuals who won't mind the cold in future!

If you cannot countenance this option, you could cover the floor extensively with rugs, but have a smooth, bare surface underneath. The drawback with this option is that it creates a lot of housework, as the rugs need regular airing and beating outside to keep them mite-free. In a country with an unpredictable climate such as Britain, passing showers will make life doubly difficult. However, if you have a tumble-drier, where the airing process can be carried out artificially, a large number of rugs (made of a heat-resistant fabric such as cotton) may be a practical proposition.

Another possibility is to stick with fitted carpets and spray them with acaricides (see p184) or substances that denature the mite allergens (see p182) – but then there is the slight worry of health risks to the child from the sprays, since there will be plenty of contact with the sprayed area. No *long-term* tests have been carried out to show that these sprays are absolutely safe, although the substances used are of very low toxicity and the risks are probably negligible.

Fortunately, there are several answers to this problem that can banish mites from fitted carpets with no risk of toxicity. The first, and simplest, is to increase the ventilation in the home by opening the windows every day so that moisture levels fall. Alternatively, you could use a dehumidifier to reduce moisture levels. If such measures are not effective, you could treat the carpet with liquid nitrogen to kill the mites (see p179). Another possibility is to use a special high-powered dehumidifier that can get the air in a room so dry as to kill most of the mites (see p306). This device is designed to be used when the room is unoccupied, and could be left on at night in the living room. As with other treatments that kill mites, you must follow up with intensive vacuum cleaning to remove the dead mites and their droppings. With regular use of the powerful dehumidifier, the overall number of mites should steadily decline, so vacuum cleaning will not be needed as often. This particular device also includes an air filter.

Special measures may be needed for the teddy bear or favourite soft toy, as it is difficult to part a child from this source of comfort, even if it *is* home to a million mites! The best solution is to give the soft toy a 'holiday' once a week, which it spends wrapped in a plastic bag in the freezer. Twenty-four hours of this treatment knocks the mite population back considerably, although it does not kill all of them. Shorter sessions will be less effective but are still worthwhile. At the outset, it is advisable to wash the toy to remove the dust-mite allergens, then to dry it as quickly as possible, preferably in a tumble-drier. (Be sure, first, that the eyes of the toy are not made from the kind of plastic that melts easily.) Two days on the washing line in bright sun should follow. This treatment will reduce the mites to a fairly low level, and weekly sessions in the freezer should then keep the problem under control. If you have a tumble-drier at home, you can follow the weekly freezer session by a hot spin for forty-five minutes, which will demoralize the mites even further.

Bunk beds are not a good idea for children who may be prone to allergy – the child in the lower bed has dust-mite allergens showered on them from above, doubling their nightly dose. If you already have bunk beds, and only one child with dust-mite allergy, he or she should sleep in the top bunk. However, both mattresses should have special allergen-proof covers to protect the other child from developing the same sensitivity. In general, where children share a bedroom, it is a good idea to treat all the mattresses in the room, not just the one belonging to the allergic child.

WHAT DUST MITES LIKE

There is a great deal of information and advice on dust-mite control now available. A lot of it comes from companies selling mite-control products, and while most of the information is excellent, some is contradictory or confusing. In particular, you are likely to read conflicting statements about the sort of temperature conditions dust mites like best. This is because their reaction to temperature conditions is quite complex. The story is roughly as follows.

What dust mites like best is a high temperature, 25–30°C (77–86°F), and very moist air with a relative humidity of 75–80 per cent. (This means that the air is holding 75–80 per cent of the maximum amount of water vapour it could hold at that temperature.) This is a high moisture level, unlikely to be encountered in a well-ventilated house, except for brief periods. However, levels of 70 per cent are found in many modern homes where draught-proofing has been ruthlessly applied and ventilation reduced to a minimum.

At high temperatures (30°C or 86°F), the lowest relative humidity a dust mite can tolerate is about 65 per cent, which is commonplace in modern energy-saving houses. The humidity can also reach these levels quite easily in a mattress that is not aired regularly, and in a pillow, as this receives moisture directly every night

Are air filters or ionizers useful for dust-mite allergy?

Air filters and air ionizers will remove particles from the air. Details of the different kinds and how they work are given on pp298–302.

Whether they are of any use to those who are allergic to house-dust mite is debatable. They are certainly not recommended as a first step in reducing your exposure to dust-mite allergens, because the main sources of allergens are likely to be your mattress, your pillow or your armchair. You have such intimate contact with these items that you are inhaling the allergens 'at source' and an air filter will make little difference. (The exception here are some special filters fitted to the headboard of a bed which provide a stream of filtered air over the sleeper's face. These work quite well, but are not widely from the sleeper's breath. Given these high temperatures and moist air, the dust mite thrives. Warmth makes all its life-processes speed up – it lays more eggs, eats more food and produces more droppings, which is bad news for anyone allergic to the little beast.

However, if the humidity is not allowed to build up in the house, high temperatures will produce dry air, and this can kill off many mites. Very dry air kills them directly, while moderate dryness keeps mould growth down, making the skin particles on which the mites feed tough and rather indigestible. This keeps the mite population at a fairly low level.

At cool temperatures, such as 15°C or 59°F, the dust mite can tolerate much drier conditions. A relative humidity of 45 per cent (which is considered fairly low for a house, and is the target for a standard dehumidifier) is tolerated well. Because the temperature is lower, the mites do not breed as fast, but they still produce a fair number of young. Each mite lives much longer, which partially offsets the lower breeding rate. Consequently, a cold empty room will have quite plentiful house-dust mites, while a holiday home that is left empty and unheated during the winter months will be developing a steadily growing population. This can precipitate a severe attack of rhinitis or asthma in a susceptible person at the start of a holiday.

sold now, as encasing the mattress in an allergen-proof cover is a much cheaper alternative.) There is no point in trying an air filter if you have not:

- put the mattress and pillow in microporous covers (see p178)

- washed the other bedding regularly, or put it into microporous covers (see pp180–81)

- aired the bed, and the bedroom, regularly

- dusted with a damp cloth, rather than a dry one, for at least the past two weeks

- fitted a disposable filter to your vacuum cleaner, so that allergens do not become airborne during vacuum cleaning

The first three measures will reduce the amount of allergen being breathed 'at source'. The last two will reduce the amount of allergen being made airborne by housework.

While there may still be plenty of allergen left lurking in your carpets and elsewhere, this will not create problems unless it actually becomes airborne in sufficient quantities. Allergens being generated at floor level by dust mites do not become airborne all that easily. In a quiet household, without much activity and air movement, the allergen will probably remain where it is, in which case an air filter will not serve much purpose.

If you have taken the five measures listed above, and are reluctant to make further changes to the bedroom (e.g. spraying the carpet with acaricide or tannic acid, or removing the carpeting altogether) yet you still suffer symptoms at night or first thing in the morning, then a filter might be worth trying. Several firms will hire out air filters, or let you have them on approval, so you can see if they help you or not. Suppliers and approximate prices are given on p302.

In the living room, before considering an air filter, at least try:

- vacuum cleaning the upholstered furniture

- wet dusting for a minimum of two weeks

- fitting a filter to the vacuum cleaner

You might also try spraying cushions and upholstered furniture with tannic acid (see p182) as a way of rendering these sources harmless. If there are still symptoms when you are in the living room, and you are unable to make further changes, then an air filter might be useful.

Only HEPA filters (see p298) have been shown to have any beneficial effects for people with house-dust mite allergy. Tests have shown no benefits from air ionizers, and in one study there was actually an increase in nocturnal coughing among asthma sufferers using ionizers, perhaps due to ozone (see p304).

MOULD SPORES

Moulds are familiar to us as the furry covering that develops on old fruit and vegetables, or the green dust on last week's bread. Moulds belong to the group of living things called fungi, which also includes mushrooms, toadstools and puffballs. Fungi are neither plant nor animal, but a distinct lifeform. (It used to be thought that they were descended from plants, but this is not the case.)

Fungi cannot make food for themselves, as plants can, so they feed on other living things, usually ones that are already dead (although some fungi are parasites and attack living things). In the wild, fungi colonize the discarded leaves of trees and plants, over-ripe fruit, or the wood of dead trees. In your fridge, moulds are simply living out the same sort of lifestyle, digesting forgotten bits of food, just as they would digest fallen leaves and berries in a forest.

But how did the moulds get into your fridge in the first place? The answer is that they went in as spores, minute specks, visible only with a microscope, that can each grow into a new mould. Those spores are on the surface of every fruit and vegetable we buy, and on most other things as well. *There are more mould spores in the air than anything else.* The record count in Britain is over 160,000 per cubic metre of air, whereas the record pollen count is only 2,800 per cubic metre. Fortunately, mould spores are not particularly allergenic.

A spore is to a fungus what a seed is to a plant, but very much smaller. To maximize the chance of some spores reaching a favourable spot, moulds produce millions upon millions of them. Most come to nothing, but a few hit the jackpot and land on a spot where they can grow into an adult mould which then produces spores itself. Like pollen, mould spores are very light, so they disperse easily and remain airborne for a long time.

There are many different species of mould, each feeding in a different way. Some can make do on the most meagre diet, scraping a living on damp paintwork or glass, or the rubber seal on a refrigerator door. You may wonder what food supply these moulds can possibly have, and the answer is that the abundant food found in 'fresh air', as described at the beginning of this chapter, is keeping them alive. Ironically, the proteins released by pollen grains when they land on a damp surface (see p10) may be an important part of the diet for these moulds. (Wallpaper paste on a damp wall is an absolute bonanza for them, and it usually contains fungicides to prevent mould growth.)

Fungi can also feed on wood, and those well-known pests, dry rot and wet rot, if they have infested the timbers of a house, can both produce spores. While not everyone who is mould-sensitive will react to them, some will.

Detecting mould-spore allergy

An allergy to mould spores can produce symptoms all year round, especially in a damp house, but most sufferers find that their symptoms are seasonal, occurring mainly in the late summer, autumn and early winter. In temperate climates, this is when the air is damp and there is plenty of food available in the form of rotting fruit and vegetation – 'mists and mellow fruitfulness' are exactly what moulds like best. The release of spores is generally timed to coincide with this most fungus-friendly season of the year.

Some mould spores are present in the air all year round, however, such as those of the blue-green *Penicillium* mould, often seen on bread and oranges. One mould, *Cladosporium herbarum*, begins spore production in June in Britain, and can roughly coincide with the grass pollen season. Allergy to this mould can easily be mistaken for hayfever (see p220). If there is doubt, a skin-prick test (see p78) should reveal whether pollen or mould spores are the culprit.

In the case of moulds, however, the skin-prick test is unlikely to include all the possible mould allergens. Over twenty different moulds are known to produce allergic reactions in Britain alone, and there are probably many more worldwide. The allergic person may be sensitive to several different moulds, or just to one, and if that one is not included in the extract used for the skin-prick test, no reaction will occur, even though the person is sensitive to some mould spores. This will not happen often, but it is a possibility.

Fortunately, mould allergy can usually be identified by the circumstances in which symptoms arise, or in which they get worse. Compost heaps are alive with moulds, and handling compost, leaf mould or fallen leaves may well bring on symptoms. Glasshouses, conservatories, basements and cellars (moulds do not need any light), old damp houses, churches and church halls are often full of spores. Damp straw or hay breeds moulds, as do grass clippings if not collected up. In the latter case, mowing the lawn again will stir up the moulds on the old clippings and release a cloud of spores, so this may be the moment when symptoms arise. (However, a reaction on mowing the lawn can also indicate grass pollen allergy, see p25.) Potted plants and bowls of pot-pourri around the house may be breeding moulds, and so may humidifiers and air-conditioning systems, which then pump the spores out into the air. Moulds that have been in a cold situation and then experience warm air are likely to release their spores suddenly, which is why Christmas trees often provoke symptoms – there are microscopic moulds on their needles. Installing central heating in an old house can have a similar effect, warming up the moulds and causing a major release of spores.

In the countryside, damp areas near rivers or lakes are likely to be rich in moulds, and symptoms may begin when camping in such places. Forests in autumn, or orchards that are carpeted with rotting fruit, are also likely spots. In late summer, fields of cereals or oil-seed rape can become infested with moulds just before harvest time, and this can cause symptoms in those living nearby, or out on a walk. Any crop that goes mouldy in the field can have the same effect. Mould spores are plentiful after the first frost of autumn, when they are released in large numbers by moulds in the soil. Damp weather and ground fog will promote fungal growth, although rain itself will wash the spores out of the air.

Dealing with mould spores
Avoiding situations where moulds abound (see above) is an obvious first step. Persuade someone else to rake up the fallen leaves, spread the compost, and cut the dead leaves from garden plants. The number of mould spores in the air is sometimes given along with the pollen count (see p127), mainly by telephone information services (see p316). If you are severely affected, you may wish to stay indoors on days with high spore counts.

Be very careful about where you choose to live, avoiding anywhere damp. Have a survey done before buying a house, to ensure that there is no dry rot or wet rot. If there is, have the problem thoroughly treated, and stay completely clear of the house until the renovation work is completed: huge numbers of spores will be released when old timbers or partitions are removed, or floors pulled up. Spores are small and may take many hours to settle from the air (see p202). It is probably wise to steer clear of any old house where extensive structural work is going on.

KEEPING DAMP OUT OF THE HOUSE
Should the house you live in already be damp, there are various steps you can take to remedy this. If the house is old, and built of stone or brick, it may have no damp-proof course: this is a horizontal waterproof layer, near ground level, which prevents moisture from soaking up into the walls from the soil. Houses built before about 1920 generally did not have a damp-proof course, but one can now be created, even in an old building, by drilling a row of small holes in all the outside walls, just above ground level, and injecting a silicon compound which hardens to form a waterproof layer within the wall. This acts as a barrier to 'rising damp', and is not particularly expensive.

A thin, invisible layer of silicon can also be sprayed on to the outside of the walls, to prevent rainwater coming directly through them. This may be

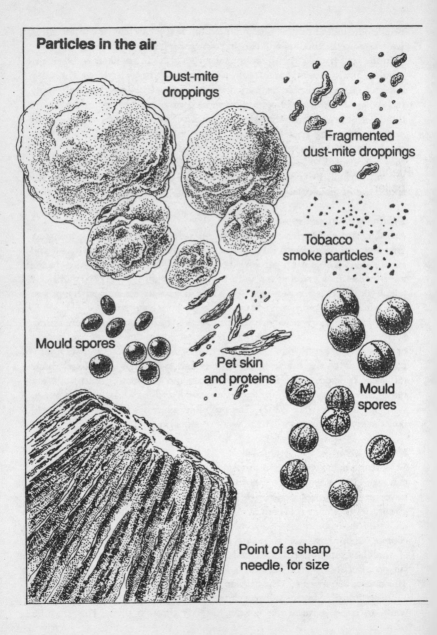

Particles in the air

Dust-mite droppings

Fragmented dust-mite droppings

Tobacco smoke particles

Mould spores

Pet skin and proteins

Mould spores

Point of a sharp needle, for size

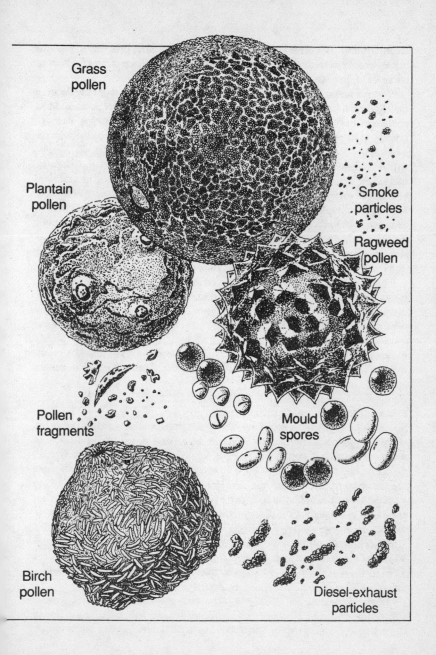

Grass pollen

Plantain pollen

Smoke particles

Ragweed pollen

Pollen fragments

Mould spores

Birch pollen

Diesel-exhaust particles

useful around the corners of windows, where rain often penetrates, but it is not advisable to treat whole walls in this way. The advice of an architect or surveyor should always be sought.

Within a house, if water is seeping up from the ground through the floors, a new floor can be laid with a layer of waterproof material incorporated. Most roofs now have a layer of waterproof 'sarking felt' under their tiles, slates or boards, but some older buildings may lack this. It can be a useful addition in making the house more watertight.

If these remedies are too expensive or troublesome, then damp must be tackled in some other way. Any damp spot should be kept warm and well ventilated, using electric space-heaters, which are cheap to run. Fan-heaters are not recommended as they churn up any mould spores in the vicinity. Silica crystals, which absorb water vapour and are then dried out in the oven for reuse, may prove helpful in a damp cupboard where heating is impossible. Dehumidifiers (see p306) are another possibility, and air-conditioning units will also reduce the moisture in the air.

If you live in rented accommodation, and there is a serious damp problem, it may be possible to force your landlord to put the problem right. In a recent court case in Britain, damages were awarded to a small boy with asthma who had lived in a damp home since birth. It was decided that the local council, who owned the property, were partially responsible for the child's ill-health by not carrying out necessary damp-proofing. This case has established a legal precedent, which could prove useful to other families in rented accommodation.

Reducing moisture production indoors

So much for moisture coming into the house from outside – that is only part of the story. Human activities within the house also generate a great deal of moisture. Steaming kettles, potatoes boiling on the stove, clothes drying in the bathroom, a hot shower or bath, liberally watered house plants – all these are pumping moisture into the air. In addition, the average human being gives off about 1 litre (2 pints) of water in sweat every night, and more during the day. A family of four is estimated to produce 10–20 litres (18–36 pints) of water vapour every twenty-four hours.

The problem will become visible as condensation, which occurs because warm air can carry far more water vapour than cold air. The water vapour is a gas in the warm air, but as soon as the air cools it turns to water again – fine droplets of water that we see as 'steam'.

The major part of the solution is to reduce the amount of water vapour going into the air, by switching off the kettle as soon as it boils, using lids to cover pans of vegetables or other boiling liquids, and having baths rather than showers. Do not dry clothes indoors unless there is no alternative. If you can, get a tumble-drier or clothes-drying cabinet, making sure that the exhaust is vented outdoors.

Whenever the air is dry outside (hot and dry preferably, but cold and dry will do), give the house an airing. Open several windows and get a draught through. It is the lack of ventilation that creates much of the dampness in modern homes. By airing the house regularly (preferably every day) you will give the moisture a chance to escape.

Ventilation is particularly important in a newly built house, or one that has been renovated. A huge amount of water, up to 1,360 litres (300 gallons), is used in construction, mainly for plastering. This takes at least *nine to twelve months* to evaporate under normal conditions. A dehumidifier may be worthwhile during this period, especially if there is a lot of wet weather, and some high-capacity models are available for this specific purpose (see p306 for suppliers). Beware of speeding up the process too much (e.g. by overheating the house) as this can cause plaster and concrete to crack, or timber to warp.

Fighting condensation

The other part of the solution, if you are sensitive to moulds, is to combat condensation, because wherever there is condensation on a surface, moulds will flourish. Condensation forms on any surface that is colder than the air around it, particularly cold windowpanes or cool walls in bathrooms and kitchens.

To combat condensation, you must remove temperature variations in the house as far as possible, keeping it warm throughout. Metal window-frames, which are always cold, create a lot of condensation and should be replaced by wooden or PVC frames if at all possible. Double glazing is also helpful, as it makes the inner surface of windows warmer. Mop up any condensation that does occur on windowsills every day. Watch for black mould growth and remove it promptly if it appears.

Heat all parts of the house well, and do not leave any rooms permanently cold or unventilated. Check in cupboards and behind furniture for any damp spots. Loft insulation will help to keep ceilings warm.

Where some condensation is inevitable, as in bathrooms and kitchens, never make the walls or ceiling impermeable with vinyl wallpaper or gloss or eggshell paint. This will trap the condensation so that it runs down to the base of the wall, creating a wet area where moulds will flourish. A permeable wall (one coated with ordinary wallpaper or emulsion paint) can absorb a certain amount of water and gradually 'breathe it out' again, either to the outside air, or back indoors again. Sometimes, for those with a serious mould problem, fitting an extractor fan in the kitchen or bathroom is the only way to reduce condensation effectively.

Combating moulds

Having kept moisture out, and reduced condensation within, the third step in the programme is to combat moulds directly. Any fabric or furniture that smells of mould or mildew must go. Although they may now be 'bone dry', that smell is indicative of old mould spores, millions of them, lingering within the article.

Clean the rubber seals around fridges and freezers with great care, going into all the crevices to get out the black mould that lives there. This process needs to be repeated regularly, and should be done by someone other than the allergy sufferer, as exposure to spores will be high during the cleaning process. Shower curtains should be replaced entirely, or thoroughly washed. If there is black mould on walls or window-frames, it can be cleaned off with white spirit, which removes it without making the wall damp, and thus delays its regrowth. Alternatively, use a mixture of one part bleach to four parts of water, with a little washing-up liquid added. Never brush off mould growth, or tackle it with a dry cloth, as this simply disperses the spores into the air. Sprays are available to help control mould growth (see p310).

House plants should be reduced to a bare minimum, and any that need to be wet all the time should definitely go. Learn to love cactuses if you can. The plants that remain should have their dead leaves and flowers removed regularly, and the top layer of the soil should also be scooped off occasionally and replaced.

Eat bread, potatoes, vegetables and fruit promptly and do not leave ripe fruit about for long.

There may be a lot of mould spores in house dust, especially in an old house, or one that has been damp in the past. Anyone who is allergic to the spores should not have to dust, vacuum clean, sweep floors or make beds. Wear a mask (see p295) if this sort of housework is unavoidable.

Air filters and mould spores

There have been no actual tests on the usefulness of air filters for mould spore allergy. However, common sense suggests that they may be valuable in this context. Many mould spores are very small, and this means that they stay suspended in the air for several hours, rather than settling rapidly (see p202). An air filter that is adequate for the size of the room (see p300) should reduce the number of mould spores significantly. But you need also to substantially reduce any mould growth in the house.

Saying goodbye to your humidifier . . .

The idea that central heating makes the air very dry, and that this irritates the nose and airways, is a popular one. Many people have bought humidifiers in an attempt to combat this supposed problem. In most cases, a humidifier is the last thing they need, since dry air is not the actual problem unless the heating is turned up high and the ventilation in the house is particularly good. The air in most modern homes is actually far too moist (see p175) and this has led to the upsurge in asthma (due to dust mite and mould spores) that all developed countries have seen in the past twenty years. Humidifiers add to the moisture in the air and, to make matters worse, can provide ideal breeding grounds for moulds.

Scientific tests in which the humidity of the air was gradually decreased from 70 per cent to 10 per cent (a very low level) showed that people felt no ill-effects, except for noticing a slight dryness in the mouth at the lowest levels. In another test, patients inhaled very dry air (only 9 per cent relative humidity) for over three days and nights. There were no changes in the membranes of the nose, or the amount of mucus they produced.

If your nose feels uncomfortable when at home, try simply turning the thermostat down and putting on a sweater – it may be the heat that is affecting you. Another possibility is that 'indoor pollution' is to blame. The scientific tests with dry air described above were carried out with very clean air, and it is conceivable that warm dry air *does* affect the nose if it is also polluted.

Most of us are subjected to far worse levels of pollution indoors than out (see p215), and reducing this is often remarkably easy. If your discomfort seems to be connected with having the heating on, it is possible that the radiators are very dusty and that the dust is burning off, producing irritants in the air. Clean the radiators thoroughly, and keep them covered with a piece of sheeting or other fabric during the summer months, to prevent dust accumulation.

PETS AND OTHER ANIMALS

Pets are a frequent, and sometimes unsuspected, source of rhinitis. They can also cause asthma and eczema. For people who are highly sensitive, small amounts of allergen carried on the clothing of pet-owners may be enough to spark off symptoms. In such cases, desensitization treatment (see Chapter Nine) may be the only solution. People with an allergic disposition who work with animals, such as vets, farmers, jockeys, animal breeders and laboratory workers, are highly susceptible to developing allergic reactions. Again, desensitization treatment may be an option, but some find that they have to change their job because the symptoms cannot be controlled.

PARTICLE SIZES

The size of a particle makes an enormous difference to its role in causing allergies. Size affects how quickly particles settle, for example, and how easily they become airborne.

Particles larger than 40 microns (40 thousandths of a millimetre) settle from the air rapidly, so there are very few in the air that we breathe. (Pine pollen is an exception here, as it has air sacs that make it more buoyant, despite its large size.) If particles are not airborne in any great number, they are unlikely to cause allergies because too few are inhaled.

Particles of 30 microns, such as grass pollen grains, also settle relatively rapidly in still air (e.g. inside a house with doors and windows closed). But they are released from the grass plant when warm air currents will carry them skywards, and rising air often takes them high into the atmosphere, to rain down on the earth later. So there are plenty available to be inhaled.

Particles of 20 microns, such as ragweed pollen grains, take a little longer to settle, but in still air even they can fall 3 metres (10 feet) in just four minutes. An average room will be clear of the pollen in this time. However, if there are tiny fragments of pollen in the air (see p23) these will take longer to settle.

At the lower end of the scale, settling times increase dramatically. For a particle 2 microns in diameter (which includes some mould spores, cat allergen particles, the smallest fragments of dust-mite droppings, and some pollen fragments) it takes a full six *hours* to drop 3 metres (10 feet). This means that the allergen load in a room with still air is unlikely to settle out except overnight. The particles may begin to settle in the daytime, but before

Cats

'Such clean animals,' people say as they watch a cat carefully licking itself. Little do they know that this feline obsession with cleanliness fills the air with microscopic specks of dried saliva. The saliva contains a protein that is the main allergen for those affected by cats. It is absolutely everywhere in a house that has a cat, forming a coating on the walls, windows and furniture, and staying airborne for hours.

they do so the air is disturbed again.

With small allergen particles that are actively propelled into the indoor air (such as mould spores or cat saliva particles), this slowness in settling means that the air is unlikely to be free of the particles for long. However, good ventilation will rapidly blow these tiny particles out of the house, so they only build up to problematic levels in houses with extensive draught-proofing.

Small allergen particles that are not actively propelled into the air are less of a problem. Thus, the fragmented droppings of dust mites that are generated by mites in a carpet tend to stay at or near floor level, unless actively dispersed (by a standard vacuum cleaner, for example). However, a small child, whose nose is a lot closer to the ground, may be inhaling air containing far more of these allergenic fragments.

Particle size also determines how far the allergens penetrate the airways. Larger particles, when inhaled, are caught by the hairs and mucus in the nose, or by mucus in the windpipe, and do not reach the bronchi. This is the case for any particle bigger than 10 microns, although there is a reflex reaction (see p21) which can produce narrowing of the bronchi when large allergenic particles land in the nose.

Particles of between 4 and 10 microns can reach the bronchi and may provoke an asthma attack directly. Only those smaller than 4 microns are likely to go beyond the bronchi, into the lung itself. Here they can accumulate and eventually cause a more serious disease called **extrinsic allergic alveolitis** (see p211).

The ubiquitous presence of the cat allergen means that people with an allergy to cats are usually well aware of it – their symptoms tend to appear promptly when they enter a house with a cat. The fact that cats are more likely to provoke allergies than dogs may also be explained by the constant presence of salivary proteins in the air.

Cat salivary protein can be found in houses where no cat has lived for many years, and occasionally there are traces of it in houses that have never

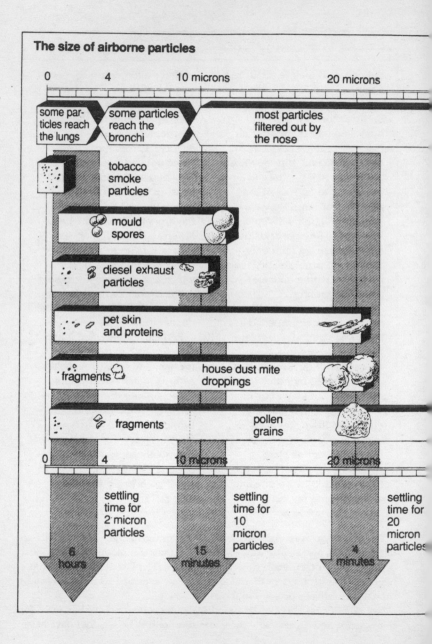

The size of airborne particles

some particles reach the lungs

some particles reach the bronchi

most particles filtered out by the nose

tobacco smoke particles

mould spores

diesel exhaust particles

pet skin and proteins

fragments — house dust mite droppings

fragments — pollen grains

settling time for 2 micron particles — 8 hours

settling time for 10 micron particles — 15 minutes

settling time for 20 micron particles — 4 minutes

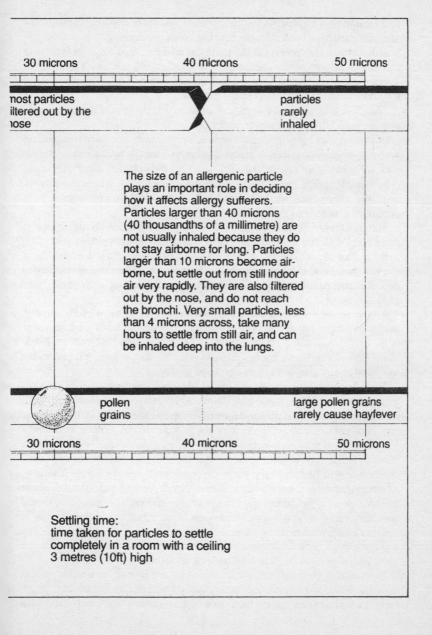

30 microns   40 microns   50 microns

most particles
filtered out by the
nose

particles
rarely
inhaled

The size of an allergenic particle
plays an important role in deciding
how it affects allergy sufferers.
Particles larger than 40 microns
(40 thousandths of a millimetre) are
not usually inhaled because they do
not stay airborne for long. Particles
larger than 10 microns become airborne, but settle out from still indoor
air very rapidly. They are also filtered
out by the nose, and do not reach
the bronchi. Very small particles, less
than 4 microns across, take many
hours to settle from still air, and can
be inhaled deep into the lungs.

pollen
grains

large pollen grains
rarely cause hayfever

30 microns   40 microns   50 microns

Settling time:
time taken for particles to settle
completely in a room with a ceiling
3 metres (10ft) high

had a cat at all – an observation that science has yet to explain, although the allergies may have been brought into the house on clothing.

Although salivary protein is the main cat allergen, skin particles from cats can also cause symptoms. The fur itself is not allergenic, although it can carry salivary proteins. Thus a short-haired cat will not be less allergenic than a long-haired cat, contrary to popular mythology.

The allergic symptoms to cats can include rhinitis or asthma. Eczema is another possibility, especially in children.

In theory, eliminating cat allergens is very simple compared to dealing with something like pollen or house-dust mite – simply find a new home for your furry friend. Of course, this can be a very difficult decision, but it is the only sensible option, particularly if asthma is among the symptoms caused, or if the allergy sufferer is a child, whose problems could worsen with continued exposure to the allergen.

Think twice before replacing your lost pet with a dog, as cat allergens can cross-react with dog allergens (see p219). This may not happen in your case, but if it does you will be faced with another heart-wrenching decision about the new pet. Another animal, such as a hamster or guinea pig, is unlikely to provoke cross-reactions, but a new sensitivity could develop when it has been in the house for a while (see p210).

A thorough spring clean is needed once the cat has gone, with all curtains and other fabrics being washed, carpets shampooed and walls washed down. If the carpets and armchairs are fairly old, and you have had a cat for many years, consider replacing them with new ones. When cleaning, pay particular attention to any areas where the cat used to sleep.

The allergy sufferer should be out of the house while this clean-up is in progress and for a day or two afterwards. Alternatively, a mask can be worn, but it must be of the right kind (see p295) and it should be kept on all the time, not just while cleaning, because the particles will remain airborne for a long time. As a minimum precaution, the allergic individual should wear a mask at home and sleep somewhere else. If this is impossible, omit cleaning the bedroom at first and keep the bedroom door closed during the clean-up. Clean the bedroom a week or two later, while the allergic individual sleeps in another room. If the cat has slept in the allergy sufferer's bedroom, tackle the problem the other way round: clean that first, while the patient sleeps in another room, preferably one where the cat rarely went. After a few days, the patient can go back to sleeping in the bedroom. The rest of the house can than be cleaned, keeping the bedroom door closed.

Even after a clean-up, some cat allergens may persist for a while, and it may therefore be a few months before symptoms subside completely.

As an additional measure, you could spray carpets and upholstery with

JERRY

Jerry suffered from hayfever in the summer, as he had done since his teens. On top of this, he had asthma attacks accompanied by a runny, congested nose all year round, particularly at the weekends. Skin-prick testing (see p78) produced several positive reactions, making it difficult to know which ones were actually causing the symptoms, so the doctor began questioning Jerry about the pattern of his symptoms. It seemed that the asthma and rhinitis built up slowly over the weekend and then cleared when he returned to work. The doctor questioned Jerry closely and found that he had suffered from 'recurrent bronchitis' as a child, which had ended abruptly when he was about fifteen. Knowing that the terms used for asthma had changed over the years, and that methods of diagnosis had changed too, the doctor suspected that this childhood 'bronchitis' might actually have been asthma. 'Did you move house when you were fifteen?' asked the doctor, 'or did anything at home change?' The only thing Jerry could remember was that the family cat had died. It seemed irrelevant to Jerry, but the doctor was interested and asked whether there were any cats in his present house. 'Yes, my girlfriend has two,' Jerry replied. The cause of the weekend asthma and rhinitis now seemed clear, and a check with the results of the skin-prick tests showed that there had been a positive reaction to cats.

Jerry's doctor suggested ways in which cat allergens could be cut down – a thorough spring clean, followed by a weekly bath for both cats. In the meantime, Jerry was given an inhaler to help stave off the asthma attacks. Once the anti-cat-allergen measures were in action, Jerry was able to stop the inhaler without ill-effects.

Jerry is not typical of cat-allergic people, who generally know that cats cause their problem because the reaction to them is so dramatic and immediate. As Jerry's case shows, skin-prick tests are often only a rough guide, and some careful detective work may be needed to pinpoint the culprit allergen.

tannic acid (see p182) to denature any lingering cat allergens. In situations where a major clean-up is difficult, or it is impossible for the allergy sufferer to be elsewhere for a few days, tannic acid could also be used as a substitute for cleaning.

Research shows that a surprising number of people keep their cat, despite the health problems it causes. Sometimes our emotional welfare and our physical welfare make conflicting demands, and the emotions win. If you really cannot bear to part with your pet, then the allergen levels can be kept down in other ways.

Firstly, the cat should be excluded from the allergy sufferer's bedroom at all times. If it has slept there in the past, all bedding should be thoroughly washed. Duvets on which the cat has slept should be washed or replaced.

Secondly, if the house is well sealed against draughts, you need to increase the ventilation. In houses with snugly fitting doors and windows, the tiny particles from a cat can build up to very high levels. Even a modest increase in the amount of air flowing through your home will help to blow away the cat allergens. For some people, these two steps may be enough on their own.

If regular ventilation to the outside is impossible, you could use a HEPA air filter instead (see p298). However, research has shown that, with the very small particles from cats, the air currents set up by the fan in the air filter will churn up allergens from the floor and furnishings. This effect can partially offset its effectiveness in filtering the air. Placing the air filter well away from the floor will help, but a better solution is to clean carpets and furniture thoroughly at the outset, thus reducing the reservoir of cat allergen. (During cleaning, the allergy sufferer must go elsewhere or be protected from the allergen that is disturbed – see p207.) You should also remove as many cushions and upholstered items as possible, as this will reduce the surfaces that can act as reservoirs for cat allergens.

Thirdly, try persuading your cat to spend more time outdoors. This will reduce the amount of allergen being generated in the house. Providing a warm and comfortable place to sleep outside, in a shed, porch or conservatory, may be helpful.

The next step is a big one for you, and an even bigger one for the cat – give it a thorough wash with shampoo once a week. This substantially cuts down the amount of allergen that is shed with its fur and skin and so decreases the amount of allergen in the air. Some cats get used to this treatment in time, others decide that the house next door is more congenial after all. (If its affections seem to be wandering, you can try improving the food on offer.)

Make sure the cat's bedding is also washed regularly, at least once a week. Research shows that a well-used blanket can contain as much allergen as the fur of seventy cats.

Cutting the cat's claws every week is also said to reduce the amount of allergen in the air, presumably because it sheds less skin when scratching. Unless you have a particularly docile individual, this is likely to be even less popular than the weekly shampoo.

If these measures are not enough to eliminate the symptoms, you could try replacing your fitted carpets with rugs, as for house-dust mite control (see p185), vacuum cleaning armchairs and sofas regularly, and using a high-quality air filter (see p298). Research in the USA has shown that these measures, combined with washing the cat, will reduce the amount of cat allergen in the air considerably. Fitting a filter to the vacuum cleaner would be advisable as the allergen particles could go through the bag and become airborne again (see p185).

Another approach is to designate the living room as a cat-free zone, spray the upholstery and carpets with tannic acid, and instal an air filter. This will keep the allergens in the air at a low level, but only as long as the cat stays out of the room. (With tannic acid sprays, the cat will probably collect quite a bit on its paws, which it will then lick off. No one has investigated the effect of this on the cat, but it may be detrimental, so you should not use the spray regularly on an area that the cat inhabits.)

Someone highly sensitive to cats should avoid buying a house where cats have lived in the past, as their allergens will linger on.

Dogs

Dogs are less likely to cause allergic reactions than cats, but they are a fairly frequent source of problems, particularly for children. Rhinitis, asthma or eczema are the common symptoms.

The allergens occur mainly in the skin particles and saliva. As with all animals, the fur is not allergenic in itself, but allergenic proteins can become attached to the hair. The urine and faeces of dogs can also contain allergens. A few people react to one breed of dog only (see p157), but most are allergic to all dogs, and may react to cats too.

Parting with the dog is the best solution, but it can be heartbreaking, and many people prefer to live with the problem. Washing the dog every week can help, or it may be easier to vacuum clean it. Some of the special vacuum cleaners sold to allergy sufferers (see p308) have brush attachments designed for this purpose. A stiff upholstery-cleaning brush from an ordinary vacuum cleaner may work equally well.

Regular vacuum cleaning of carpets and armchairs will be helpful in reducing the level of allergens in the air, and tannic acid (see p182) may also be useful. Replacing fitted carpets with rugs (see p185) will reduce the reservoir of dog allergens in the house, provided you mop or vacuum clean the bare floors regularly, and beat rugs outdoors to remove the skin particles.

The dog's bedding should be washed every week, and the animal itself should be strictly excluded from the allergy sufferer's bedroom. If it has ever slept on the bed, all the bedding should be thoroughly washed to remove the allergens, or replaced.

Small animals

Any animal can produce an allergic reaction, and rabbits, guinea pigs, mice, hamsters, gerbils and rats are no exception. Unfortunately, these allergies are often overlooked by doctors, who enquire about cats and dogs but forget to ask about smaller pets. An allergy to such a pet can be investigated with a skin-prick test (see p78), and you should ask for this test if it has not been carried out already. (People working with small animals can be similarly affected, see p216.)

Skin particles, or proteins from the animal's urine, are probably the allergen involved. Rhinitis or asthma may occur as a result of the allergy, and these can come on gradually, beginning some time after the pet has arrived in the home.

The only real solution is to move the animal's cage outside, or at least into a porch or conservatory.

It is possible that where houses are infested with mice or rats (a growing problem in Britain and many other countries), allergic reactions to these animals could develop. To date, this possibility has not been investigated. As with cockroach allergy (see p83), those most likely to be affected are those least likely to get the medical treatment they need. A constant runny nose is very common in children living in poor housing, and is often attributed to repeated infections. Anyone living in poor housing who has a 'perpetual cold' could perhaps be tested for allergies to rats, mice and cockroaches, particularly if they have given negative tests to moulds and house-dust mite.

Birds

Feather particles, or proteins from the droppings, are the main allergens in the case of birds. They can cause rhinitis, asthma, or a lung complaint known as bird-fancier's lung (see p211).

The particles are very small and therefore difficult to control. You could try keeping the cage in a room which the allergy sufferer does not enter, but this is unlikely to help as the particles will be wafted into the rest of the house whenever the door is opened. The best solution is to find another home for the bird.

If this is impossible, a HEPA filter (see p298) would probably keep the

ALLERGENS DEEP IN THE LUNG

Very small particles that go deep into the lung can cause **extrinsic allergic alveolitis** (see p203), but only if they are inhaled in large amounts. Farmer's lung and bird-fancier's lung are two examples of this disease, the first caused by mould spores from mouldy hay and the second by feather particles or proteins from bird droppings. Cagebirds such as budgerigars can bring on this disease, but it is most often seen in those who keep pigeons.

The disease produces attacks of a flu-like illness, with feverishness, pains in the limbs, breathlessness and a dry cough. The symptoms tend to last a few days, then disappear, only to come back later. They may not develop immediately after exposure to the allergen, but many hours later, so the link is not obvious. The disease is produced in a different way from hayfever and other common allergies, and unlike them it carries a risk of serious long-term damage. If you have any symptoms of this sort you should see your doctor immediately. (There is a widespread medical belief that you cannot suffer from rhinitis or asthma to an allergen *and* have extrinsic allergic alveolitis to the same allergen. Recent research shows that this is not correct.)

particle levels down, but it must be sufficiently powerful for the size of the room. Even with a filter running, the affected person will probably be unable to enter the room where the bird is kept.

Whether the bird is removed from the house or not, a general clean-up to remove the existing reservoir of allergens may be valuable. Follow the cleaning guidelines described for cat allergy (see pp207–8).

Sheep's wool

Until recently, the medical profession had been largely unaware that some people have an allergy to sheep's wool. A recent British study, however, revealed that many people with an allergy to house dust, but not to house-dust mites, were actually sensitive to wool particles in the dust. It is not clear what the allergen is in this case, since fur and hair (of which wool is one form) are thought not to be allergenic. And there is another puzzle regarding wool allergy: for reasons that are not understood, very few of those affected give a positive reaction when skin-prick tested with wool extract itself. However, they give strong reactions to a nasal provocation test (see p79) with wool. Some are already aware of the source of their problems since they experience symptoms (rhinitis or asthma) from sheepskin jackets and rugs, from woollen blankets and carpets, or when knitting with wool.

The obvious treatment for this allergy is to avoid woollen clothing, bedding and carpets. A thorough spring clean may be necessary to remove the existing pool of wool fibres in the household dust. Unfortunately, avoiding wool can be difficult, as the fibres are almost everywhere. If medicinal drugs do not control the symptoms adequately, a desensitization treatment may be helpful (see Chapter Nine).

Horses

Few people have much contact with horses these days, yet these animals seem to cause reactions very frequently, suggesting that they produce powerful allergens. Fortunately, avoidance of horses is relatively easy. If you are very sensitive, you may find that old sofas and armchairs stuffed with horsehair affect you. The clothes of someone else who has been riding may contain enough allergen to affect you, and in some cases *this source can sensitize a person who has no direct contact with horses themselves*. Where one person in a family is a keen rider, and another is allergic to horses, the best compromise is for the non-allergic person to change his or her riding clothes before coming indoors.

Insects

The discovery of insects as a major and widespread cause of rhinitis and asthma – that is, one affecting more than 10 per cent of those with allergic disease – is a relatively recent development. Such allergic reactions have been found in a surprising number of countries, and the true extent of the problem is still unknown.

Widespread insect allergy generally comes to light only where it is specifically looked for, as with cockroach allergy in the southern USA (see p83). More recently, both mosquitoes and cockroaches have been found to cause rhinitis and asthma in India. Silkworm moths are a problem in Japan and some parts of central Asia, while midges and caddis flies are also a cause of rhinitis in Japan. Around the Great Lakes in Canada, the moulted skin of mayflies can cause asthma and rhinitis in the breeding season. The green nemitry fly of Egypt and Sudan causes widespread seasonal rhinitis, and may aggravate asthma, mainly in the hot summer months. In several countries allergies to maggots are found among fishermen using them as bait, and the symptoms may include rhinitis.

In Britain no one has yet looked for widespread allergies to insects. However, there are well-documented cases of people who react strongly to house flies, or to carpet beetles. In the case of carpet beetles, the larvae (often called 'fuzzy bears') are covered with tiny hairs. It is these hairs that are likely to provoke allergic reactions. There have also been occasional cases of allergy to daphnia (not insects, but crustaceans) used to feed fish; inhaled particles from these can cause rhinitis or asthma.

Cockroach allergy is a distinct possibility in Britain, although the cooler climate does not allow cockroaches to flourish as much as they do nearer the Equator. Anyone living in poor housing conditions, or in accommodation where cockroaches are known to be present, and who has a 'perpetual cold', may be suffering from an allergy to cockroaches. The extracts for skin-prick testing are available (see p318) and a family doctor should be able to carry out this test. Alternatively, cockroaches could cause seasonal symptoms that might be mistaken for hayfever (see p220).

With insects that infest houses, such as cockroaches, their droppings may carry the allergen. Alternatively, it can be hairs that they shed, bits of broken-off wing and skin, or tiny fragments of their bodies which have disintegrated after death. With largely outdoor insects, such as midges and caddis flies, it is hairs and body fragments floating in the air that cause problems. Bees, butterflies and moths can also cause problems in this way, but allergies to these insects are very rare.

One potential hazard that has yet to be investigated are the electric fly killers used in butchers' shops. These attract flies and kill them instantly by electrocution. Researchers have found that the flies explode into minute particles, small enough to stay airborne for up to 100 hours. As yet, allergy to these insect fragments has not been identified, but it is a possibility.

Treatment for insect allergy, where the insects are household pests, involves eradication. There are various commercial companies that can advise and assist with this (see p311). The eradication process could involve pulling away panelling (around baths, or at the back of cupboards for example) or removing carpets if they are heavily infested with carpet beetle. This will release a great deal of allergen into the air, and it is therefore vital that the allergy sufferer is out of the house at the time and for several hours afterwards. (On one occasion, an asthmatic with cockroach allergy suffered a fatal asthma attack when cockroach allergens were released during an eradication treatment.) Insecticidal sprays, or the solvents in which they are dissolved, can in themselves cause symptoms, and it is really best to leave the house for several days after spraying, particularly if there are children in the household. (This advice also applies to standard treatments for woodworm and dry or wet rot.)

IRRITANTS IN THE AIR

A few of the items found in the air can act as irritants to the nose. If they affect the nose, they generally affect the bronchi as well, except for large particles that cannot reach the bronchi (see p202).

Anyone can be affected by these irritant particles or gases, not just those of an allergic disposition, but some people are more sensitive than others. Those with hayfever are often more susceptible during the pollen season. Someone whose nose is highly sensitive to a variety of airborne irritants, but who has *no* allergic responses, may be considered to have vasomotor rhinitis (see p229).

The irritants may have their effect just by stimulating nerves in the nose, so that the parasympathetic nervous system (see p226) reacts. Some irritants, however, do provoke genuine inflammation – a response that involves parts of the immune system. This is the case with sulphur dioxide, for example.

Most of the airborne irritants are man-made, but some are natural substances produced by plants or animals. Natural forces can also produce significant amounts of irritants in certain areas.

Irritants in outdoor air

Pine pollen may act as an irritant because of its large size, the enormous quantity inhaled, and certain chemicals carried on its surface (see p7). The tiny hairs produced by plane trees, which are scattered in spring and summer, irritate the eyes of some people. The hairs from peaches are also a major irritant and may affect anyone close to a peach tree in fruit; the symptoms are similar to hayfever.

Volatile substances produced by plants can also act as irritants, and certain plants, such as oil-seed rape, produce these in abundance (see p120). The scents of flowers can irritate the nose in some people.

Many man-made substances act as irritants, notably smoke. The smoke that we see consists of tiny unburned or partially burned particles, plus droplets of moisture in some cases. These particles and droplets act as irritants, but there are also many invisible constituents in smoke, including acrolein, a gas that is highly irritating to the airways. The more moisture there is in the material being burned, and the less ventilation at the base of the fire, the more smoke particles and acrolein will be produced. A really hot fire produces no smoke at all. Garden bonfires, particularly those burning damp wood or leaves, are an unrecognized hazard, particularly for anyone with asthma. Plastics and other synthetic materials, when burned on a bonfire, can make matters worse by producing a variety of powerful irritants.

Ozone, a gas produced by the action of sunlight on car exhausts, is also irritating to the airways, and has been shown to aggravate both rhinitis and asthma (see p70). Nitrogen dioxide, which is produced by car exhausts, can also be an irritant when it builds up to sufficiently high levels (see p60).

A variety of gases produced by industrial processes, and expelled from factory or power-station chimneys into the surrounding air, can act as irritants. Sulphur dioxide and sulphuric acid droplets (see p62) are notable offenders. As with many irritants, those worst affected will be asthmatics.

Advice on reducing exposure to outdoor pollutants can be found on p322.

Airborne irritants indoors

One major indoor irritant is tobacco smoke, which can make both rhinitis and asthma worse. Some people are far more susceptible to this irritant than others.

The smoke produced by frying, particularly if the oil or fat is overheated, is also a powerful irritant to the airways. An oven that has not been cleaned for some time will produce a similar type of smoke when heated.

Nitrogen dioxide is produced by burning most fuels and is an irritant when it reaches a certain concentration in the air. With gas cookers, and old-fashioned paraffin heaters, nitrogen dioxide may build up to high levels in poorly ventilated rooms (see p61).

Many household products – such as polish, some cleaning fluids, paint, white spirit, turpentine and bleach – can act as irritants to susceptible individuals, particularly those whose nose or bronchi are already inflamed by an allergic reaction. Air fresheners can irritate the eyes, nose and chest.

Formaldehyde is an indoor pollutant of which people are often quite unaware. It can cause dryness and irritation in the nose and throat, and may affect the eyes or the bronchi as well. One source of this gas is injected cavity wall insulation. Some of the materials used in this process generate formaldehyde, and will continue to do so for months after it has been injected. Chipboard is the other major source, but if it has been painted with gloss paint this will keep the formaldehyde locked inside. Plywood and blockboard give off lesser amounts of formaldehyde. Other minor sources are foam rubber, new textiles and carpets, paper (including newsprint), photographs, leather luggage, anti-perspirants, some cosmetics and some shampoos. Mobile homes and caravans are often rich in formaldehyde, because plywood and chipboard are used extensively in making them. Modern buildings such as offices and hotels can also have high levels of formaldehyde in the air. Formaldehyde is also used to sterilize soil and glasshouses, and there may be an unhealthy level of exposure if these processes are not carried out carefully. There is a personal monitoring system that can show how much formaldehyde you are being exposed to (see p311).

Sprays used to kill house-dust mites (see p179) have sometimes produced symptoms in those suffering from asthma. Advice on reducing exposure to pollutants in the home can be found on p321.

ALLERGENS AND IRRITANTS AT WORK

Any particles that are inhaled all day in large quantities may affect the airways. Often it is clear that the workplace is the cause of symptoms, particularly with irritants. With an allergen, however, late-phase reactions (see p41) are often important, and these can make the allergic reaction continue all weekend. This frequently obscures the source of the problem, although symptoms should clear up during a longer holiday. With asthma the symptoms may continue over the weekend, even though the substance responsible is merely an irritant.

Particles encountered at work which are known to act as allergens include wheat flour, rye flour, soya-bean flour or dust, castor-bean dust (see p45), and tiny droplets of egg sprayed on to pies and pastries. Farmers in Australia often show an allergic reaction to wheat dust, and this may well affect farmers elsewhere.

Some of the complex salts of platinum can also act as allergens, having first combined with proteins in the body, and there is a high level of airway disease in the platinum-refining industry. (Platinum salts are also believed to act as adjuvants for IgE, see p45.)

Natural pyrethroid insecticides, and the flowers they are made from, can also produce an allergic reaction.

Mould spores can act as allergens (see p193), and a variety of workers have a very high exposure to these, including farmers, builders and decorators (when stripping out fittings in old houses or those with damp problems), mushroom growers and those working in breweries.

Sometimes wood dusts act as allergens, but they are more likely to be irritants (see below). Those with hayfever to a tree pollen may show a cross-reaction to wood dust or pulp (see p166) but this is unusual.

Laboratory workers who look after rats, mice and other small mammals can readily develop an allergy to the proteins found in their urine, or to skin particles. Powered respirator helmets (see p297) are sometimes used to protect such workers from the allergens.

Those working on maggot farms may become allergic to maggots, and people rearing locusts, fruit flies, silkworms, butterflies, stick insects or bees can be similarly affected. Concern has been expressed about fly killers in butchers' shops (see p213).

As already noted, anyone working closely with plants may become allergic to the pollen, even though it is a pollen that does not normally cause hayfever (see pp5–7).

With all allergens, a skin-prick test can be used to confirm that this is indeed the cause of the problem. However, a negative skin-prick test does not entirely rule out an allergic reaction, as false negatives are possible (see p81).

The potential irritants encountered in industrial processes are too numerous to mention here. The industries where large numbers suffer from symptoms in the airways include platinum smelting, electronics, plastics manufacturing, detergent manufacturing, the textile industry and any industrial process using formaldehyde, toluene, diphylmethane, hexamethylene, naphthalene, phthalic acid or trimellitic acid. For the majority of people, it will be obvious that something in the workplace is producing symptoms in the nose or bronchi. Sometimes, as in platinum smelting and electronics, there may be both irritants *and* allergens in the air, and a single chemical may even take both roles. The irritant effects will generally be known to other workers, trade union officials, the company medical service, or local doctors, who can advise on long-term effects. Everyone is different, and if a substance affects others far less than it affects you, this is no reason to ignore the irritation it causes. Taking the early signs seriously may help to avoid more serious long-term consequences.

In general, those with an allergic disposition should avoid going into jobs where there is high allergen exposure, such as in bakeries, or looking after animals. If asthma is already present, they should not work with known irritants.

With non-industrial jobs, there is often assumed to be little or no hazard. While this is largely true, there are certain problems which have been generally ignored in the past. For example, permanent-wave solutions can produce rhinitis in hairdressers, and hair spray can produce the lung disease thesaurosis. Carpenters and wood-turners may be affected by wood dust, as may goldsmiths who use wood dust for drying jewellery. Laser printers may occasionally affect the nose too, due to the styrene-butadiene toners used. Photocopying machines produce small amounts of ozone, and if there are several machines in a poorly ventilated area, this irritant gas may build up to a level where it can affect people with rhinitis or asthma.

Ozone can also be produced by electrostatic air cleaners, although this problem has been overcome with newer devices. If the electrostatic plates are left on over the weekend, but the fans turned off, there can be a build-up of ozone, which then floods into the building when the ventilation system is switched on at the beginning of the week. This can produce severe symptoms of coughing and nasal irritation in a large proportion of the workforce. The problem is relatively rare, but it can occur in older office buildings. There are now companies who can investigate and remedy health problems caused by buildings (see p311).

Sick building syndrome

This controversial problem, which often affects workers in large office buildings, probably has several different causes. One may be formaldehyde in the air (see p215), produced by office furniture and fittings. There may also be other gases in the air that act as irritants, gases which are slowly being given off by plastics and other materials used in carpeting or office fittings. The dryness of the air may make exposure to such pollutants more irritating to the nose. Ozone from photocopiers and fumes from laser printers (see above) can sometimes add to the problem, as can cleaning solutions such as bleach. Increasing the ventilation usually dispels such pollutants.

Another cause of sick building syndrome may be allergic reactions to mould spores. The moulds are usually growing in the air ducts or water tanks, and then being circulated around the office. More seriously, mould spores and other microbes growing in water tanks can cause **humidifier fever** or **humidifier lung**, but this only occurs when there is a serious infestation producing large numbers of spores and microbes in the air. Anyone can be affected by this, not just those of an allergic disposition. The symptoms are fever, cough, a general feeling of malaise, tightness in the chest and aching muscles. They develop within a few hours of starting work and are worse on Monday mornings, when the ventilation system is turned on, releasing a large dose of spores and microbes that have built up in the system over the weekend. This disease is similar to **extrinsic allergic alveolitis** (see p211) and requires prompt treatment.

Tobacco smoke may also be a factor in sick building syndrome, and studies show that people vary greatly in their sensitivity to this pollutant. Occasionally house-dust mites turn out to be the problem (see p174). Sometimes fluorescent lighting is at the root of sick building syndrome, but if this is the sole cause, the symptoms are unlikely to affect the nose. Psychological factors, including monotonous work, and the feeling of being trapped in a building where the windows cannot be opened nor the heating system controlled, may contribute to sick building syndrome.

SEASONAL SYMPTOMS FROM ALLERGENS OTHER THAN POLLEN

If you appear to have hayfever, but give no positive skin-prick tests to pollen, then there are other possibilities you should consider.

Mould spore allergy, where the main source of spores is outdoor air, can produce seasonal symptoms, usually in late summer and autumn. (Indoors, winter is a more mouldy time of year, because windows are opened less, people are at home more, clothes are dried indoors and more hot meals are prepared. House-dust mite allergy often peaks in winter too, and cat allergy could get worse due to less ventilation – see p208.)

CROSS-REACTIONS INVOLVING AIRBORNE ALLERGENS

There are few cross-reactions between pollen allergens and the airborne allergens described in this chapter, although mugwort pollen can cross-react with the dust from wood of the spindle tree. It is possible that grass pollen might cross-react with inhaled wheat flour or wheat dust.

For those who are sensitive to house-dust mites, there are often cross-reactions to other mites, such as those found in stored grain, or those which live as parasites on dogs, cats or horses. There is also a most peculiar cross-reaction between dust mites and two fruits: kiwi fruit and papaya (see p165).

For those sensitive to dog allergens, there can be some cross-reaction to cats, and vice versa, because certain allergens are similar. However, these cross-reactions are unusual.

People who are highly sensitized to feather allergens, or to protein from bird droppings, sometimes develop a cross-reaction to egg proteins, and may react badly when they eat eggs. The same can be true, naturally enough, for those sensitized to inhaled egg droplets from working in the food industry (see p216). Those who are highly egg-sensitive sometimes react allergically to vaccines, because these are often cultured in eggs and minute traces of egg protein remain.

A few people with mould allergy show a cross-reaction to fungi found in some wines. Occasionally, people who seem to be sensitive to strawberries are actually reacting to the grey mould known as *Botrytis* that grows on them. A cross-reaction with edible fungi, such as mushrooms, is also possible.

Those allergic to horses may react to old mattresses, armchairs or settees stuffed with horsehair, while anyone sensitive to birds may obviously react to feather stuffing in furniture, pillows or duvets. (These are not true cross-reactions, just reactions to the same allergen from a different source.)

In Britain, one mould, *Cladosporium herbarum*, releases its spores from June to September. Someone who is allergic to this species, and not to other moulds, may seem to have grass-pollen hayfever, but their symptoms will be entirely out of step with the pollen counts. Another mould, *Alternaria*, sporulates mainly in July and August. Skin-prick tests that are specific for these moulds, and not for other types, are possible.

In cool climates, cockroaches may produce allergic symptoms only in summer (see p83). Similarly, house flies will be much more common in summer. In both cases, symptoms will be worse indoors, unlike hayfever.

Many outdoor insects such as midges, mayflies and caddis flies will only produce symptoms in summer, and such symptoms could be mistaken for hayfever. These insects are more common in damp places, and by water.

Mosquitoes are obviously more common in summer, and might produce symptoms indoors, outdoors, or both.

Volatile substances from plants (see p120) could also act as seasonal irritants, and some people may show a non-allergic reaction to pollen. Non-allergic seasonal reactions are considered in more detail on p243.

If none of these explanations seems likely in your case, you could ask for a nasal provocation test (see p79) with pollen. This may reveal a positive reaction when a skin-prick test has given a false negative.

Chapter Thirteen

OTHER FORMS OF RHINITIS

So far we have looked at pollen and the various other allergens and irritants found floating in the air. These have direct access to the nose, and are prime suspects when symptoms occur there, but there are several other ways in which problems in the nose can be caused.

INFECTIONS

The most frequent cause of problems is, of course, infection. Indeed, the common cold, produced by a viral infection, brings most of us a short sharp dose of **rhinitis** (inflammation in the nose) each winter. Here the immune reaction that causes inflammation (see p34) is doing its proper job – fighting off infectious microbes. That is why you should never use corticosteroid drops (see p100), which you may have been prescribed for hayfever, when suffering from a cold or other infection – they will reduce your resistance to the microbe.

Colds generally last less than a week, and if one continues for more than three or four weeks, you should see your doctor. Asthmatics should see the doctor if their attacks become more frequent or more severe during a cold, as they frequently do.

INFECTION-PLUS-ALLERGY

Very rarely, patients develop a damaging allergic reaction against certain infectious bacteria in the nose. This causes a prolonged rhinitis, with a great deal of unpleasant mucus coming from the nose. Because the condition is rare, your doctor may not recognize it at first. Antibiotics are needed to kill off the bacteria, and desensitization (see Chapter Nine) to control the allergic reaction.

Allergic reactions to infectious fungi are also possible, and can sometimes cause rhinitis. This is known to happen with the fungus that causes athlete's foot, *Trichophyton*. As well as infecting the skin, the fungus can sometimes make its home in the nose, and an allergic reaction there then causes rhinitis. Occasionally, asthma is due to an allergic reaction to the same fungus.

REPEATED INFECTIONS

A long succession of infections in the nose can leave its delicate inner structure damaged, with the membranes thickened and the blood vessels congested. This will produce a constant stuffiness in the nose, and may impair the sense of smell. The condition is known as **hypertrophic rhinitis**. Surgery may help but is only used for the more severe cases.

PROBLEMS IN THE NOSE CAUSED BY DRUGS

Certain drugs can affect the nose badly, and the rather pompous Latin term **rhinitis medicamentosa** is used to refer to the problems they can cause. The most common culprits are decongestant nose drops containing **sympathomimetics** (see p96), to which the nose readily becomes addicted. To avoid this problem, such drops should not be used for more than a few days (see p97). Cocaine, when 'snorted', has a similar effect to sympathomimetics, and can therefore produce rebound congestion in the same way. Cocaine can also cause problems simply by acting as an irritant.

Very occasionally, sympathomimetics taken by mouth (e.g. *pseudoephedrine*, *phenylephrine* and *phenylpropanolamine*) can have the same effect, but the doses used in tablets that combine a sympathomimetic with an antihistamine (see p98) are low enough to be very safe. Certain drugs used to lower blood pressure can cause rhinitis, although this again is rare. They include *bethanidine* (Bethanidine), *guanethidine* (Ismelin), *indoramin* (Baratol), *phentolamine* (Rogitine), *propanolol* (Betadur) and *reserpine*.

Nose drops containing **corticosteroids** can also cause problems such as crusting, dryness and nosebleeds (see p101). Much more rarely, contraceptive pills can cause a mild rhinitis (see below).

HORMONAL EFFECTS

The female hormones, oestrogen and progesterone, can affect the nose, causing runniness or congestion. This can cause problems for a minority of women during pregnancy. All the usual treatments for rhinitis have been tried but nothing seems to help in this situation. As soon as the baby is born, however, the rhinitis disappears.

This hormonal interference with the nose can also affect women taking contraceptive pills, or going through the menopause, although these effects are most unusual.

People with underactive thyroid glands may also suffer a blocked nose until they are treated.

FORMS OF RHINITIS WITH NO OBVIOUS CAUSE

The diseases dealt with so far in this chapter (and in earlier chapters) are those where the factor causing the problem has been identified and largely understood. From this point on we are entering much murkier waters, where the cause of disease is not fully understood by the medical profession. Nevertheless, doctors can identify certain types of disease, on the basis of characteristic features, and they can often provide quite effective treatments.

In trying to understand sickness and find cures for it, classifying diseases and naming them is all-important. When a field of medicine is still evolving, the classifications tend to change rather often, as doctors realize that what they previously thought of as one disease is actually two quite different ones. Several changes of this kind have happened in non-allergic rhinitis in recent years, and if you were diagnosed as having 'vasomotor rhinitis' several years ago, that diagnosis may no longer be considered appropriate for your condition. Medical science may have caught up with you, and can perhaps offer more appropriate treatments than before, so it might be worth seeing a specialist again. If your 'vasomotor rhinitis' is still being treated with a sympathomimetic-antihistamine mixture (see p98) or with sympathomimetics alone, then this is almost certainly the case, and you should see your specialist again. You can look up the name of the drug you are using in Appendix 6, and this will show what type of drug it is.

Before diving into these murky waters where causes are largely unknown, let us first look back at the well-mapped terrain we are leaving behind. That terrain has a large enclosure on it with a sign saying 'allergic rhinitis'. You will have been excluded from that enclosure if you had no positive skin-prick tests and no positive blood tests for IgE (see Chapter Six). These tests are generally good, but unfortunately they do exclude a few people who should rightly be in the allergic enclosure. This problem is discussed at the end of this chapter, on p243.

There are several other enclosures available, that have already been described. These include infection or its consequences (see pp221–2), exposure to irritants at work or at home (see pp214–8), rhinitis medicamentosa (see p222), and hormonal effects (see p222).

When all these possibilities have been excluded, then you will be consigned to the murky waters, where causes cannot be identified but treatment is still possible.

At this point, the ear-nose-and-throat specialist will generally take a tiny sample from the lining of the nose and send it to a laboratory for examination. If the laboratory finds that there are a large number of immune cells known as **eosinophils** present then the diagnosis will be **non-allergic rhinitis with eosinophilia**, sometimes abbreviated to **NARES**. If there are few eosinophils, the diagnosis will probably be **vasomotor rhinitis**, although some doctors prefer a different term for reasons that will be explained later. A third possibility, but one which occurs only rarely, is that the nose will be rich in mast cells. The diagnosis in this case is **nasal mastocytosis**. We will look at each of these three conditions in turn.

NARES

Non-allergic rhinitis with eosinophilia or NARES (also called eosinophilic non-allergic perennial rhinitis) is a disease that has only been identified properly in the last few years. In the past, people with this problem were usually diagnosed as having 'vasomotor rhinitis'.

NARES is the diagnosis given when large numbers of eosinophils are found in the nose, but the patient has not given any positive test reactions for allergy. As well as a congested and runny nose, with bouts of sneezing, patients with NARES often lose their sense of smell.

The fact that eosinophils have converged on the nose in their thousands shows that some kind of immune reaction is going on there. Exactly why is at present unknown. Mast cells are also releasing some mediators in the nose of a patient with NARES.

Hand-in-hand with this immune reaction, there is an imbalance in the autonomic nervous system producing hyperreactivity in the nose (see box article on p226). Recent research shows that there are many subtle interactions between the autonomic nervous system and the immune system, and it is difficult to say which is the fundamental problem in NARES – the inflammation, or the malfunctioning nervous controls. Either of these could be the underlying problem, which has sparked off the other disorder.

You may remember that eosinophils also flock to the nose during the late phase of an allergic reaction (see p41). But with an allergic reaction there are also many basophils (another type of immune cell) there as well, so the laboratory finding will be a little different for someone with allergic rhinitis. It is possible, however, that a few patients diagnosed as having NARES are actually suffering from allergic rhinitis, which has somehow been overlooked by conventional allergy tests (see p243).

With the realization that NARES is distinct from 'vasomotor rhinitis' (see p230) and involves inflammation, an effective treatment has been found. Nose drops containing corticosteroids (see p100) damp down the inflammation and produce very good results in most patients, but must not be over-used (see pp101–2). Cod-liver oil may also be valuable (see p229).

ASPIRIN SENSITIVITY, ASTHMA, RHINITIS AND NASAL POLYPS

For many years, allergists have been noticing a set of patients with a rather odd combination of problems: they usually have asthma and perennial rhinitis, they are very prone to nasal polyps (see p228), and they are extremely sensitive to aspirin, so that a couple of ordinary aspirin tablets will produce an unpleasant reaction. The most severe reactions to aspirin are similar to anaphylactic shock (see p139). However, the patient does not produce any IgE molecules (see p31) to aspirin, so this is no ordinary allergic reaction. Some of these patients also have urticaria (nettle rash).

This condition became known as the **triad**, because of the three typical symptoms: asthma, polyps and aspirin sensitivity.

Recently it has been realized that there is a link between NARES and this triad syndrome. People diagnosed as having NARES *sometimes* go on to become triad patients. And triad patients show an influx of eosinophils into the nose very like that in NARES, although there may be other immune cells as well.

This link may point the way to explaining both NARES and triad. Aspirin affects the production of substances called **prostaglandins**. (This action by aspirin is largely beneficial in the normal person, helping to reduce inflammation in the joints for example.) Prostaglandins can be produced by almost any cell in the body, although they are also among the mediators released from mast cells (see Chapter Three). There are at least twenty different types of prostaglandin and they are involved in the regulation of inflammation, but in a very complex way: the actions of different prostaglandins often oppose one another. They interact with each other, and with other parts of the immune system, through a complicated network of checks and balances.

Researchers in this area now suspect that both NARES and triad may be disorders in the production or regulation of the prostaglandins, although they have no idea what produces the disorder. Prostaglandins are known to affect the autonomic nervous system, and vice versa, which might explain why inflammation and autonomic imbalance (see p227) go together in NARES. The arrival of eosinophils in the nose could just be a response to the initial inflammation, but a response that would aggravate the inflammation.

In triad patients, presumably, the prostaglandin disorder has become serious enough to make the interplay of prostaglandin reactions fundamentally different from that in normal people. This in itself causes symptoms such as asthma, rhinitis and nasal polyps, but it also makes the prostaglandin

NERVES IN THE NOSE

The brain helps to control what is going on in the nose, by means of the **autonomic nervous system**. The autonomic nervous system is the equivalent of 'autopilot' in an aeroplane – a system that can run things by itself, without any conscious thought on our part. The autonomic system regulates the heart, ensures that we breathe in and out, and organizes the breakdown of food, without our even being aware of these activities.

The autonomic system has two separate networks of nerves. One is called the **parasympathetic system** and its basic message to the body is, 'Don't panic, everything is fine.' The other is called the **sympathetic system**, and its basic message is, 'Action needed'. Having these two opposing systems allows the body to adapt to different situations. When danger threatens, or when we simply have to run upstairs, the heart must beat faster, the lungs work harder and the airways let in more air. The sympathetic system gears up the body for these more energetic moments of the day. The parasympathetic is involved in calming things down again afterwards, and making sure that important maintenance tasks are carried out – tasks such as digestion and the clearing of dust from the airways.

The parasympathetic promotes secretion of many important substances in the body, including mucus in the nose and bronchi. The mucus helps to pick up dust and microbes, so that they can be swept out of the nasal passages and down the throat. When something irritates the nose, a message goes to the brain and stimulates the parasympathetic system, which in turn steps up the production of mucus.

When it comes to the control of the blood vessels in the nose, both the sympathetic and the parasympathetic are involved.

balance fragile, and susceptible to interference from outside – so that the action of two aspirin tablets is highly disruptive and damaging.

These explanations are entirely speculative at the moment, but research is

There are many small blood vessels in the lining of the nose, and if they enlarge, the lining itself grows thicker as a result, which makes the air passages narrower. The parasympathetic has this effect. The sympathetic system makes the blood vessels smaller, which widens the nasal passages, so that more air can get through.

In the healthy nose, the sympathetic system opens up the airways when more air is needed, while the parasympathetic restores the status quo afterwards.

The **hyperreactive** nose is one where the parasympathetic system has become much too busy, and the sympathetic a little lazy. Instead of restoring the blood vessels in the nose to their normal width, the parasympathetic can make them expand and expand, until the nasal passages are uncomfortably narrow. The sympathetic, meanwhile, does not do enough to compensate. Instead of producing a useful amount of mucus to clear out the nose, the parasympathetic produces an excessive amount, so that the nose runs constantly. And rather than reacting to irritants such as smoke when they reach potentially damaging levels, the parasympathetic reacts to them in mere traces.

This process (also called **autonomic imbalance**) plays some part in almost all the diseases described in this book. Any nose that is inflamed is also hyperreactive – the nervous controls are disturbed by the Inflammation process in the membranes. That is why people with hayfever can find strong scents, tobacco smoke or paint fumes unusually troublesome to the nose during the pollen season.

Autonomic imbalance can be an important feature in asthma, too, with an overzealous parasympathetic system narrowing the bronchi and stimulating too much mucus production.

continuing in this area, and clearer answers may be available in the next few years.

The treatment of triad involves several different measures aimed at the different symptoms. Corticosteroid nose drops (see p100) are often effective in

NASAL POLYPS

Nasal polyps are small soft bulbous outgrowths from the lining of the nose. Except in a few, very rare cases, they have nothing to do with cancerous tumours. These polyps are entirely harmless, and cause concern only when they block the nasal passages. This can make nose-breathing difficult, or reduce the sense of smell.

Many healthy people have nasal polyps, but they are far more frequent in those suffering from rhinitis. At the end of a long hot summer, people with severe hayfever may develop nasal polyps, although they are far more common in year-round rhinitis. The group with the greatest tendency to polyps are triad patients (see p225) closely followed by those with NARES (see p224).

Polyps that develop during the hayfever season will probably go away again of their own accord. For those with year-round rhinitis, polyps are usually treated by removing them surgically, but they tend to reappear. Corticosteroid drops are useful in keeping new polyps at bay after the old ones have been removed. It is important to allow the drops to penetrate as far as possible into the nasal passages, and the 'head down' position shown on p229 is the best way to achieve this. Sometimes small nasal polyps can be persuaded to shrink away by the use of corticosteroid drops alone.

treating the rhinitis seen in triad patients, but must be used carefully (see pp101–2). Corticosteroid inhalers are valuable for controlling the asthma. Polyps are often treated surgically, or with corticosteroids (see above).

Anyone who has ever reacted badly to aspirin should be careful about taking painkillers in future. Many contain, if not aspirin itself, then an aspirin-like drug that can have much the same effect. Several drugs used to treat rheumatoid arthritis also belong in this family. A list of the medicines you should avoid is given on pp70–71.

Several doctors have tried out diets that are low in salicylates for their triad patients, salicylates being the natural counterparts of aspirin. They are found in a variety of fruits, vegetables, herbs and spices. The diet is quite difficult to stick to, and rarely produces any major benefits, so this treatment is probably not worth trying.

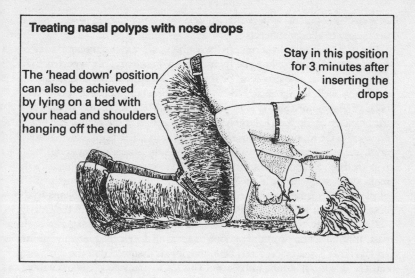

Treating nasal polyps with nose drops

The 'head down' position can also be achieved by lying on a bed with your head and shoulders hanging off the end

Stay in this position for 3 minutes after inserting the drops

With the growing understanding of NARES and triad, it is likely that new forms of treatment may become available in the future, such as drugs that address the basic problem of the prostaglandin disorder. One intriguing discovery is that some triad patients show an improvement in their asthma and polyps if they take a tiny amount of aspirin every day. However, you should *definitely* not try this for yourself without the agreement of your doctor, because the reaction to aspirin is potentially dangerous.

One treatment that you can try for yourself is to take cod-liver oil. Some substances found in this oil influence the production of prostaglandins by the body, tending to reduce their pro-inflammatory action. They may therefore be particularly useful to NARES and triad patients. Only two teaspoons a day should be taken – too much can be toxic. Eating oily fish such as herring or mackerel at least twice a week will have a similar effect.

VASOMOTOR RHINITTIS

This is a term which can mean a variety of different things, and tends to create considerable confusion, not to say controversy. To begin with, we will explain what vasomotor rhinitis *should* mean.

As already explained, nerves in the nose play a crucial part in narrowing or widening the air passages, and in producing mucus (see p226). A **hyperreactive nose** is one where the parasympathetic system is overactive, making the nose blocked and runny most of the time, or making it respond too readily to irritants, or both. This hyperreactivity occurs in any inflamed nose, adding to the misery of allergy sufferers.

For some patients, hyperreactivity in the nose, due to autonomic imbalance (see p227) is thought to be their primary problem. This hyperreactivity may even be the sole problem, or it may be accompanied by some inflammation as well. If hyperreactivity is the fundamental problem, then a diagnosis of **vasomotor rhinitis** is entirely appropriate: 'vasomotor' implies that the blockage of the nose is largely due to the action of the autonomic nerves on veins in the lining of the nose. Where the fault arises is unknown. It could originate in the part of the brain that controls the autonomic system.

With true vasomotor rhinitis, a runny and congested nose is usually the main symptom, with little sneezing or itchiness in the nose. Sometimes the blockage shifts from one nostril to another. Unlike allergic problems in the nose, vasomotor rhinitis usually comes on in adulthood, often in the elderly.

Unfortunately, the term 'vasomotor rhinitis' has been much abused in the past. If no infection or allergy could be identified in someone with rhinitis, and no other explanation could be found, it was assumed that the symptoms must be due to autonomic imbalance. This led to many people being wrongly diagnosed as having 'vasomotor rhinitis'. Some had what we would now call NARES (see p224). Others were allergic to something, but this had not been picked up by allergy tests for various reasons (see p243). Some had food intolerance (see p232).

Techniques of diagnosis have improved greatly in the past ten years, and this mislabelling is far less common now. Even so, it can still occur, since there is no way to show that a disorder is truly vasomotor rhinitis: a foolproof test cannot be devised because there is some degree of hyperreactivity in most forms of rhinitis. The doctor simply assumes that the patient has vasomotor rhinitis because all the other possibilities have been ruled out. For this reason, some specialists prefer to use the term **non-allergic rhinitis without eosinophilia**. It may be a mouthful, but at least it is an honest way of saying, 'We don't know what you've got, actually.'

Anyone diagnosed as having vasomotor rhinitis some years ago should ask to see a specialist again, especially if the treatment is not helping a great deal, or new problems have developed, such as asthma. If you have never had a sample taken from the nose, then the possibility of NARES (see p224) has not been ruled out.

For true vasomotor rhinitis, the modern form of treatment is an **anticholinergic drug**, one which largely blocks the action of the parasympathetic nervous system (see p226). The main drugs used are *atropine* and *ipratropium* (Rinatec), both given as nasal drops. In severe cases, which do not respond to this treatment, parasympathetic and sympathetic nerves leading to the nose can be cut, which gives complete and prompt relief. Sadly, the nerves grow back again within a year or two, so the operation has to be repeated. As it is quite a difficult operation, this treatment has fallen out of favour.

A simple form of self-help is to take some strenuous exercise. Any vigorous activity requires the sympathetic nervous system to come into play, and this has a beneficial side-effect in unblocking the nose. Obviously, you should take your exercise in clean air, away from potential irritants such as smoke.

These are the irritants that can provoke a reaction when there is hyperreactivity in the nose:

- cigarette smoke and other pollutants

- cold air, hot air or changes in temperature

- a change from damp to dry air, or vice versa

- some foods, particularly hot spicy ones

- alcoholic drinks

- bright lights

- strong smells such as those of perfume, flowers, wet paint or smoke

- emotional upsets

Although these are important in vasomotor rhinitis, remember that such hyperreactivity can also occur in any form of nasal disease.

There are certain specific diseases that seem to be forms of vasomotor rhinitis. One of these is **skier's nose**, a response to the cold dry air of the mountains. Although there are some inflammatory mediators released, the main reaction is probably hyperreactivity by the parasympathetic system. *Atropine* or *ipratropium* nose drops work well. A somewhat more embarrassing problem is **post-coital rhinitis**, which may be accompanied by post-coital asthma. This rare condition is apparently linked with anxieties and inhibitions about sex. The emotional disturbances seem to be responsible for triggering off reactions in the nose or bronchi. One patient had to be rushed to hospital late at night on several occasions, due to such an asthma attack. Counselling on sexual relationships is often helpful in the long term, but drugs can also be prescribed to cope with the immediate effects, particularly those of asthma.

NASAL MASTOCYTOSIS

This problem is thought to be very rare. It occurs in people with no sign of allergy whatever, yet they have very high numbers of mast cells in the nose. The problem may come on suddenly, and seem like 'a cold that never goes away'. For other people it begins gradually.

The rhinitis suffered by people with nasal mastocytosis is often made worse by drinking alchohol, or by exposure to smells such as turpentine and perfume. All these seem to act by triggering off the many mast cells in the nose, but again this is not an allergic reaction.

Antihistamines do not seem to work well for this disease, but *sodium cromoglycate* (see p87) may help.

RHINITIS CAUSED BY FOOD INTOLERANCE

Some people who have been told that they are suffering from 'perennial non-allergic rhinitis' or 'vasomotor rhinitis' are actually being affected by the food they eat. Because this relationship between food and the nose is not widely recognized by most conventional doctors, few patients with this problem get satisfactory treatment. And because the symptoms do not come on as soon as they eat the food, the patients themselves are generally unaware of the connection. However, they can diagnose themselves, and get rid of the symptoms, pretty easily.

The term that covers this reaction, and a number of other reactions to food (including asthma, migraine, irritable bowel syndrome and joint pains) is **food intolerance**. It should not be referred to as food allergy, although it often is, particularly by alternative practitioners. 'Allergy' should not be used since the mechanism is not clear – it could involve some allergic response, but other factors are likely to be at work as well. Skin-prick tests (see p78) for the foods are almost always negative, which sets it apart from true allergic reactions. Calling the reaction food allergy only perpetuates the problem of non-acceptance by mainstream medicine, since food allergy (see p160) is a clearly defined disease whose symptoms come on immediately and are largely different from food intolerance.

Food intolerance, as an explanation for your perennial rhinitis, is worth considering if:

- you have no positive skin-prick tests (see p78)

- you have positive skin-prick tests to pollen, but not to other allergens, yet your rhinitis continues to some extent all year round

MARY

Mary's allergic disposition showed up as a small child, when she suffered from eczema. The cause was never discovered, but she 'grew out of' the eczema within a few years. In her teens Mary developed hayfever and sinusitis, with the sinusitis persisting and becoming very painful, particularly in winter. In her early thirties, the sinusitis became much worse and reached a crisis on returning from a holiday abroad. An X-ray showed a build-up of fluid in the sinuses, which was causing the intense pain, and an operation was performed to drain the fluid away.

Despite this improvement, Mary was now suffering symptoms similar to hayfever all year round. There were occasions when the symptoms changed, or got worse, and Mary began to notice a certain pattern to these. Drinking wine, for example, was always followed by a badly blocked nose the following morning. A course of vitamin B tablets seemed to make her nose far more blocked and uncomfortable than usual. As an experiment, she tried stopping the tablets, and then restarting them a few days later – the severe symptoms in her nose followed suit. Her doctor could not make sense of these observations and referred her to a specialist. He realized that vitamin B tablets are often made from dried yeast, and wine is also rich in yeast. He suggested that Mary try a yeast-free diet for a while, cutting out bread, yeast extract, mushrooms, beer, wine, cider and certain other foods (see p237 for a complete list). The effect pleased Mary greatly: her nose was no longer blocked or runny, and she found that she also felt far more energetic than before.

By accident, she ate some gravy in a restaurant, not realizing that it would contain yeast extract. Within a few hours, she had developed severe symptoms in the nose, which lasted until the following day. Clearly, her year-round rhinitis was due to yeast sensitivity, and on the yeast-free diet Mary remained well. Later, she was able to return to a more normal diet by using neutralization therapy (see p141) for yeast. During the pollen season, her hayfever returned, but was not as severe as before.

- you are definitely not suffering from a prolonged infection (see pp221–2)

- there is no possibility of rhinitis medicamentosa (see p222) or any hormonal effect (see pp222–3)

- you have ruled out the possibility of irritants or allergens in the workplace causing your rhinitis (see p216)

- you are not suffering from the 'triad' of asthma, nasal polyps, and aspirin sensitivity (see p225)

You can test for food intolerance quite simply with an elimination diet. The diet suggested here is not a particularly restrictive one, and there is no need to consult your doctor before starting it, unless you are already under-nourished or seriously unwell. If you have ever suffered from *anorexia nervosa* you should have medical supervision when on the diet. Children can safely be put on this diet for a few weeks, as long as they are healthy and well fed at the outset, but if you identify problem foods, and decide to keep the child off them permanently, check with your doctor that the diet being eaten is adequate. It is all too easy for children to suffer nutritional deficiencies.

There are several other forms of elimination diet used, some of which permit very few foods at the outset, with the aim of identifying every possible food sensitivity, even the most unusual ones. (One of the best known is the lamb-and pears-diet.) While a diet of this type has its uses, we feel that a less restrictive diet will help almost everyone with food-induced rhinitis. Should the diet outlined here not help you, and you wish to try a more stringent diet, one is given in *The Complete Guide to Food Allergy and Intolerance* (see p318).

Exclusion phase
This is the first phase of the diet. For a week or so you cut out many of the foods you commonly eat – it is the everyday foods that are the usual offenders in food intolerance. The important point here is that you must stick to the diet absolutely. It is not like a slimming diet where the odd lapse is allowed. Not a molecule of the excluded foods must cross your lips.

The foods you must eliminate are:
Yeast and all yeast-containing foods (see Table 1)
Mushrooms and any other fungi
Wheat (which means anything made from flour, unless potato or rice flour)
Rye and oats

Maize (corn)
Milk
Cheese, butter, yoghurt and all milk products
Eggs
Fish
Citrus fruits (oranges, tangerines, lemons, grapefruit, etc.)
Peanuts
Tea
Coffee
Chocolate
Anything containing preservatives or colourings
Anything containing sulphur dioxide (see Appendix 8)
Sugar and honey, or any food containing them
Alcoholic drinks

You should add to this list any food that you are really 'addicted to', something you eat every day and cannot imagine going without. This may be the hardest part, but it could make all the difference: for some strange reason, those with food intolerance are often 'hooked' on their problem food.

These are the allowed foods:
Any kind of meat
Most fruit if peeled (but not citrus fruits, dried fruits or anything over-ripe because of yeast contamination)
Freshly squeezed fruit juice
All vegetables
Beans and lentils
Soya milk
Potatoes
Rice
Rice cakes (available from health-food shops and good as a temporary substitute for bread)
Rice noodles (try Chinese stores)
Buckwheat and buckwheat spaghetti (try health-food shops)
Yams
Sweet potatoes
Eddoes and Jerusalem artichokes
Milk-free margarine (also available in health-food shops; ordinary brands contain some milk)
Cooking oil, olive oil, nut oils
Almond butter, cashew butter (health-food shops)

Nuts, other than peanuts
Sunflower seeds and pumpkin seeds
Herb teas, other than redbush (rooitbosh) and maté

There is plenty here for a good healthy diet, and you are unlikely to be hungry if you approach the matter intelligently. Don't be in a rush to start – you need to plan for the diet in advance, and stock up on suitable foods, otherwise you can suddenly find yourself hungry and with nothing to hand that you are allowed. Bananas, nuts and seeds make good snacks to replace biscuits and cakes. Make sure that no great social events, such as Christmas or a wedding, are going to occur within the next ten weeks.

The best way to avoid mistakes is to cook your own food and keep meals plain and simple, using pure ingredients that are exactly what they seem. When eating out, have something simple like steak, chips and a salad. Anything 'instant' can be a source of forbidden food. Stock cubes, Bovril and packet soups contain yeast, for example, sauces contain flour or cornflour, while eggs and milk turn up in a variety of ways, and are often not named as such on the label. Certain packet foods, such as rice cakes, are acceptable because they contain just one ingredient. Avoid gluten-free breads and similar products at this stage.

For lunches at work, take food in a plastic container (e.g. a mixture of potatoes and stir-fried vegetables with beans or meat). Breakfast can seem problematic, especially if you dislike soya milk. One good substitute for conventional breakfast foods is pre-cooked rice, heated gently in a mixture of almond butter and cooking oil, with apples, bananas or other fruit added.

Pay special attention to avoiding yeast, as this is often the guilty party in rhinitis caused by food. Look at Table 1 and scrupulously avoid everything on it during the exclusion phase.

Be careful not to eat huge amounts of any one food, and try to keep meals varied. If you have a large appetite normally, overdoing one of the starchy foods is a risk. Try out some of the exotic substitutes, such as sweet potatoes, yams or millet. They are best if boiled first and then fried. Boiled millet can be mixed with a nut butter while still warm, then shaped into cakes and fried – another good breakfast food.

Possible outcome of the exclusion phase
Feeling much worse
This can happen, particularly in the first few days. Keep going: it is usually a sign that food intolerance is indeed your problem.

If you still feel terrible after ten days, then try reintroducing all the foods, but not tea, coffee, alcohol or sugar. Stay on this diet for several weeks and you will probably improve.

TABLE 1 FOODS CONTAINING YEAST

Main sources of yeast
Bread, including some pitta bread and pizza, but excluding soda
    bread, matzos and chapattis
Buns and cakes made with yeast, e.g. doughnuts
Yeast extract (Marmite, Vegemite, etc.)
Oxo cubes and most other stock cubes
Bovril
Anything labelled 'hydrolysed vegetable protein'
Beer, wine and cider
Vinegar and pickles
Sauerkraut
Vitamin tablets containing B vitamins, unless labelled 'yeast-free'

Secondary sources of yeast
Dried fruit
Over-ripe fruit
Any unpeeled fruit
Commercial fruit juices
Anything labelled 'malt'
Yoghurt, buttermilk and sour cream
Synthetic cream
Soy sauce
Tofu
Any leftover food, unless eaten within 24 hours, or 48 hours if in a
    refrigerator
Whisky, vodka, gin, brandy and other spirits

Other sources of fungi which may affect some people
Mushrooms, puffballs, truffles and other edible fungi
Quorn, mycoprotein (meat substitutes derived from fungi)
Cheese, especially Brie and Camembert

Yeasts and moulds in the air
You should stay away from damp houses, greenhouses (unless very
    dry and clean), compost heaps and rotting leaves. After you have
    been on the diet for a while, you can test whether such exposure
    makes you ill.

Feeling about the same
Keep going for two weeks. If at the end of that time your symptoms are unchanged, then it is unlikely that food is anything to do with them. (However, you could try a more stringent elimination diet to check other foods – see p234.)

Feeling partially better
Keep going for two weeks. If at the end of that time there is still only a partial improvement, try cutting out potatoes and any other food that you normally eat every day. Stay on the exclusion phase for another week. If there is no further improvement, you could try testing some foods (see below, under reintroduction phase). If your improvement is only slight, return to your ordinary diet and assume that food is not involved.

Feeling a lot better
This is a pretty clear sign that food is at fault, unless your symptoms tend to come and go a great deal anyway. When you have been feeling fine for four days, go on to the reintroduction phase. Do not delay for too long, or you may not get clear results.

Reintroduction phase
Continue with the same diet as during the exclusion phase, but reintroduce the following foods, recording those tested and any reappearance of symptoms in a notebook.

First test
Take two yeast tablets, or a spoonful of yeast extract. If you get no reaction, repeat every day for three days, stopping if a reaction occurs. Then leave a day without testing any food.

If nothing happens, you can relax the restrictions on yeast to some extent – you can eat unpeeled fruits, drink commercial fruit juices, and not worry about over-ripe fruit or leftovers (see Table 1). But do not reintroduce any major yeast-containing foods or alcoholic drinks.

Do not begin the second test if you still have any symptoms from the first. Allow at least one symptom-free day in between tests. This applies to all subsequent tests as well.

Second test
Drink a glass of milk, or eat some plain cottage cheese or cow's milk yoghurt. If you get no reaction, repeat every day for three days, stopping if a reaction occurs.

Leave a day without testing any food. Even if nothing happens, cut milk out again for now.

If you experience a very strong reaction to either yeast or milk, then you may prefer to cut short the testing programme. Among foods, these two are the most common cause of rhinitis, and often the sole offenders. If yeast provoked a reaction, consult Table 1 again to see which foods contain yeast, and omit all those for the moment. (You can experiment later with the ones that are only secondary sources of yeast, or only affect some people.) If milk brought on symptoms, consult Table 2 (see p241) for synonyms of milk used on packet labels and avoid these too. Apart from these restrictions, you can go back to a normal diet. In the unlikely event that your symptoms recur, you will need to cut everything out again, wait for the symptoms to die down, and then resume testing.

Third test
Eat four pieces of rye crispbread (it should be pure rye). If you get no reaction, repeat every day for three days, stopping if a reaction occurs.

Leave a day without testing any food. Even if nothing happens, cut rye out again for now.

Fourth test
Eat something that is pure wheat, such as pasta (check the label for other ingredients), Puffed Wheat or Shredded Wheat (you can moisten them with fruit juice, if necessary). Bulgar wheat could also be used for this test. If you get no reaction, repeat every day for three days, stopping if a reaction occurs.

Leave a day without testing any food. Even if nothing happens, cut wheat out again for now.

Fifth test
Eat some fish. If you get no reaction, repeat every day for three days, using a different type of fish each time, but stopping if a reaction occurs.

Leave a day without testing any food. Even if nothing happens, cut fish out again for now.

Sixth test
Eat two or more eggs, cooked in any way you like. If you get no reaction, repeat every day for three days, stopping if a reaction occurs. Leave a day without testing any food.

At this point you have tested most of the likely culprits and you can reintroduce any food that caused no problem when tested, to give yourself a more normal diet. (If you proved sensitive to yeast but not to wheat, you can eat soda bread, matzos and chapattis. Consult Table 1 again to see which foods are a source of yeast and should therefore be avoided. At a later date you can experiment with the secondary sources of yeast, to see if you are able to tolerate these.)

Eat this new and more relaxed diet for a week. You should remain well, in which case you can continue testing foods. (If you relapse, which is most unlikely, then you need to cut all the foods out, wait for the symptoms to clear again, and start retesting. This time, test each food for a week before going on to the next.)

During this week you should, at some point, test out sulphur dioxide. This is a mild irritant given off by several foods, which can provoke rhinitis in sensitive people. Assuming you are not sensitive to yeast, try chewing some uncooked dried apricots or sultanas (not if they are labelled 'unsulphured' or 'no preservatives', nor if they are very dark in colour, which is a sign that sulphur dioxide has not been used). If you are sensitive to yeast, then buy Campden tablets (sold to home wine-makers) from the chemist, dissolve in warm water, and sniff the fumes coming off. Should either of these tests produce your symptoms, you are almost certainly sensitive to sulphur dioxide and you should refer to Appendix 8 for the foods that can produce this gas.

Assuming you have stayed well while eating your expanded diet for a week, continue testing the remaining foods, with three days for each. Once they have been tested, cut the foods out again, even if they caused no reaction.

Seventh test

If you did not react to rye or wheat, you can reintroduce oats without testing them. If you *did* react to rye or wheat, test oats either using porridge, or using oatcakes (make sure they contain no forbidden ingredients). If you never normally eat oats, don't bother to test them, unless you are keen to have them as a substitute for wheat.

Eighth test

Test oranges, satsumas, tangerines and clementines. If you have discovered that you are yeast-sensitive, use fresh fruit only. Should you prove tolerant of oranges and their kin, introduce lemons and grapefruit the next day. If there is no reaction, then leave one test-free day and continue.

Ninth test

Test peanuts using plain salted peanuts (not dry-roasted) or plain peanut butter as sold in wholefood shops. Eat a good handful of nuts, or a thick spread of peanut butter.

TABLE 2 SYNONYMS FOR FOOD INGREDIENTS

The following synonyms may be used on food labels:

Baking powder	May contain maize (corn)
Casein, caseinate	Milk
Cereal binder	Usually wheat
Cereal filler	Usually wheat
Cereal protein	Usually wheat
Cereal starch	Usually wheat or maize (corn)
Corn meal	Maize
Corn starch	Maize
Corn syrup	Maize
Dextrose	A type of sugar, derived from maize
Edible starch	Usually wheat or maize (corn)
Flour	Usually wheat flour
Food starch	Usually wheat or maize (corn)
Fructose	A type of sugar
Glucose syrup	A type of sugar, usually derived from maize (corn)
Hydrolysed protein	Usually yeast
Hydrolysed vegetable protein	Usually yeast
Lactalbumin	Milk
Lactose	Milk sugar
Leavening	Yeast
Lecithin	Usually egg or soya
Maltose	A type of sugar
Miso	Soya
Modified starch	Usually wheat or maize (corn)
Ovalbumin	Egg
Starch	Usually wheat or maize (corn)
Sucrose	Sugar
Textured vegetable protein	Soya
Tofu	Soya
Vegetable gum	Can be soya or maize (corn)
Vegetable oil	Usually a mixture of oils, often including corn (maize) oil
Vegetable protein	Usually soya
Vegetable starch	Can be soya or maize (corn)
Whey	Milk

In some foods labelled 'no added sugar' apple juice could be considered as a synonym for sugar because highly concentrated apple juice has been used to sweeten the product.

Tenth test
If you were not affected by milk, yoghurt or cottage cheese, then test ordinary cheeses (but not Brie or Camembert if you have proved to be yeast-sensitive; you can experiment with these later).

Eleventh test
Test maize by eating a large portion of frozen sweetcorn.

Twelfth test
Whether or not you were sensitive to yeast, test mushrooms, trying different kinds (button, field, etc.).

Any of this second batch of foods that proved harmless can now be reintroduced. This means that (with the exception of foods that produced symptoms) you are on a normal diet apart from alcohol, sugar, tea, coffee, chocolate, and certain additives (preservatives and colours). Add each of these back into the diet at the rate of one a week.

With alcohol, try a small tot of pure spirit such as vodka or white rum on the first day, whisky on the second, sherry on the third, wine on the fourth, beer on the fifth, and so on. Obviously, if you are yeast-sensitive, beer, wine and cider are unlikely to be tolerated, but you may wish to test spirits. If you proved sensitive to sulphur dioxide, you may also have problems with these drinks (see Appendix 8).

At the end of the reintroduction phase you should know what foods bring on your nasal problems (and you may have found that some other ailments were also related to food). Avoid those foods for at least six months, using Table 2 to spot hidden ingredients in packaged foods. After about six months, you can retest each of the incriminated foods, to see if you still react to them. If you do react, then try again six months later. If not, you can begin eating them once every four days or so. Continue in this way for a year, then increase the frequency a little if you like. Some people can go back to eating the food normally, but most find that they can never eat the food every day again, nor in large amounts. If symptoms recur, cut out the culprit foods entirely for a couple of months.

If you find it very difficult to avoid your problem foods, you could try neutralization therapy (see p141) or enzyme-potentiated desensitization (see p139). Both of these have been tried and work well with food intolerance. Nose drops containing *sodium cromoglycate* (see p87) may also help.

The reintroduction phase for foods should take about eight weeks. If it takes any longer than this (because you get flu in the middle, for example) then there is a risk of lost sensitivity – the food-intolerant person becomes less reactive after avoiding the culprit food for a time. If you are still testing foods after eight weeks, you should eat each test food every day for a week, rather than for three days.

RHINITIS DUE TO UNDETECTED AIRBORNE ALLERGENS

This is possible with both perennial rhinitis and seasonal rhinitis (see below).

There are two ways in which allergies can go undetected. First, if patients are allergic to something that no one tests for, their sensitivity will not be detected (see pp81–4). Rare pollen allergens (see pp4–7) or insect allergens (see p83 and 212) are the most likely candidates here, and both could cause either perennial or seasonal symptoms. Second, some people with genuine allergic reactions to common allergens fail to react to the usual tests. It seems that they have the allergy antibody IgE in the nose and nowhere else, causing both skin tests and blood tests to be negative. For these patients the allergy will be revealed only by nasal provocation testing – something that a consultant allergist can carry out. Ask for a referral to someone who can do such a test.

One good (but not foolproof) sign is violent sneezing on waking up. This rarely occurs with non-allergic rhinitis but is often seen with allergy to house-dust mite.

In a situation where your opinion differs from that of the doctor treating you, there is a case for being persistent and seeking a second or even a third opinion. Occasionally, patients with genuine allergies have only got the treatment they needed by such persistence. However, you should also keep an open mind about the possible cause of your illness, and be prepared to accept that it may, after all, be non-allergic.

SEASONAL NON-ALLERGIC RHINITIS

This is a disease that does not appear in the medical textbooks, since in theory it does not exist! All seasonal rhinitis is assumed to be allergic. However, researchers in Sweden have found people with all the symptoms of spring hayfever, but no allergic response to pollen or other likely allergens. There are occasional reports from other parts of the world as well. The possible explanations for this problem (apart from undetected allergy – see above) are as follows:

• the nose is hyperreactive (see p227), particularly to volatile chemicals (see p120) given off from plants, e.g. from birch twigs, tree buds or perfumed flowers

- there is no allergy to pollen, but the grains are acting as an irritant; this has been demonstrated with pine pollen, which has large grains and is very abundant in the air, allowing large amounts to be inhaled

- pollen grains are carrying pollutants which irritate the nose

- there is food intolerance (see p232) to something eaten only in summer (such as fresh strawberries) or to something eaten much more then (such as additives or colouring in orange squash)

- there is a reaction to an irritant that is more common in the air in summer, such as ozone (see p319). This explanation is just speculative at present.

Chapter Fourteen

AVOIDING ALLERGIES IN YOUR CHILD

Most people want a better life for their children, and those with severe hayfever will surely hope that their children can be spared the same fate. Unfortunately, you cannot take any measures that will guarantee a hayfever-free future for your child, but you can reduce the chances of their developing the same disease.

To try and prevent hayfever alone is not a logical approach, however. What is passed on from parent to child is a general tendency to allergy, called **atopy** (see p39). Your children will not necessarily inherit this allergic predisposition, but if they do, it could appear in a variety of ways – as eczema, for example, or perennial rhinitis, asthma or food allergy. If you have hayfever, there is a *slightly* greater chance that your children (if atopic) will have hayfever rather than one of these other allergic diseases, but it would make no sense to take precautions against hayfever alone. For this reason, the measures outlined here are those that will minimize the chance of allergic reactions in general, not just reactions to pollen.

What is the chance of your child inheriting the allergic tendency? It is impossible to say exactly, but where one parent has allergies, the child has roughly a 20–40 per cent chance of developing them. The chance is higher if it is the mother who is allergic. Where both parents have allergies, the figure is 40–60 per cent, but higher if it is the same *type* of allergic reaction in both, that is, both have asthma, or both have hayfever: for these children the risk is 60–80 per cent. Where neither parent has allergies, but one of their children does, then a new baby has a 25–35 per cent risk. Should there be a large number of other close relatives with allergies, you can assume that the risk is higher.

A difficult birth may make allergy more likely, while low birth weight with a slow increase in weight just after birth can be a sign of greater susceptibility to allergy.

You need to make a rough assessment of the risk to your baby, bearing all these factors in mind, and then decide just how careful you should be in protecting the child from allergens. Few people will feel able to take all the precautions described here, but do what you can.

There is a test that can be done at birth, where some blood is taken from the umbilical cord, and the amount of IgE measured. IgE is the antibody that plays a key role in allergy (see p31) and a high level indicates that the child is definitely at risk. This test is not done routinely in Britain, but if you ask the hospital it may be possible to arrange. Blood tests for IgE can also be carried out on the baby after birth. A high level of IgE would indicate that it was worth taking the more difficult measures described here.

Some forward planning is helpful in allergy avoidance, and it is valuable to start thinking about the matter well before you get pregnant. (However, there is still a great deal you can do if you are pregnant as you read this, or even if the baby has already been born.) The most crucial period for allergy prevention is from birth to about one year of age. Reducing exposure to allergens during this time can drastically reduce the risk of allergies. One recent study, which employed only some of the measures described here, saved two out of three susceptible children from developing allergies in their first year of life.

MEASURES TO TAKE BEFORE BECOMING PREGNANT

First, you can plan the timing of your child's birth. There is some evidence that being born during or just before the pollen season increases the risk of hayfever. The effect is strongest for tree pollens, notably birch, but it may also be a factor in allergy to grasses and ragweed. Low-risk months are those just after the pollen season. High-risk months are the season itself and two to three months beforehand. It seems that babies are most vulnerable to sensitization by pollen in the first three to six months of life. Use Appendix 1 to check when the main pollen seasons occur.

As the effect of birth timing is not that great, you should not worry too much if you fail to get it right. However, if you are aiming for a birth in, say, August or September, to avoid the grass-pollen season, and it actually works out at December or January, you are still giving the baby some protection from pollen. Should your plans not work out at all and the baby is born at the worst time of year, then you could consider using an air filter or other measures (see p114) which would at least reduce the pollen levels indoors.

Another aspect of forward planning is to make sure you do not move house or undertake major structural work just before the birth. A remarkable number of parents do fall into this trap by realizing that they will need more living space only after the baby is conceived. The hazards of renovation include the stirring up of house dust, which contains a rich variety of allergens, and the release of many mould spores into the air. There are ways of partially combating these hazards, by using air filters and cleaning up carefully (see p186), but it is much better not to create the problem in the first place. Plastering or laying concrete floors will establish a reservoir of water in the house that continues to ooze moisture into the air for up to a year afterwards (see p199). This affects both new and renovated houses. If you have already got into this situation, and the baby is due during the autumn or winter, a dehumidifier may be the only option to keep the humidity down. Moisture promotes the growth of both moulds (see p193) and house-dust mite (see p172).

Should your house be suffering from damp penetration or condensation, sort such problems out as soon as you can (see p195). Bringing a baby home to a severely damp house is taking an unnecessary risk with its health.

Mothers who smoke should stop before becoming pregnant. Smoking has a variety of bad effects on an unborn child, but one of them is to increase the risk of allergies. Since there must be no tobacco smoke in the house once the baby is born, it is as well for the father to give up at the same time. Advice on this is given on p321.

The drug *metoprolol* is also thought to increase the risk of allergies in children if taken by their mothers while pregnant. The drug is sold under a variety of trade names: Betaloc, Co-Betaloc, Lopresor and Lopresoretic.

Finally, mothers with allergies should also bear in mind certain other risks to the baby. If you suffer from asthma, it is important that you get the best possible treatment for it during pregnancy (see p108). Some antihistamines carry a small risk of causing deformities in unborn children, so you should stop taking them several weeks before becoming pregnant (see p108).

MEASURES TO TAKE DURING PREGNANCY

There is no need for the expectant mother to avoid any allergens while pregnant – various studies have looked at this and shown that it has few benefits. Some babies do become sensitized while in the womb to foods eaten by the mother, but this occurs so rarely that it is not considered worth putting pregnant mothers on a special diet. The important thing to do at this stage is to prepare the house for its new inhabitant, reducing the allergens to levels that will not sensitize the baby.

With airborne allergens, the levels needed to sensitize someone (that is, to start up an allergic reaction) are much higher than the levels needed to produce symptoms in someone who is already sensitized. So the actions you need to take against dust mites, for example, are not as drastic as those needed by someone with a severe allergy to mites.

Reducing damp in the house

Minimizing damp is an important part of the battle against both dust mites and moulds. Once the baby is born, there will be a lot of washing to dry, which can increase the amount of moisture in the house at the very moment when you most want to keep it down. Before the baby arrives, organize a good method of drying clothes, particularly if the baby is due in the autumn or winter, or if you have nowhere to dry clothes outside. A spin-drier is helpful, as it spins faster than the spin cycle of a washing machine and will therefore take out far more water. If you can afford either a tumble-drier or a clothes-drying cabinet, this would be a good investment. Make sure it is vented to the outside. A cheaper alternative is to dry clothes in a porch, conservatory or utility room, but it must have good ventilation so that the moisture goes outside rather than coming in. If this is not possible, dry clothes in a room that has some heating and a partially open window, keeping the door closed to prevent the moist air travelling into other rooms.

If your house is well insulated and draught-free, get into the habit of increasing the ventilation so that the air inside is drier (see p175). The sooner you begin to do this the better.

Specific action against dust mites

For a baby, dust mites are a major source of allergic problems. Reducing mite allergens to a minimum will be one of the most worthwhile measures you can take in lowering the risk of allergy.

Making sure that the newborn's mattress and bedding are free from mite allergens is a simple matter (see p188), and if you can manage no other changes around the house, at least take this step.

It is also valuable to reduce mite allergens in carpets, since the child will start to play on them when a few months old. Simply increasing the ventilation in the house and taking other measures against damp, will do quite a lot to combat mites. If you have begun this early on in pregnancy, the mite levels will have been declining for many months before the baby arrives. Thorough vacuuming must also be carried out to remove the existing reservoir of mite allergens. Fitting a filter to the vacuum cleaner (see p308) is advisable to ensure that the allergens are not dispersed into the air.

If you have increased the ventilation, and are reluctant to take further steps unless absolutely necessary, you could test the carpets after a few months to see how high the levels of mite allergen are. There is a special test kit available for this (see p310). Use it to look at the living-room carpet, and any carpets or rugs in the room where the baby will sleep. At the same time, test the upholstered furniture. If the level of infestation is any greater than 'light', then you should take further measures against dust mites. The best kinds of treatment for houses with babies and small children are described on p188.

Avoiding animal allergens

Being exposed to a cat or dog during the first year of life greatly increases the chance of developing an allergic reaction to these animals. The same is almost certainly true of cagebirds, rabbits, guinea pigs, mice and other small animals, although no specific surveys have been carried out.

If you already have a pet you should either part with it, or at least keep it out of house for the first year. This may be a very difficult decision, but it could make an enormous difference to your child's future. An allergy to pets can be a great social problem for a child, making it impossible to visit friends or relatives who have pets. Sometimes the sensitivity is so great that the child even reacts to the clothing of people who have a cat or dog.

If you really cannot face the idea of losing your pet, or exiling it to the garden shed for a year, then there are other measures you can take, although these are much less satisfactory (see pp208–211).

In the case of cats, once they have departed, a thorough clean-up of the house is recommended (see p207), as the allergens get everywhere. With a dog, removing or washing its bedding followed by vigorous vacuum cleaning of the carpets and upholstery should be sufficient.

Whether an allergy-prone family should acquire pets later, once the youngest child has passed its first birthday, is a matter of debate. Some doctors would say that they definitely should not. However, the risks are lower for older children, so you may want to take a chance, accepting that, if one of the children develops an allergy to the pet, it will have to go to another home.

Reducing pollutants in the home

Any decorating that needs doing should be completed some months before the baby is due. All too often fathers decorate the nursery while the mother is in the labour ward, and the baby comes home to a room smelling of fresh paint. If the decorating has to be done less than eight weeks before the baby is due, use a low-odour paint – these are now widely available.

Tobacco smoke is one of the worst pollutants that a baby can be exposed to, making asthma far more likely. Even though both parents have stopped smoking, there may be problems with guests. The best way to deal with this is to designate a 'smoking room' well away from the baby. An ionizer or air filter (see p298) in this room will clear the smoke from the air and prevent it seeping into the rest of the house.

A gas cooker in a poorly ventilated kitchen can be a source of nitrogen dioxide. This gas, if it becomes sufficiently concentrated, may increase the chance of a child developing an allergic reaction to an allergen in the air (see p61). Consider installing an extractor fan. Old-fashioned paraffin heaters also generate nitrogen dioxide, and should be replaced with some other form of heating.

Formaldehyde acts as an irritant to the airways, and you should consider whether there may be high levels in your home (see p215). Unpainted chipboard, blockboard and plywood could be painted to reduce the amount of formaldehyde being given off. Simply increasing ventilation will reduce the level of this pollutant.

There are other potential sources of irritants to the nose and airways, such as air fresheners, polish, white spirit and cleaning fluids. Eradicate these as far as possible (see p321).

Preparing yourself for breastfeeding

Breastfeeding is thought to help in preventing allergies in babies, particularly a bad reaction to cow's milk. There is a great deal of controversy about how much difference breastfeeding makes, so the advice given here is based on the best evidence available at present.

On one point there is no doubt: the practice of giving 'supplementary' or 'complementary' bottle feeds to newborn babies while in hospital carries a risk of sensitizing them to cow's milk. Unfortunately, this practice is still routine in some hospitals, and the mother is usually unaware that the bottle feed has been given. Sometimes cow's milk is the first food a newborn baby receives.

As early as possible in your pregnancy, find out about the policy on supplementary feeds in the hospital where you will give birth. Make it very clear to the midwife that you do not wish your baby to have anything but breast milk. Ask whether you will be able to have your baby with you and feed it on demand – that way you will be able to ensure that it is not given a bottle. Feeding on demand is also far more conducive to establishing successful breastfeeding than a system that is ruled by the clock. Putting the baby to the breast soon after birth, within four hours at most, is also important in establishing successful breastfeeding, and you should ask about hospital policy on this.

If the hospital will not allow the child to sleep beside you, then you should ask that a notice be put on the baby's cot, stating that bottle feeds must not be given. In a recent British study, doctors who were trying to compare the effects of breastfeeding with bottle feeding found their efforts unintentionally thwarted by nurses giving bottles to babies who should have been breastfed only. Giving bottles to all babies was just part of the normal routine. They discovered that notices on the cots were the only way to ensure this did not happen – so be prepared to stick your neck out a little, if necessary, and insist on your rights.

Where there is a hospital policy of not putting babies to the breast during the night, breast milk can be 'expressed' and stored, to be given from a bottle by a nurse. However, this is a somewhat unsatisfactory solution for the newborn baby, because it is easier to suck milk from a bottle than a breast, so the baby learns to suck less hard. Since the intensity of sucking influences the amount of milk produced, a mother may begin to produce less milk under this system (see below).

If your enquiries about feeding policy at the hospital are not being treated sympathetically, ask to speak to the head of the maternity unit.

As well as finding out about the hospital, you should learn as much as you can about breastfeeding before you give birth. Since breastfeeding is a natural process, it is often assumed that it 'comes naturally'. Unfortunately, this is not always the case, and many mothers give up because they have not been shown how to breastfeed properly, or because they have sore nipples, or as a result of other problems. These problems can be overcome, but nursing staff generally find it more convenient to fall back on bottle feeds. The idea that some mothers 'don't have enough milk' is a prevalent one, but the truth is that the supply is established by the demand – that is, by the intensity with which the baby sucks. If the breastfeeding relationship between mother and baby has been established properly, there is unlikely to be any problem with the amount of milk produced. Several voluntary organizations, which are committed to helping women breastfeed, can give you advice and support. Some have local advisers who will happily visit you at home. Contact one of these before you give birth; addresses are given on p318.

MEASURES TO TAKE AFTER THE BIRTH

If breastfeeding is not possible, for whatever reason, you should not feel guilty about the situation. Fortunately, there are alternatives which carry less risk of allergy than standard infant formulas. These are feed mixtures known as **hydrolysates** which are available on prescription. They are made from either cow's milk or soya protein which has been treated to break up the allergens. When broken up into smaller pieces, the proteins are far less allergenic. Consequently, these hydrolysates are far safer than ordinary cow's milk formulas, although a tiny minority of children do react to them. Note that soya hydrolysates are *not* the same as standard soya formulas, where the soya allergens have not been broken up: children can become sensitized to these intact soya allergens in time.

If you have established successful breastfeeding, continue it for as long as you can, preferably for six months, although continuing for four or five months is also valuable. Do not give any solids until the baby is at least four months old. Should the baby seem to need extra food, a hydrolysate formula can be used (see above). Learning to express and store breast milk will give you some much needed freedom during this time; breastfeeding advice groups can help with this.

When you do introduce solid foods, do so gradually, so that breast milk still supplies most of the child's needs. If some breastfeeding can be continued until the child is a year old, so much the better.

When it comes to introducing new foods, those with low allergenic potential should be given at first, and the foods that most often produce allergic reactions withheld for a time. The main problem foods are eggs, milk (including all milk products such as butter, yoghurt, cheese and cottage cheese), fish, peanuts, wheat, rye, barley, nuts, soya (including all soya products such as tofu and soya milk), citrus fruits and chocolate. Delay introducing the baby to these foods until at least nine months old, and then introduce them slowly, one per week. If there are any reactions to the foods, or if the child shows an intense dislike of them, take them off the menu again. Keep eggs and foods containing peanut until last.

Another measure that can have some benefit in reducing allergies is for a breastfeeding mother to avoid certain foods herself, especially those containing the most powerful allergens. Small amounts of food allergen do pass unchanged from the mother's stomach into her breast milk, and these can sensitize some children who are prone to allergy. The foods to avoid are milk and all milk products, eggs, fish and peanuts.

Restricting your diet in this way while breastfeeding and caring for a baby can prove too much of a burden, but try it for a while and see if you can cope. To get the maximum benefit you should continue avoiding these foods until the child is eating them as solids. If you cannot manage this, simply avoiding the foods for a month or two may be helpful. Always check packaged food to see that it does not contain milk or eggs (and see the synonyms for these foods, given in Table 2, p241). Calcium gluconate tablets can be prescribed to make up for the lack of calcium in a milk-free diet.

A breastfed baby who develops colic may be reacting to traces of food allergens in its mother's milk. If you are breastfeeding, but not restricting your diet, and the baby becomes colicky, try cutting out milk, eggs, fish and peanuts for a week. This will often cure the colic. If there is no improvement, eliminate soya, chocolate, all nuts, wheat and citrus fruits as well.

The measures for reducing dampness and combating house-dust mite, already described in Chapter Twelve, should continue for the first year of the baby's life, and longer if possible. When soft toys are bought, make sure that they are ones which can be laundered easily.

For as long as possible, keep the baby away from areas of high traffic pollution when outdoors.

APPENDIX 1
Pollen seasons around the world

The authors would like to acknowledge the help of Dr Jean Emberlin, of the Pollen Research Unit at the University of North London, in compiling these lists, and to thank Professor Eugenio Dominguez-Vilches of the University of Cordoba for supplying information on behalf of REA (Spanish Aerobiology Network). Special mention should also be made of Professor Walter H. Lewis and Dr Prathiba Vinay of Washington University, whose excellent publications on allergenic pollen, both in the USA and around the world, have been immensely useful as a source of reference.

THE REGIONAL LISTINGS

The regions of the world are dealt with in the following order:

USING THIS APPENDIX

The information given here can be useful in several different ways, as follows. For most people, planning hayfever-free holidays will probably be the most important consideration.

Diagnosis

By comparing the time when you suffer symptoms with the pollen seasons given for the area where you live, you may be able to identify the particular pollen or pollens responsible for your hayfever. This can help in everyday pollen avoidance (see Chapter Eight), although it is not essential.

Identification of the pollen allergen *is* essential before any type of desensitization treatment (see Chapter Nine), but in this case a skin-prick test (see p78) or other diagnostic test must be used beforehand for precise diagnosis.

In trying to pinpoint the source of your problems, bear in mind that you may be sensitive to more than one type of pollen. Sensitivity to mould spores (see p193) can also confuse the picture as these sometimes produce seasonal symptoms. You could be sensitive to mould spores alone, or to both mould spores and pollen. Mould spores are not included in these lists, but spore counts are given on some pollen information telephone lines (see p316).

Allergies to other airborne allergens, such as house-dust mite (see p172) or animal proteins and skin particles (see pp201–213) can produce year-round symptoms. These are frequently milder than hayfever. If your 'hayfever' drags on for much of the year, but is worst in one of the pollen seasons identified below, this may be the explanation.

The information given here is fairly

generalized, and local features (such as mountain ranges or forestry plantations) can make enormous differences to the pollen in the air. A local doctor or allergist may have more specialized knowledge of potentially allergenic pollens in your immediate area. See your doctor if you feel you need more guidance, or a skin-prick test to confirm the diagnosis.

The dates given here may not hold true in every year. Changes in the seasonal weather can affect the timing of pollination; in temperate climates, for example, a warm spring will advance the grass pollen season by as much as three weeks.

Bear in mind that there are also 'minority interest' pollens, which cause problems for a few people only. These are not included here. However, you are very unlikely to react to a pollen of this type unless you are *also* sensitive to another pollen that *is* a major allergen (that is, if you are already disposed to react allergically to pollens). The exception to this rule arises when people are breathing in huge amounts of a 'minority' pollen, either at home or at work. This can happen when people work with plants or cut flowers or live close to fields or orchards where a single crop is grown (see pp5–7). It can occasionally affect gardeners who are keen growers of one type of plant.

Getting away from your problem pollen

The lists in this appendix can also be used to show where you will find lower concentrations of your problem pollen, if you need to 'escape' during the pollen season. Again, keep in mind that this information is generalized and does not cover local variations. In some countries there are specialized sources of information which can supply more details about pollen seasons in different parts of the world (see p316 for addresses of these).

Also remember that an unusual variation in the weather can change the timing of the pollen season in your 'retreat' area. These changes should not be more than a week or two, however. Allow a margin of error of two weeks on any of the dates given below.

People with very severe hayfever are sometimes driven to moving house, or even emigrating. The list following can

help you to choose a new home area, but more specialist advice is definitely advisable in this case. If you are already very allergic to one pollen, the chance of developing a new sensitivity to a different pollen is fairly high. Such sensitivities generally appear within two to three years of arriving in a new area. The more potently allergenic the pollen, the more likely a new sensitivity, so areas with high pollen counts for particularly notorious allergens (e.g. ragweed, birch, grasses or pellitory) should be avoided.

Planning holidays

Before making any travel arrangements, always check the regional lists. Choosing the right time of the year can make all the difference to your holiday.

Local variations are again important here, and are not covered in the lists below. For example, one side of a holiday island may have much higher pollen counts than the other, while mountain areas may be lower (or higher) in certain pollens. If you are in any doubt, seek more detailed information from specialized sources (see p316).

Using the lists

The grasses, including grass crops, are dealt with first in all regions. These are followed by trees and tree crops, then shrubs and hedging plants. Next crops such as sunflowers are listed in the few countries where these are relevant. Finally 'weeds' (wild plants other than trees and grasses) are dealt with.

Within these categories the most likely allergens are dealt with first, to help you pinpoint your culprit pollen, if this is your objective. More detailed information is given about the major allergens, less about the minor ones.

If travelling you should look for your problem plant using the common name first, then using the scientific name. Many common names differ around the world, especially in the USA. For example, sagebrush is a cause of hayfever in parts of the USA. It belongs to the same genus (*Artemisia*) as the mugworts and wormwoods found elsewhere in the world, and almost certainly shares their allergens. By looking down the list for *Artemisia* you would be able to locate this plant. Where possible, alternative common names have been included.

Sometimes travellers who are already sensitized to a plant in their home country may react to small amounts of that pollen abroad, whereas the levels are too low to sensitize local people. (The presence or absence of a powerful allergen which can provoke cross-reactions, such as ragweed, may also make a difference. This is the case with dandelion and goldenrod, for example – see p158.) To help travellers, plants that are common allergens worldwide have generally been included in the lists, even if they cause little or no hayfever in the region where they are listed. While every effort has been made to give complete coverage in this respect, there may be a few omissions due to lack of information, because pollens that are locally unimportant as allergens may not be recorded. Additionally, pollens that are known as allergens in certain countries but do not cause much hayfever worldwide – e.g. those of willows, poplars, elms, maples, limes (lindens and basswoods), chestnut trees, horse chestnut trees, plane trees, walnut trees, elder, privet, heather, goldenrod, cocklebur and dandelion – are not always included. They appear in those areas where *are* significant allergens, and in the list for the British Isles if there is a chance of the pollen being encountered (to help readers who may have been sensitized elsewhere), but not in other lists. If you are allergic to the pollen of one of these plants, you may want to check further with a specialist advice service (see p316). This is also advisable for areas where a brief summary, rather than a list of plants, is given.

BRITAIN AND IRELAND

Grasses (Gramineae or Poaceae)

May to July
Grasses are the prime cause of hayfever in the British Isles. About twelve major species seem to be responsible, and most patients react to several of these.

The grass pollen season usually begins first along the warm coasts of Cornwall, west Cork, west Kerry and southwest Clare, sometimes at the beginning of May. A week later, southern Britain, the Midlands, Wales, East Anglia, and the southwestern counties of Ireland, follow suit. Much of the north of England, and all the rest of Ireland begin a week later still. Another week passes before pollination begins in Durham, Northumberland and much of Scotland. The highlands of Scotland follow on a week later, but the extreme north, beyond Loch Shin, waits another week. In all, there may be a five-week difference between the southwest tip of Cornwall and Ireland, and the extreme north of Scotland. However, the pollen season ends in the north only a week or two later than in the south, so the season in the extreme north is substantially shorter. In southern Britain the pollen peak is usually in the second week of June, and this is when most people suffer symptoms. A warm spring, with temperatures above average in March, April and the first half of May, will bring the pollen season on earlier.

There are some variations from one region to another. Cities surrounded by countryside, such as Cardiff and Glasgow, show higher pollen counts than extensive conurbations such as London. Pollen counts are usually lower at the tops of mountains, and on breezy coasts.

Birches (*Betula*)

April to May
Birches are the trees most likely to cause hayfever. They include downy birch, silver birch, and various introduced species grown in gardens. Some people show cross-reactions (see p154) with alder and hazel, which belong to the same plant family (see below).

Alder, hornbeam and hazel (*Alnus, Carpinus* and *Corylus*)

February to April
Birch-sensitive people who also react to alder and/or hazel may experience symptoms before the birch season begins. For hazel, pollination is usually in March, but can be as early as the beginning of February, or even January in a mild winter. (In a few sheltered gardens, it can begin in December.) Alder pollen comes out later than hazel, in March or April. Hornbeam pollen is very scarce in some years, abundant in others.

Oaks and beeches (*Quercus* and *Fagus*)

April to May
These trees affect a certain number of people in Britain. The allergens in the pollen can cross-react with those of birch (see p154).

Ash trees (*Fraxinus*)

April to May
Not a particularly strong allergen, but those already sensitive to olive pollen may become allergic to it through a cross-reaction (see p155).

Poplars and willows (*Populus* and *Salix*)

March to May
Pollen counts are generally moderate. Probably affect relatively few people in Britain, but considered important allergens in the USA.

Plane trees (*Platanus*)

April to May
Particularly common in London and some other cities where they may cause a certain amount of hayfever. In general, however, pollen counts are low and they affect relatively few people. Planes are considered important allergens in parts of France and around the Mediterranean.

Maples and sycamore (*Acer*)

April to May
Not considered a source of hayfever in the British Isles (unlike the USA) and pollen counts are low. The most allergenic of the maples, the wind-pollinated box elder or ash-leaved maple (*Acer negundo*), is grown in parks and gardens but is not thought to cause hayfever in Britain; it flowers in early March.

Lime trees (*Tilia*)

June to July
Not a common cause of hayfever, although a few people may be sensitized. Pollination is by insects and the pollen does not generally travel very far on the wind. Pollen counts are low to moderate, but may be high near the trees.

Horse chestnuts (*Aesculus*)

April to May
Not considered a source of hayfever in the British Isles, but gives some positive skin-prick tests among birch-sensitive patients in Scandinavia, and reported as an allergen in Turkey. Pollen counts are moderate and may be high in the vicinity of the trees.

Elms (*Ulmus*)

February to March
Not thought to cause any hayfever in Britain, but elms are considered allergenic in the USA and (to a lesser extent) in the Netherlands. Pollen counts in Britain are low to moderate.

Walnut trees (*Juglans*)

May to June
Not believed to cause any hayfever in Britain, and pollen counts are low. Walnuts do cause problems in the USA, probably due to cross-reactions from the more allergenic pollens of hickories and pecans.

Chestnut trees (*Castanea*)

June to July
Pollination does not begin until late June. Chestnuts are not believed to cause hayfever in Britain, though they do in parts of Europe, owing largely to cross-reactions with birch. Cross-reactions with oak and beech are also likely. Chestnuts are fairly widespread in southern England, less common elsewhere. Pollen counts are low.

Pines (Pinaceae)

April to May
Unknown as a cause of hayfever in Britain, but there is ample pollen in the air, which might affect visitors from other countries who are already sensitized.

Cypresses (Cupressaceae)

April, June
Although these grow widely in Britain, there is very little pollen in the air. Not a cause of hayfever locally and unlikely to affect those sensitized elsewhere.

Japanese red cedar (*Cryptomeria japonica*)

February
Grown as an ornamental tree in some parks; has also been tried as a timber tree and a few small plantations remain in parts of Devon, for example. The tree is uncommon except in the west of Britain. Pollen counts are negligible except in the immediate vicinity of the trees.

Privet (*Ligustrum*)

May to June
One species grows wild and another is used very widely for hedging (although regularly clipped hedges do not flower). Pollen counts are very low. A rare cause of hayfever in the British Isles, though it does affect a significant number of people in other countries (e.g. New Zealand). It may provoke symptoms in people who have been sensitized to olive pollen abroad, owing to a cross-reaction (see p155). Those sensitive to privet may react while hedge cutting (see p25).

Elder (*Sambucus*)

May to July
A very common shrub in Britain, and some pollen becomes airborne, but pollen counts are low and there are no reports of resultant hayfever. Seems to cause some allergic reactions in Sweden, particularly among birch-sensitive individuals, and may cause a certain amount of hayfever in the Netherlands.

Heathers (*Erica* and *Calluna*)

July to September
Not reported as a cause of hayfever in Britain, but heathers seem to affect some people in Scandinavia, particularly if they are already sensitive to birch. Tree heather is reported as a potent allergen in Turkey. Heathers grow mainly in moorland areas. Pollen counts are low to moderate in areas such as Scotland where heather is abundant, very low elsewhere.

Bog myrtle (*Myrica gale*)

April to May
Not considered a source of hayfever in Britain, and pollen counts are very low or nonexistent as the plant is scarce throughout most of the country. However, boggy moorland country in northern Scotland and the west of Ireland often has extensive colonies of this plant, and pollen counts could be higher in such areas. Bog myrtle has been identified as a strong allergen in Canada (where it is known as sweet gale) and Scandinavia; it seems to cross-react with birch.

Nettles (*Urtica*)

June to July, August to September
Common weeds with two separate spurts of pollination. Not particularly allergenic, but they do cause some summer hayfever.

Plantains (*Plantago*)

July to September
Do not usually begin pollinating until late July. Only small amounts of pollen are produced, but the pollen is very allergenic, causing some summer hayfever.

Mugwort and wormwoods (*Artemisia*)

July to September
Do not usually begin pollinating until late July. Probably not a common cause of hayfever in Britain, though they are elsewhere. The pollen could affect sensitized visitors from other countries.

Pellitory-of-the-wall (*Parietaria*)

June to September
A weed introduced from southern Europe. It may cause a few cases of hayfever in southern England. Could affect sensitized visitors from southern Europe.

Docks and sorrels (*Rumex*)

May to July
Do not usually begin pollinating until mid-May, and there is relatively little pollen in the air after the end of June. Pollen counts are generally low, so not considered to be an important cause of hayfever in Britain. (If such hayfever does occur, it would probably be mistaken for grass allergy.)

Goosefoots and amaranths (Chenopodiaceae and Amaranthaceae)

May to October
Various species grow widely, but there is relatively little pollen in the air and they are not considered a cause of hayfever in Britain. Rural areas can have slightly higher pollen counts. Whether these would affect someone from another country already sensitized to this type of pollen is unknown.

Ragweeds (*Ambrosia*)

June to September
Pollen counts are very low and do not seem to cause any symptoms either in residents or visitors. There may, however, be localized areas with higher levels of pollen, especially near sea ports, and on wasteland with ragweed colonies, e.g. around London and East Anglia.

Goldenrod and dandelion (Compositae or Asteraceae)

April to September
These and other plants belonging to the Asteraceae may cause problems through cross-reactions for visitors who are highly sensitive to ragweed (see p156). They are not thought to cause hayfever among those who have never been sensitized to ragweed.

AUSTRALIA

WESTERN AUSTRALIA

Grasses (Gramineae or Poaceae)

September to March
The peak is from September to November. However there can be some grass pollen in the air at any time of the year. While the pollen count is generally lower from March to September, there is a small peak in June.

White cypress pine (*Callitris columellaris*)

August to October
A conifer but not a true pine. Commonly a cause of hayfever in this area. Planted for shelter, and found growing wild.

She-oak or 'Australian pine' (*Casuarina*)

July to November
Neither an oak nor a pine, so no cross-reactions with these trees are likely. Pollination shows a peak during July and August, then a lull, followed by a second peak in November. Planted for shelter, and found growing wild.

Wattles (*Acacia*)

May to February
The highest pollen counts are from July to October. Note that cross-reactions are likely with cultivated mimosas.

Olive trees (*Olea*)

November to December
Not a particularly common source of hayfever here, but may affect those sensitized elsewhere.

Cypresses (Cupressaceae)

August to October
Widely planted for shelter.

Pines (Pinaceae)

July to November
Planted for shelter in some areas. The pollen may produce allergic reactions, or simply act as an irritant (see p7).

Gum trees (*Eucalyptus*)

October to March
A rare cause of hayfever.

Privet (*Ligustrum*)

August to November
Planted for hedging in some areas and may cause some hayfever. Cross-reactions with olive are possible.

Sunflower (*Helianthus*)

October to February
May cause local problems where cultivated.

Paterson's curse or Salvation Jane
(*Echium plantagineum*)

October to November
A shorter season than in some other parts of Australia.

Plantains (*Plantago*)

August to February
The most allergenic species pollinates in October.

Docks and sorrels (*Rumex*)

September to January
Common weeds but not a major cause of hayfever in this area.

Goosefoots (Chenopodiaceae)

September to February
The native species are known as salt bushes. Common in dry and windy places.

Capeweed (*Arctotheca calendula*)

July to November
The pollination peak is during September and October. A common allergenic weed.

NORTHERN TERRITORY

Very little information available. In the north, grass pollen is likely in summer (October to March).

QUEENSLAND

Grasses (Gramineae or Poaceae)

September to May
There is likely to be some grass pollen in the air all year round in many areas. Pollen counts are much higher in the south of the state, lower on the northeast coast.

White cypress pine or Murray pine
(*Callitris columellaris*)

September to November
Peak pollination occurs in October. Only grows in the south of the state (below the Tropic of Capricorn).

She-oak or 'Australian pine'
(*Casuarina*)

September to February
Confined to the central and southern part of the state.

Wattles (*Acacia*)

May to October
Some pollen in the air all year round. Pollen counts higher inland, in areas of wattle scrub and woodland. Also grown in gardens.

Gum trees (*Eucalyptus*)

All year
A rare cause of hayfever.

Privet (*Ligustrum*)

September to November
Not considered a particularly important allergen in this area, but may affect those sensitized elsewhere. Only in the south of the state; planted for hedging.

Sunflower (*Helianthus*)

December to May
A frequent cause of hayfever where it is cultivated.

Plantains (*Plantago*)

August to March
An important type of allergenic pollen in the south of this region.

Docks and sorrels (*Rumex*)

September to February
The pollen count is lower after the end of November. Mainly in the south of the state.

Goosefoots (Chenopodiaceae)

September to April
The peak is from December onwards. Considered an important allergen in the south.

Capeweed (*Arctotheca calendula*)

September to December
Not particularly common except in the south of this state.

NEW SOUTH WALES

Grasses (Gramineae or Poaceae)

August to May
There will be some grass pollen in the air all year round. The peak season is from September to March.

White cypress pine or Murray pine (*Callitris columellaris*)

August to November
Pollen counts are lower after the end of October. An important allergenic tree. Less common in northern areas.

She-oak or 'Australian pine' (*Casuarina*)

July to April
Neither an oak nor a pine, so cross-reactions with these trees are unlikely. An important allergen in the central and southern areas; often planted for shelter. The season varies from one part of the state to another.

Silver birch (*Betula pendula*)

September to October
A tree introduced from Europe; grows mainly in cooler areas.

Wattles (*Acacia*)

June to December
High pollen counts in wattle scrub and woodland; also grown in gardens.

Olive trees (*Olea*)

October to November
The peak is in November, when pollen counts can be high near olive-growing areas in the south of the state.

Gum trees (*Eucalyptus*)

All year
A rare cause of hayfever.

Privet (*Ligustrum*)

September to November
The pollen count can be high in October and November. Can cross-react with olive pollen and people may become allergic to it in this way.

Cypresses (Cupressaceae)

August to November
Not a particularly important allergen locally but may affect those sensitized elsewhere. Planted for shelter in the south.

Paterson's curse or Salvation Jane (*Echium plantagineum*)

September to December
A weed that commonly causes hayfever. Only found in the south and in inland areas.

Plantains (*Plantago*)

June to February
The season varies from one part of the state to another. A very common weed and an important source of hayfever.

Docks and sorrels (*Rumex*)

September to February
The pollen peak is from September to November.

Goosefoots (Chenopodiaceae)

December to February
The pollen is in the air all year round, but peaks in late summer. Common throughout the state.

Pellitory-of-the-wall (*Parietaria judaica*)

June to April
Only found in the Sydney area, mainly on the lower North Shore, but also now colonizing the inner city. The weed has been found growing in Melbourne, Adelaide and Freemantle, but not yet in sufficient numbers to cause hayfever.

Capeweed (*Arctotheca calendula*)

September to November
High pollen counts except in the north.

Wormwood (*Artemisia*)

December to January
Mainly in inland areas.

VICTORIA

Grasses (Gramineae or Poaceae)

September to May
There is some pollen in the air all year round.

White cypress pine or Murray pine (*Callitris columellaris*)

June to October
The season varies from one part of the state to another. Found mainly in the north and not particularly common.

She-oak or 'Australian pine' (*Casuarina*)

March to April, July to August
Pollination season may vary. Confined to the north of the state and not common except where planted for shelter. Neither an oak nor a pine, so cross-reactions with these trees are unlikely.

Silver birch (*Betula pendula*)

September to October
Planted for shelter in southern areas.

Wattles (*Acacia*)

July to January
The peak of the season is in August and September. Common throughout the area; also grown in gardens.

Olive trees (*Olea*)

October to November
Grown mainly in the north of the state.

Cypresses (Cupressaceae)

April to September
Widely planted for shelter in the south.

Pines (Pinaceae)

August to September
Commonly planted for shelter in the south.

Gum trees (*Eucalyptus*)

All year
A rare cause of hayfever.

Privet (*Ligustrum*)

October to December
Commonly used for hedging and considered a likely cause of hayfever.

Clover (*Trifolium*)

September to February
Peak is in October and November. May cause some hayfever where common.

Paterson's curse or Salvation Jane (*Echium plantagineum*)

August to December
The peak is in October. Not common except in the northeast.

Plantains (*Plantago*)

October to March
Peak pollen counts are from November to January. A very common weed throughout the state.

Docks and sorrels (*Rumex*)

August to February
The peak is in October and November. Common throughout the state.

Goosefoots (Chenopodiaceae)

December to April
Common in the north only.

Capeweed (*Arctotheca calendula*)

August to December
Common throughout and an important allergen.

SOUTH AUSTRALIA

Grasses (Gramineae or Poaceae)

July to March
Plentiful pollen in the air for much of the year; airborne in lesser amounts even in May and June.

White cypress pine or Murray pine (*Callitris columellaris*)

August to October
Planted for shelter; also grows wild.

She-oak or 'Australian pine' (*Casuarina*)

August to September, March to July
Pollination season very variable. Grown for shelter, and found in the wild. Neither an oak nor a pine, so cross-reactions are unlikely.

Silver birch (*Betula pendula*)

September to November
Planted for shelter in some cooler areas.

Wattles (*Acacia*)

July to November
Very common in the wild, and planted in gardens.

Olive trees (*Olea*)

September to November
Peak is in November. Pollen counts are only high where olive groves are found.

Gum trees (*Eucalyptus*)

August to March
A rare cause of hayfever.

Privet (*Ligustrum*)

September to November
Cross-reactions with olive may produce sensitivity.

Cypresses (Cupressaceae)

August to October
These conifers can be a source of hayfever where planted for shelter.

Paterson's curse or Salvation Jane (*Echium plantagineum*)

July to December
The peak is in October and November. A common cause of hayfever when found in abundance.

Plantains (*Plantago*)

August to March
The peak is from September to January. A widespread weed that often causes hayfever.

Docks and sorrels (*Rumex*)

September to December
A common weed throughout the area.

Goosefoots (Chenopodiaceae)

December to April
The peak is at the end of the season in March and April. Native species are known as salt bushes.

Capeweed (*Arctotheca calendula*)

August to November
The peak is in September and October. A very common weed throughout the state, and an important allergen.

TASMANIA

Grasses (Gramineae or Poaceae)

September to April
The peak is in December. Pollen counts can be high.

She-oak or 'Australian pine' (*Casuarina*)

June to December
Grows wild; also planted in some areas.

Silver birch (*Betula pendula*)

September to November
Widely planted.

Wattles (*Acacia*)

August to February
Pollen counts higher in the north.

Cypresses and pines (Cupressaceae and Pinaceae)

July to November
Planted for shelter. Cypresses are only likely to cause hayfever in hot dry areas. Pines are more likely to act as irritants than allergens.

Gum trees (*Eucalyptus*)

August to February
A rare cause of hayfever.

Plantains (*Plantago*)

October to March
A common weed in most parts of the island and an important allergen.

Docks and sorrels (*Rumex*)

September to May
The peak is in November and December.

Capeweed (*Arctotheca calendula*)

September to January
Pollen counts are lower after the end of October. Considered an important allergen.

NEW ZEALAND

Grasses (Gramineae or Poaceae)

October to February
Grasses are the largest pollen producers and the major cause of springtime hayfever.

The grass pollen season starts earlier in the north than in the south, with a four-week difference between the northern end of North Island and the southern end of South Island. The season also ends earlier in the far south, so that the whole pollen season is two months shorter. In Kaikohe, near the tip of North Island, for example, grass pollen is in the air from mid-November to late February, in Wellington from early December to late February, and in Gore, at the southern end of South Island, from mid-December to the end of January.

There is a lot of variation in concentration from place to place. Cities and large towns are often surrounded by grazing lands, and therefore experience higher concentrations of grass pollen. The pollen counts are highest in inland pastoral areas such as Hamilton and Palmerstone North, which can have relatively severe seasons. Concentrations are lower in coastal areas such as Christchurch.

Wattles and mimosas (*Acacia* and *Albizia*)

August to November
These are potent allergens, but the pollen concentration is only high in the immediate vicinity of the trees.

Birches (*Betula*)

August to October
A tree introduced from Europe, and therefore only found in a few areas. However, pollen is produced abundantly, so these localized pockets can cause problems for sensitized people.

Cypresses (Cupressaceae)

July to November
Only a small percentage of people react to this pollen. Problems mainly occur in drier areas if people live near dense banks of cypresses.

Oaks (*Quercus*)

August to October
Introduced from Europe, and therefore only found in a few areas. These localized pockets can cause problems for a few sensitized people.

Pines (*Pinaceae*)

July to October
Huge amounts of pine pollen come from forestry plantations of *Pinus radiata*. As with all pines, the pollen is not highly allergenic, and only a small proportion of patients with hayfever and asthma are genuinely allergic to it. However, by virtue of its size, quantity and certain chemicals carried on the pollen wall, this particular pine pollen may cause some irritation in the nose if a very large amount is inhaled. The reaction is not an allergic one.

Privet (*Ligustrum*)

October to March
Produces plenty of pollen, but most of it does not travel far. Only a modest allergen, and the number of people affected is small.

Docks (*Rumex*)

January to March
These are not very heavy pollen producers. They are very common as weeds, and while relatively few people react to them, those who do tend to react vigorously.

Plantains (*Plantago*)

October to February
Only small amounts of pollen are produced, but the pollen is very allergenic.

CANADA

ALASKA (USA) AND NORTH CANADA

Grasses (Gramineae and Poaceae)

May to September
The season is shorter in northern Canada, from July to August. In Alaska, the season usually ends in early September; peak pollen counts occur early on and are over quickly. There can be high concentrations of pollen in some areas.
The season is later and shorter further north, and at high altitude. Pollen counts are low in forest areas, higher on the tundra (where sedges also contribute to symptoms) and in transitional vegetation zones.

Birches (*Betula*)

May to June
The peak is in April. The season is later in the north and at high altitudes. Pollen counts can be very high.

Alders (*Alnus*)

April to May
Can cross-react with birch, lengthening the hayfever season for those with birch sensitivity. Most abundant in mountain areas to the west.

Poplars and willows (*Populus* and *Salix*)

April to May
Found throughout the forest zones. Balsam poplar (*Populus balsamifera*) and quaking aspen (*Populus tremuloides*) are among the species growing here, and are the most likely to cause hayfever.

Bog myrtle or sweet gale (*Myrica gale*)

April to June
The same species grows in Scandinavia

where it is known to cross-react with birch. May also cause symptoms in birch-sensitive patients in Canada. Cross-reactions with the bayberries or wax myrtles of southern USA are likely.

NORTHEAST CANADA

Northern Ontario, northern Quebec, Labrador and Newfoundland.

Grasses (Gramineae or Poaceae)

July
Pollen sparse in northern Ontario. May be prolific in the northeast but the season is very short. Sedges may also cause symptoms due to cross-reactions.

Birches (*Betula*)

May to June
The season is short, usually from late May to early June only.

Spruce, fir and larch (Pinaceae)

July to August
Prolific pollen producers but very rarely produce allergic reactions. Might cause some irritation.

Bog myrtle or sweet gale (*Myrica gale*)

April to June
The same species grows in Scandinavia where it is known to cross-react with birch. May also cause symptoms in birch-sensitive patients in Canada. Cross-reactions with the bayberries or wax myrtles of the southern USA are likely.

SOUTHEAST CANADA

Southern Ontario and Quebec, New Brunswick and Nova Scotia

Grass (Gramineae or Poaceae)

May to August
The peak is in June and July. In Ontario the season is shorter, from the end of June to the end of July, starting later in the north. There is extensive grassland in some areas around the St Lawrence seaway.

Birches (*Betula*)

May to June
The season does not begin until late May in most parts, but south of the St Lawrence, and around Montreal, it may start in early May. Pollen production can vary from year to year, with very high counts in some years.

Alders (*Alnus*)

April
Can produce cross-reactions in those sensitized by birch.

Oaks and beeches (*Quercus* and *Fagus*)

May to June
Not an abundant pollen except in Ontario and along the St Lawrence seaway. Can pollinate as early as April in the south of this state. Cross-reactions are possible with birch.

Hickories (*Carya*)

May to June
Only found in the most southern parts of Ontario and Quebec. A highly allergenic pollen, but the grains are large so it does not disperse widely.

Mulberry (*Morus*)

April to June
Found in the air in the Toronto region. A highly allergenic pollen.

Willows and poplars (*Salix* and *Populus*)

April to May
The season is later in the north, from May to June. Can produce high pollen counts in some parts of the region.

Maples (*Acer*)

May to June
Can be as early as April in the south. Maples growing in this area are all insect-pollinated and probably of low allergenicity. Box elder (*Acer negundo*), the most allergenic species of maple, is not found here.

Lindens and basswoods (*Tilia*)

July
These trees are known as limes in Britain.

Pines and spruces (*Pinaceae*)

June to August
The season is earlier in the south. Not considered to be a common cause of true allergy, but can act as an irritant.

Elms and hackberries (*Ulmus* and *Celtis*)

May to June
The season is later in the north.

Ash trees (*Fraxinus*)

April to May
Not a potent allergen; may affect those sensitized by olive pollen.

Privet (*Ligustrum*)

May to June
Only in the southern part of this region and the number of people affected is small. Those affected have often been sensitized by olive pollen, which cross-reacts with privet.

Bog myrtle or sweet gale (*Myrica gale*)

April to June
The same species grows in Scandinavia where it is known to cross-react with birch. May also cause symptoms in birch-sensitive patients in Canada. Cross-reactions with the bayberries or wax myrtles of the southern USA are likely.

Ragweeds (*Ambrosia*)

August to September
Mainly found around settlements and on disturbed ground. Pollen counts can be very high in the south. They decline sharply with the first frosts.

Mugwort and wormwoods (*Artemisia*)

August to September
Very high counts in some areas, such as around Montreal. Mainly on disturbed sites and near settlements.

Goosefoots, pigweed and 'Russian thistle' (Chenopodiaceae)

July to September
May cause some hayfever in the Great Lakes region.

Plantains (*Plantago*)

July to October
Only in the Great Lakes region and along the St Lawrence seaway.

BRITISH COLUMBIA

Grasses (Gramineae or Poaceae)

May to September
The peak is in June and July, but there are variations with altitude. The season starts two weeks earlier in the south than in the north, and is longest in the coastal areas. Pollen counts are not particularly high since grassland areas, except in some coastal regions, are mostly restricted to small areas.

Birches (*Betula*)

May and June
Pollen counts are highest near the tree line on mountain slopes, but birches are found throughout the area.

Alders (*Alnus*)

April to May
Can show a cross-reaction with birch. West of the Rockies, alder pollen is a more important allergen than birch.

Poplars and willows (*Populus* and *Salix*)

April to May
The willow season is later, from May to early June, in the north and at high altitudes.

Maples (*Acer*)

May to June
The most common cause of hayfever among the maples, box elder (*Acer negundo*), does not grow in this area. Local species are not particularly allergenic.

Cypresses, junipers and 'cedars' (Cupressaceae)

February to June
The peak is in April. Rarely a cause of hayfever in this area, but the pollen may affect those sensitized in warmer climates.

Bog myrtle or sweet gale (*Myrica gale*)

April to June
The same species grows in Scandinavia where it is known to cross-react with birch. May also cause symptoms in birch-sensitive patients in Canada. Cross-reactions with the bayberries or wax myrtles of the southern USA are likely.

Ragweeds (*Ambrosia*)

August to September
The season begins earlier here than in eastern Canada. Pollen counts are highest in the south and near to settlements.

GREAT PLAINS OF CANADA

Alberta, Saskatchewan and Manitoba.

Grasses (Gramineae and Poaceae)

May to August
The peak is in June and July. Grass pollen can be very abundant in parts of the southern prairies during this season. Pollen counts are generally moderate in the north because areas of grassland are limited, but they can be high locally, such as in the Peace River valley in the northwest where there is more pastureland.

Birches (*Betula*)

April to May
Birches are scattered throughout this region and are more widespread in southern Manitoba.

Poplars and quaking aspen (*Populus*)

April to May
Balsam poplar and quaking aspen (*Populus balsamifera* and *Populus tremuloides*) are believed to be prime offenders in hayfever and are found

throughout this area. Aspens are most common in southern Manitoba.

Maples (*Acer*)

May to June
The highly allergenic box elder or ash-leaved maple (*Acer negundo*) is found in the south of this area, notably in southern Manitoba.

Oaks (*Quercus*)

May
Southern Manitoba only.

Elms (*Ulmus*)

May to June
Found in the southern prairies only.

Cypresses, junipers and 'cedars' (Cupressaceae)

March to June
The peak is in April. These trees are mainly found in the Rocky Mountains to the west of this area. Rarely a cause of hayfever locally, but the pollen may affect those sensitized in warmer climates.

Bog myrtle or sweet gale (*Myrica gale*)

April to June
Not found in the far south of this region. The same species grows in Scandinavia where it is known to cross-react with birch. May also cause symptoms in birch-sensitive patients in Canada. Cross-reactions with the bayberries or wax myrtles of the southern USA are likely.

Ragweeds (*Ambrosia*)

August to September
Only found in the far south of this region, mainly within 200 km (125 miles) of the US border.

Goosefoots and plantains (Chenopodiaceae and *Plantago*)

August to September
The season may end earlier in the north. These weeds grow only where there are settlements, and are therefore more scattered in the north.

Mugwort and wormwoods (*Artemisia*)

August to September
These weeds grow mainly around settlements, and are therefore more common in the south.

USA

WASHINGTON AND OREGON

The seasons tend to be later to the east of the Cascade Mountains. All seasons are about two weeks longer in the south than in the north.

Grasses (Gramineae or Poaceae)

April to September
The peak is in June and July. Pollen counts are moderate in most regions.

Alders (*Alnus*)

February to April
A common cause of hayfever due to very high pollen counts, particularly in March. Alders are allergenically more important than birches in this area.

Birches (*Betula*)

April to May
Can cross-react with alder and thus prolong the season.

Poplars and willows (*Populus* and *Salix*)

March to May
Two of the more allergenic poplars, balsam poplar and quaking aspen (*Populus balsamifera* and *Populus tremuloides*) both grow here.

Oaks (*Quercus*)

April to May
Oak pollen has the potential for cross-reactions with birch and alder.

Maples (*Acer*)

April to May
Considered a fairly common source of hayfever.

Coast redwood (*Sequoia*)

March to May
Moderately allergenic pollen.

Cypresses, junipers and 'cedars' (Cupressaceae)

March to May
May cause some hayfever, but not to the same extent as in California owing to the cooler climate.

Ragweeds (*Ambrosia*)

July to October
Pollen counts are not as high as in other states. They are generally lower to the west of the Cascade Mountains.

Docks and sorrels (*Rumex*)

May to September
The peak is in early summer, coinciding with the grass pollen season, so that allergies to docks and sorrels can easily be misdiagnosed.

Plantains (*Plantago*)

May to November
High pollen counts in July and August, lessening a little in September. Considered moderately significant as a cause of hayfever.

Goosefoots and amaranths (Chenopodiaceae and Amaranthaceae)

June to October
The amaranths are known locally as redroot pigweed and spiny pigweed. Widespread weeds in this area.

CALIFORNIA

Grasses (Gramineae or Poaceae)

April to October
The season peaks in May and June in the south and during June and July in the north. It ends earlier in the north – by the end of September. Parts of southern California have some grass pollen in the air all year round.

The highest pollen counts occur inland and up to the middle slopes of the mountains.

Cypresses, junipers and 'cedars' (Cupressaceae)

September to March
The peak is from January to March. One species pollinates later, in April and May. A moderately common cause of hayfever as in other warm dry climates.

Poplars (*Populus*)

April to May
Balsam poplar and quaking aspen (*Populus balsamifera* and *Populus tremuloides*) both grow in this region and are more allergenic than other poplars.

Alders and birches (*Alnus* and *Betula*)

December to May
Alders are found at higher altitudes in the north of the state. They pollinate first, from December to February, with lower counts continuing into April. Birches pollinate from April to May. Cross-reactions between the two are common.

Oaks (*Quercus*)

February to April
In the south flowering ends in March; in the north it does not begin until March and continues into April. Local species of oak are considered highly allergenic.

She-oak or 'Australian pine' (*Casuarina*)

February to May, September to November
Pollination seasons are very variable. Planted as a windbreak and for erosion control, and a cause of some hayfever as the pollen is highly allergenic. Neither an oak nor a pine, so cross-reactions with these trees are unlikely.

Walnuts, pecans and hickories (*Juglans* and *Carya*)

March to May
Where cultivated these produce high pollen counts causing many cases of hayfever, but the pollen does not travel far in the air.

Olive trees (*Olea*)

May to June
Introduced from the Mediterranean region. Can cause problems where grown as a crop.

Ash (*Fraxinus*)

February to April
The season ends in March in the south, just as the season in the north is beginning. May affect those already sensitized by olive pollen due to a cross-reaction.

Elms (*Ulmus*)

February to April, August to October
In southern California, the species of elm that flower in autumn (*U. crassifolia, U. serotina* and *U. parvifolia*) are important allergens. The season for these trees can sometimes continue to November. Cross-reactions with hackberry (*Celtis*) pollen are likely.

Japanese red cedar (*Cryptomeria*)

March to April
Planted for landscaping and windbreaks and a potential source of hayfever locally.

Paper mulberry and mulberry (*Broussonetia* and *Morus*)

March to May
Paper mulberry produces highly allergenic pollen. Cases of hayfever reported from southern California. The two groups are related and will cross-react.

Maples (*Acer*)

March to May
Considered a fairly common cause of hayfever. The most allergenic maple, box elder or ash-leaved maple (*Acer negundo*) grows in parts of California.

Palm trees (*Arecaceae*)

June to December
Those affected are mainly people pollinating the palms, or living on streets where palms are planted.

Gum trees (*Eucalyptus*)

December to March
A rare cause of hayfever.

Wattles and acacias (*Acacia*)

January to October
Widely planted as ornamental shrubs and trees. Pollen counts are only high close to where the plants are growing. May cause cross-reactions with mesquite which belongs to the same family.

Mesquite (*Prosopis*)

May to July
Found in the southeast and thought to cause some hayfever.

Privet (*Ligustrum*)

March to June
Produces plenty of pollen, but most of it does not travel far. Only a modest allergen, and the number of people affected is small. Those affected have often been sensitized by olive pollen which cross-reacts with privet.

Bayberry or wax myrtle (*Myrica*)

February to May
The south sees flowering during February and March, the north from April to May. A moderately strong allergen affecting a few hayfever patients. Note that this is the same genus as the sweet gale or bog myrtle of Canada, Scandinavia and parts of Britain. Cross-reactions may occur.

Ragweeds (*Ambrosia*)

April to December
There may be some pollen in the air all year round, from ragweed or closely related plants that cross-react with ragweed. However, pollen counts are generally low compared with other states.

Poverty weeds and marsh elders (*Iva*)

August to November
Cross-react with ragweed pollen. Common in some areas.

Goosefoots and amaranths (Chenopodiaceae and Amaranthaceae)

April to December
The pollen levels are fairly high from June onwards in southern California, and remain so until late November. The local names for species of amaranth include careless weed, redroot pigweed and spiny pigweed.

Plantains (*Plantago*)

May to November
The pollen peak coincides with the grass pollen season in many areas.

Docks and sorrels (*Rumex*)

All year
The peak pollen season is from March to August.

Sagebrush (*Artemisia*)

July to September
A powerful allergen. Will cross-react with mugwort.

Nettles (*Urtica*)

January to September
The cause of some hayfever in southern California.

Pellitories (*Parietaria*)

February to July
Found in some parts and may affect visitors sensitized elsewhere.

MONTANA, IDAHO AND WYOMING

Grasses (Gramineae and Poaceae)

May to September
The seasons are much shorter in Wyoming (ends in late July) and Montana (ends in June).

Birches (*Betula*)

April to May
An important allergenic pollen.

Alders, ironwood, hornbeams and hazels (*Alnus, Ostrya, Carpinus* and *Corylus*)

February to April
Can cross-react with birch, producing symptoms before birch flowers. Hazel pollen declines in March, and alder pollen in April. Hornbeams and ironwood flower from April to May.

Willows and poplars (*Salix* and *Populus*)

March to May
Most species finish pollinating by the end of April. Two of the more allergenic poplars, quaking aspen and balsam poplar (*Populus tremuloides* and *Populus balsamifera*) grow here; both flower from April to May.

Oaks (*Quercus*)

April to May
Can cross-react with birches and related trees.

Cypresses (Cupressaceae)

January to February
May cause some hayfever locally, and could affect those sensitized elsewhere.

Ragweeds (*Ambrosia*)

August to September
The most important allergenic pollen.

Docks, sorrels and plantains (*Rumex* and *Plantago*)

May to November
Docks and sorrels stop pollinating earlier, by the end of September.

Goosefoots and amaranths (Chenopodiaceae and Amaranthaceae)

June to October
The local species of amaranth are generally known as pigweeds, but this name may also be applied to some species of goosefoot. Burning bush (*Kochia scoparia*), which grows in dry places, also belongs to this group, and cross-reactions are common; its pollen is a potent allergen. 'Russian thistle' (*Salsola*

kali) is common in Idaho and is likewise a powerful allergen. Smotherweed (*Bassia*) and greasewood (*Sarcobatus*), found growing locally, are also members of this group.

Sagebrush (*Artemisia*)

August to September
Considered an important allergen in Idaho.

NEVADA, UTAH AND COLORADO

Grasses (Gramineae or Poaceae)

March to October
This very long season is only seen in the west of the zone. The season in Utah runs from May to July, while in much of Colorado it lasts from May to September. Pollen counts are low in dry areas, but irrigation greatly increases the amount of pollen produced. At high altitudes, where there is more rainfall, pollen counts can be high.

Cypresses, junipers and 'cedars' (Cupressaceae)

January to March
The most important allergenic trees in the mountains.

Poplars (*Populus*)

April to May
Balsam poplar and quaking aspen (*Populus balsamifera* and *Populus tremuloides*), two of the more allergenic poplars, both grow here. At high altitudes the season may start and end later.

Goosefoots and amaranths (Chenopodiaceae and Amaranthaceae)

June to October
These include various species known as pigweeds (*Chenopodium* and *Amaranthus*), saltbush or orach (*Atriplex*), smotherweed (*Bassia*), greasewood (*Sarcobatus*) and 'Russian thistle' (*Salsola kali*). The last is a particularly potent sensitizer. Extensive cross-reactions occur among the plants of this group (see p159), making them a widespread source of hayfever.

Ragweeds (*Ambrosia*)

August to September
Only Colorado has high pollen counts.

Pellitories (*Parietaria*)

July to September
The pollen of these plants is a potent sensitizer. Found growing on disturbed ground.

Docks and sorrels (*Rumex*)

May to September
Pollination coincides with the peak period for grass, so hayfever caused by these plants is easily mistaken for grass-pollen hayfever.

ARIZONA AND NEW MEXICO

Irrigation in Arizona, particularly in gardens, has allowed a greater variety of plants to be grown. As in Israel (see p289) irrigated plants in a dry area can produce very high pollen counts. The number of allergenic pollens in the air has increased considerably in the past fifty years.

Grasses (Gramineae or Poaceae)

Feburary to November
In New Mexico the season is a little shorter, from April to September.

Cypresses, junipers and 'cedars' (Cupressaceae)

September to March
Pinchot junipers produce pollen from September to November, other species from December to March.

Olive trees (*Olea*)

May to June
Introduced from the Mediterranean region. Can cause problems where grown as a crop.

Ash trees (*Fraxinus*)

February to March
An important cause of hayfever in Arizona. Olive pollen can cross-react with that of ash, making sensitivity to ash more likely in areas where olives are grown.

Mesquite (*Prosopis*)

May to July
Could provoke cross-reactions in anyone allergic to wattles (*Acacia*).

Sagebrush (*Artemisia*)

July to September
A common cause of hayfever. Will almost certainly affect those sensitive to mugwort.

Ragweeds and bur ragweed (*Ambrosia* and *Franseria*)

August to September
Cross-reactions can occur between these two closely related groups. Certain species of ragweed flower during the winter in parts of Arizona.

Goosefoots and amaranths (Chenopodiaceae and Amaranthaceae)

April to October
Several species are known locally as pigweeds and saltbushes. Most are moderate allergens, but Mexican tea (*Chenopodium ambrosioides*) and 'Russian thistle' (*Salsola kali*) are both potent allergens, and cross-reactions with other species are common. 'Russian thistle' flowers from July to October.

Docks and sorrels (*Rumex*)

March to September
Pollination coincides with the peak period for grass, so hayfever caused by these plants is easily mistaken for grass-pollen hayfever.

THE SOUTH

This area includes Texas, Louisiana, Mississippi and Alabama.

Grasses (Gramineae and Poaceae)

March to December
The season runs from March to October in Texas, with west Texas having a slightly longer season than east Texas. Some areas of southern Texas have grass pollen in the air all year round. In Louisiana the grass pollen season runs from April to November or December. In much of Mississippi, the season begins in April but ends earlier, in October. Alabama's season is from May to November.

Junipers and 'cedars' (Cupressaceae)

September to March
The main season is from January to March. Only one species, the pinchot juniper, flowers from September to November. Mountain cedar (*Juniperus ashei*) grows on neglected grassland and has become a particular problem.

Maples (*Acer*)

February to May
The main allergen is box elder or ash-leaved maple (*Acer negundo*).

Elms, hackberries and sugarberries (*Ulmus* and *Celtis*)

January to April, August to October
The peak season is from January to March, with very high counts in February, particularly in Texas.

Hickories and pecans (*Carya*)

March to May
Where cultivated or planted as street trees, these are often the second most important cause of hayfever, after ragweed. Pecans and hickories are widely cultivated in Texas.

Mulberries and paper mulberry (*Morus* and *Broussonetia*)

March to May
Paper mulberry, in particular, is highly allergenic. It is widely planted in this area.

Hedgeplant or osage orange (*Maclura*)

April to June
Used for hedging and moderately allergenic. Can cross-react with paper mulberries and mulberries which belong to the same family (Moraceae).

Privet (*Ligustrum*)

March to June
May produce a few cases of hayfever in some parts of this region. Those affected have often been sensitized by olive pollen, which cross-reacts with privet.

**Southern bayberry or wax myrtle
(*Myrica cerifera*)**

March to April
Pollination may begin in February in the
southeastern part of this region, towards
Florida. A moderately allergenic pollen
sometimes producing severe symptoms in
those affected. May well cross-react with
sweet gale or bog myrtle (*Myrica gale*),
found in Canada and Scandinavia, and in
parts of Britain.

Ragweeds (*Ambrosia*)

July to November
The pollen of some species may appear in
the air earlier, from May onwards, but
counts are low. Peak season is from mid-
August to October. Ragweeds are the
main cause of hayfever in this region.

Marsh elders and dune elder (*Iva*)

August to November
Related to the ragweeds so cross-
reactions are common. Some species may
begin pollinating as early as June. Found
mainly in coastal areas and the lower
Mississippi valley.

**Groundsel bush or tree (*Baccharis
halmilifolia*)**

August to November
Can begin pollinating much earlier in
parts of Texas. May cause hayfever
through cross-reactions with ragweed. A
great many other plants belonging to the
same family (Compositae or Asteraceae)
grow throughout this area, and can
provoke cross-reactions in those with
ragweed hayfever. There may be some
pollen in the air for most of the year, with
the lowest pollen counts in January and
February, and the highest from
August to December.

**Goosefoots and amaranths
(Chenopodiaceae and
Amaranthaceae)**

June to December
Many different species are involved, and
they can provoke cross-reactions with
other plants in these two related families.
Local names include southern water-
hemp, pigweed and tumbleweed.

SOUTH-CENTRAL STATES

This area includes Kansas, Oklahoma,
Missouri and Arkansas.

Grasses (Gramineae or Poaceae)

April to November
The season lasts for eight months in
Arkansas but is shorter elsewhere in the
region, usually from May to August.

Maples (*Acer*)

February to May
The most allergenic of the maples, box
elder or ash-leaved maple (*Acer negundo*)
grows in this region and is a major cause
of hayfever.

Birches (*Betula*)

March to May
A fairly common source of hayfever. The
most common species grows on the
banks of rivers and streams; pollen counts
will therefore be highest in these areas.

Oaks (*Quercus*)

April to May
Can cross-react with birch pollen.

Hackberries and sugarberries (*Celtis*)

February to March
Particularly common in Oklahoma.

Ash (*Fraxinus*)

February to March
Only a moderate allergen. Found growing
in wet lowland areas.

**Paper mulberry (*Broussonetia
papyrifera*)**

March to May
Grown in Oklahoma and a powerful
allergen.

Osage orange or hedgeplant (*Maclura*)

April to May
Widely planted for hedging. Can cross-
react with paper mulberry and mulberries.

Southern bayberry or wax myrtle (Myrica cerifera)

March to April
A moderately allergenic pollen sometimes producing severe symptoms in those affected. May well cross-react with sweet gale or bog myrtle (Myrica gale), found in Canada and Scandinavia, and in parts of Britain.

Ragweeds (Ambrosia)

August to September
The season can continue into mid-October in Oklahoma. The major allergenic pollen in this region. Various other members of the same family (Compositae or Asteraceae) also grow in this region and may cross-react. These can prolong the hayfever season until November or December.

Goosefoots and amaranths (Chenopodiaceae and Amaranthaceae)

April to October
Local names for these plants include pigweed and redroot.

Docks and sorrels (Rumex)

May to September
The peak pollination season coincides with that of grass, so allergy to docks and sorrels is often wrongly attributed to grass pollen.

Plantains (Plantago)

May to November
Peak pollination is from May to July.

Sagebrush (Artemisia)

July to September
Mainly found in the dry western areas. Cross-reacts with mugwort and wormwoods.

KENTUCKY AND TENNESSEE

Grasses (Gramineae and Poaceae)

May to August
The season is longer in Tennessee, continuing until early December in the south.

'Cedars' and junipers (Cupressaceae)

January to March
These cross-react with cypress pollen.

Maples (Acer)

February to March
Box elder or ash-leaved maple (Acer negundo), the most powerfully allergenic of the maples, is plentiful in this region.

Willows (Salix)

March to April
Moderate allergens. Can cross-react with poplars.

Oaks (Quercus)

April to May
Moderate allergens. Can cross-react with birch.

Ragweeds (Ambrosia)

August to October
The most important allergenic pollen in this region.

Wormwoods (Artemisia)

August to October
Will cross-react with mugwort and sagebrush. Particularly common in Tennessee.

Docks and sorrels (Rumex)

April to September
The peak season is from May to August.

Plantains (Plantago)

May to November
Only small amounts of pollen are produced, but the pollen is very allergenic.

THE MID-WEST

This area includes North and South Dakota, Nebraska, Minnesota, Michigan, Wisconsin, Iowa, Indiana and Idaho.

Grasses (Gramineae or Poaceae)

May to July
Begins in early May in the south, late May in the north. The season ends earlier in the east.

Maples (*Acer*)

April to May
The main allergen is the pollen of the box elder or ash-leaved maple (*Acer negundo*).

Birches (*Betula*)

April to May
Powerful allergens that cross-react with several other trees, notably alder, hazel, hornbeam and oak. More common in the north of this region.

Hazel, ironwood, hornbeam and alder (*Corylus, Carpinus, Ostrya* and *Alnus*)

February to April
Can provoke cross-reactions in those sensitive to birch.

Elms (*Ulmus*)

March to April
Can cross-react with hackberries and sugarberries (*Celtis*) which belong to the same family (Ulmaceae).

Oaks (*Quercus*)

April to May
Can cross-react with birch.

Willows and poplars (*Salix* and *Populus*)

March to April
Moderate allergens. Most common in the Great Lakes region and northern Minnesota. Balsam poplar and quaking aspen (*Populus balsamifera* and *Populus tremuloides*), both noted allergens, are found in this area.

Ash trees (*Fraxinus*)

April or May
The season is during April in the south of the region, during May in the north. Moderate allergens, most likely to provoke reactions in those already sensitized to olive pollen.

Privet (*Ligustrum*)

May to June
Produces plenty of pollen, but most of it does not travel far. Only a modest allergen, and the number of people affected is small. Those affected have often been sensitized by olive pollen, which cross-reacts with privet.

Ragweeds (*Ambrosia*)

July to October
The most important allergen in the region. There are many related plants that can cross-react with ragweed allergens including bur ragweed (*Franseria*) and marsh elders (*Iva*), both of which flower at about the same time.

Nettles and clearweed (*Urtica* and *Pilea*)

July to September
The season continues into October in the west of the region. Only moderately allergenic.

Pellitories (*Parietaria*)

July to September
Not reported as a common source of hayfever in this area, but may affect visitors sensitized elsewhere.

Docks and sorrels (*Rumex*)

May to September
The peak pollen season usually coincides with that of grass. Mainly in the east of the region.

Plantains (*Plantago*)

May to November
Very little in the west of this region. Counts can be high in the east particularly in July.

Hemp or cannabis (*Cannabis sativa*)

June to September
A fairly common cause of hayfever in Nebraska and the Dakotas.

Goosefoots and amaranths (Chenopodiaceae and Amaranthaceae)

June to October
Local names for these plants include pigweed, lamb's quarters and sowbane.

THE NORTH EAST AND NEW ENGLAND

This area includes Maine, New Hampshire, Vermont, Massachusetts, Connecticut, Rhode Island, Pennsylvania, New York State, New Jersey, Delaware, and Virginia.

Grasses (Gramineae and Poaceae)

May to July
Counts can be very high in June and July. The season continues until early August or even September in the Virginias and Delaware. Throughout the region, some pollen may remain in the air until October.

Birches (Betula)

April to May
Some pollen may still be airborne in June. A strongly allergenic pollen. Birches are more common in New England and the Appalachian Mountains than in any other part of the USA.

Alders, ironwood, hornbeams and hazels (Alnus, Carpinus, Ostrya and Corylus)

April to May
Some alders may begin pollinating earlier, in March or even February, particularly in the south of this region. All these pollens can cross-react with birch.

Oaks and beeches (Quercus)

April to May
Oaks are the main allergen, but in some areas, such as New Jersey, beeches seem to cause hayfever The two groups cross-react with each other and with birches.

Elms (Ulmus)

February to April
Pollen counts can be very high. The season is later in Delaware and the Virginias, from April to May. Cross-reactions with hackberry (Celtis) pollen are likely.

Maples (Acer)

February to May
The most allergenic species is box elder or ash-leaved maple (Acer negundo).

Willows and poplars (Salix and Populus)

March to April
Cross-reactions between these two groups are common. The season may begin earlier and end later in the south of the region. Willows are particularly common in the north of this region, e.g. in Maine.

Lindens or basswoods (Tilia)

June to July
Considered an important cause of hayfever in Virginia.

'Cedars' and junipers (Cupressaceae)

March to May
Can cross-react with cypresses.

Pines (Pinaceae)

April to May
New England has the highest recorded rate of genuine allergy to pine pollen in the world. The species concerned is Pinus strobus which grows in other countries as well. Why it should prove so allergenic here is a mystery.

Ash trees (Fraxinus)

May
The season can begin in April in the south of this region. Only a moderate allergen, but may affect those sensitized by olive pollen. Grows mainly on moist lowland soils.

Privet (Ligustrum)

May to June
Produces plenty of pollen, but most of it does not travel far. Only a modest allergen, and the number of people affected is small. Those affected have

often been sensitized by olive pollen which cross-reacts with privet.

Bayberry or wax myrtle (*Myrica*)

April to July
Only found on the coastal plain. A fairly strong allergen. Cross-reactions with sweet gale or bog myrtle (*Myrica gale*), which grows throughout Canada and Scandinavia, and in parts of the British Isles, are likely.

Sweet fern (*Comptonia peregrina*)

April to June
Not a true fern, but a shrub with fern-like leaves. This invasive plant is a fairly strong allergen and is spreading rapidly. A member of the same family as the bayberries (Myricaceae) so cross-reactions might occur, but this possibility has not been investigated.

Ragweeds (*Ambrosia*)

July to October
Ragweeds are the major cause of hayfever in this region. The peak season is from August to September. The season can continue into early November in the Virginias. Several other members of the same family (Compositae or Asteraceae) can provoke cross-reactions in those sensitive to ragweed pollen, and some flower at other times, thus prolonging the season.

Marsh elders (*Iva*)

August to October
These are the most common of the plants that cross-react with ragweed.

Nettles and clearweed (*Urtica* and *Pilea*)

May to October
The main season is from August to September. Moderately allergenic. Found mainly on disturbed ground and around abandoned buildings.

Pellitories (*Parietaria*)

June to October
The peak is in August and September. May cause some hayfever. A highly potent allergen but pollen counts are fairly low.

Goosefoots and amaranths (Chenopodiaceae and Amaranthaceae)

June to October
Pollen counts are never as high as in the western USA, and cases of hayfever to these plants are correspondingly fewer. Some patients who have symptoms in the ragweed season may actually be reacting to these plants, not to ragweed.

Docks and sorrels (*Rumex*)

May to September
The peak season coincides with that for grass. Counts are lower after the end of August.

Plantains (*Plantago*)

June to August
Where English plantain (*Plantago lanceolata*) grows, there may be some pollen in the air until October. In the south of the region (Delaware, West Virginia and Virginia) the season continues until November. Pollen counts are not as high as in northwest USA, and plantains are considered a minor cause of hayfever.

THE SOUTHEAST STATES

This area includes North Carolina, South Carolina, Georgia and Florida. The range of plants found growing in Florida is much wider than that of the other states, and growing seasons are longer. This is particularly true of southern Florida, and some of the plants listed below are only relevant for this region.

Grasses (Gramineae or Poaceae)

March to October
In southern Florida the season is much longer, and there is sufficient grass pollen in the air throughout the year to produce year-round symptoms in many people. The peak in Florida is from April to October.

'Cedars', cypresses and junipers (Cupressaceae)

December to March
The peak levels begin in January and last until March. Visitors sensitized to cypresses elsewhere in the world will

probably show cross-reactions to these conifers.

Oaks (*Quercus*)

February to May
In southern Florida the season starts much earlier, in December. The highest counts are during March and April in all areas, and can be very high in southern Florida. Oak pollen can cross-react with that of birch.

Elms (*Ulmus*)

March to May
The season is much longer in southern Florida, with one species, Chinese elm (*U. parvifolia*) pollinating from September to December, and other species beginning in January and continuing through to March.

Birches (*Betula*)

February to April
Pollen counts are not high, except in the Appalachian Mountains of North Carolina and northern Georgia.

Bald 'cypress' or swamp 'cypress' and pond 'cypress' (*Taxodium*)

December to March
The peak is from January to March. These are not true cypresses but relatives of the redwoods. Found in the swamp forests of southern Florida. A moderate allergen.

She-oaks or 'Australian pines' (*Casuarina*)

February to April, October to December
The pollination season is very variable and they may pollinate intermittently throughout the year in the Tampa Bay area of southern Florida. Planted in parts of Florida for windbreaks. A strongly allergenic pollen. Neither a pine nor an oak, so cross-reactions with these trees are unlikely.

Hickories and walnuts (*Carya* and *Juglans*)

April to May
In southern Florida hickory pollen can be airborne in February.

Willows and poplars (*Salix* and *Populus*)

March to May
Willows are generally less common in Florida, but the southern willow which grows in southern Florida can begin pollinating in January or February.

Maples (*Acer*)

March to May
The box elder or ash-leaved maple (*Acer negundo*) may be a problem in some areas, notably in Florida.

Everglades palm (*Acoelorrhaphe wrightii*)

April to June
Seems to cause some hayfever in the small area of southern Florida where it grows.

Paper mulberry (*Broussonetia papyrifera*)

March to June
The peak is in April and May. Not found in the northern part of this area, but widely planted in the south. It has become naturalized in parts of southern Florida. A powerful allergen. Cross-reactions with mulberry (*Morus*) are likely.

Mimosa or silk tree (*Albizia*)

April to June
Causes some hayfever in southern Florida.

Pines (*Pinaceae*)

December to June
The peak is from February to March. There are very high pollen counts in some areas, notably southern Florida. These may affect visitors who are already sensitive to pine, either as an allergen or as an irritant.

Gum trees (*Eucalyptus*)

December to March
A rare cause of hayfever in Florida.

Osage orange or hedgeplant (*Maclura*)

April to May
Widely planted for hedging. Can cross-react with mulberries and paper mulberry.

Privet (*Ligustrum*)

May to June
Produces plenty of pollen, but most of it does not travel far. Only a modest allergen, and the number of people affected is small. Those affected have often been sensitized by olive pollen, which cross-reacts with privet.

Bayberry or wax myrtle (*Myrica*)

February to April
A potential allergen in southern Florida. May well cross-react with the bog myrtle or sweet gale (*Myrica gale*) of Canada, Scandinavia and parts of Britain.

Ragweeds (*Ambrosia*)

July to November
There is some ragweed pollen in the air throughout the year, but the counts are generally low from January to March. They may be fairly high near the Florida coast, even in these months, where one species of ragweed flowers at this time.

By way of compensation, ragweed pollen counts at the height of the season (August to October) are not as high as in the northeastern USA or the states of the Mid-West.

Other plants in the same family (Asteraceae or Compositae) can provoke cross-reactions. Among those growing here is dog fennel or boneset (*Eupatorium*), which flowers from October to November and produces large amounts of airborne pollen. Groundsel bush or tree (*Baccharis halmilifolia*) and feverfew (*Parthenium*) also contribute to the pollen load.

Marsh elders and dune elder (*Iva*)

August to September
Found in the coastal areas, notably the salt marshes of Florida. Allergens are likely to cross-react with those of ragweed.

Goosefoots and amaranths (Chenopodiaceae and Amaranthaceae)

April to October
Pollen counts are never as high as in the western USA, and cases of hayfever to these plants are correspondingly fewer. However, some patients who have symptoms in the ragweed season may actually be responding to these plants, not to ragweed. In southern Florida, there may be some pollen in the air all year round, but levels are low from January to March.

Docks and sorrels (*Rumex*)

April to June
May continue producing some pollen until September.

Plantains (*Plantago*)

May to November
English plantain (*Plantago lanceolata*), the most allergenic species, is widespread.

Pellitories (*Parietaria*)

January to June
Pollen counts are low, but this is a powerful allergen and may affect those sensitized elsewhere in the world.

Nettles and clearweed (*Urtica* and *Pilea*)

August to October
Nettles are not found in southern Florida.

THE CARIBBEAN

The list below may omit some important local allergens, as the allergenic properties of the native trees have been very little studied.

Pollen is in the air during all seasons because the tropical climate allows plants to grow and flower all year round. Overall, the highest pollen counts occur from October to January, and the lowest during the dry season, from August to late September. If you are a holiday-maker visiting the islands, concentrate on avoiding pollens to which you are already sensitive. If you are highly sensitive to several pollens, stick to the dry season and stay in a coastal resort.

Grasses (Gramineae or Poaceae)

October to March, June to July
There are hundreds of different grasses and sedges, with a great range of flowering times. There will be some grass pollen in the air all year round, but the main season is from October to March. There is another burst of flowering in June and July but the pollen count is much lower then.

There are variations between lowlands and mountains, with the greatest differences on large islands such as Jamaica. The lowest pollen counts are found on coasts with onshore winds.

She-oaks or 'Australian pines' (*Casuarina*)

February to April
Introduced trees often planted in sandy coastal areas, and up to about 400 metres (1320 feet) altitude. Irregular pollen producers – very high in some years, very low in others. Neither oaks nor pines, so unlikely to produce cross-reactions with these trees.

Paper mulberry (*Broussonetia papyrifera*)

April to May
Planted in some areas for rearing silkworms. Note that silkworms themselves can produce airborne allergens (see p212)

Sugarberry or hackberry trees (*Celtis*)

June to October
Produces particularly strong allergens. Occurs in woodland, especially on limestone, as in parts of Jamaica. Belongs to the elm family, so there might be some cross-reactivity with elm pollen.

Pellitory-of-the-wall (*Parietaria judaica*)

December to August
A weed of open habitats which also grows in crevices in banks and walls. Found at altitudes up to 1200 metres (4000 feet). Only a problem in some localities.

Nettles (*Urtica*)

March to June
Some pollen is in the air at other times of year as well. A common weed on waste ground in lowland areas, especially around centres of population.

SOUTH AMERICA

Pollen information for South America is very limited, but some educated guesses can be made on the basis of the seasonal weather patterns and type of vegetation.

In countries north of the Equator, such as Venezuela, there will be a grass pollen season from April to July, peaking in May. The coastal plain of Venezuela may have some grass pollen in the air all year round.

In northern Brazil there are reports of an increase in the amount of grass pollen in some areas, due to the replacement of the rainforest by pastureland. This causes hayfever from October to December. Around Rio de Janeiro there may well be grass pollen in the air all year round with the highest concentrations likely to occur from December to March, the lowest from June to October.

Ecuador has sufficient warmth and moisture to encourage grass pollen all year round. For Peru, the peak pollen counts for grass probably occur from October to January, with low counts from February to June.

Buenos Aires has the right conditions for grass growth all year round, with peak production likely to occur from October to February. It is reported from Argentina that hayfever to hackberries (*Celtis*) is very common; this pollen may cross-react with that of elms.

NORTH AFRICA

Along the northern coast of Morocco, Algeria and Tunisia, the vegetation is very similar to the Mediterranean region (see p287) but the pollination seasons may be earlier. The grass season, for example, runs from March to May. Olives (*Olea*) pollinate mainly in May. Goosefoot (Chenopodiaceae) and mugwort (*Artemisia*) pollen can both reach high levels in some areas.

Egypt has a desert climate over large areas, with low pollen counts, but many of the most visited regions are in the Nile Delta where pollen seasons are very long. Around Alexandria, for example, grass pollen along with many other pollens is abundant from mid-February to early December. The nettle (*Urtica*) season lasts from late February or early March through to November with peak counts in April. Goosefoots (Chenopodiaceae) flower from late February to November. Cairo has much lower pollen counts owing to the very dry climate.

WEST AFRICA

Little information is available for this area, but the flowering season for grasses in the savanna regions can be given. This region stretches from the edge of the rainforests north to the Sahel and includes much of Nigeria and northern Ghana. Most of the grasses pollinate from April to July, with a peak in May. There will be some grass pollen in the air through to November.

EAST AFRICA

As for West Africa, there is little information available, but the pollen season for grasses can be quoted. The peak seasons occur in the months following the rains. Some areas have one rainy season per year, others have two, and the grass pollen seasons follow suit. Kenya's grasses flower from September to October, and again from December to January. In the savannas of Tanzania, the savanna grass pollinates from June to December with a peak in September and October. In Zimbabwe pollen is present in the air all year round, but peak grass pollen counts occur from July to August, and again from October to November. In Malawi the peak is from October to February. There are reports of hayfever-like symptoms at the time of the maize harvest in Malawi, which could be due to mould spores.

SOUTHERN AFRICA

Botswana has peak grass pollen counts from November to April. In South Africa, there may be some grass pollen in the air in most months of the year. Around Cape Town, the peak for grass pollen counts is from November to January. The area round Johannesburg and Pretoria has a shorter peak season, from December to January. The grass pollen counts are generally very high, as are counts for mould spores.

Capeweed (*Arctotheca calendula*) is a native plant here and may cause problems for Australian visitors sensitized to its pollen. Mesquite (*Prosopis*), a cause of hayfever in the southern states of America, also grows here.

SCANDINAVIA

This area includes Finland, Sweden, Norway and Denmark.

Grasses (Gramineae or Poaceae)

May to August
A more common cause of hayfever than birch in some parts of Scandinavia, but grasses rank second in the northern and central areas. Here the grass season is shorter (mid-June to mid-August) and pollen counts are low.

Birches (*Betula*)

April to June
The main season, for most of Scandinavia, is during May and the early part of June. The season begins earlier in Denmark (mid-April to early June). South and central Finland experience birch pollen from April to May. In the far north the season begins in late May and continues into July. Counts are lower here than elsewhere. The highest counts are in central Norway and Sweden, and central and southern Finland.

Birch is one of the trees that produces abundant pollen in one year, sparse pollen in the next. In recent times the odd-numbered years (1987, 1989, 1991) have experienced high pollen counts for much of Scandinavia, while the even-numbered years have had low counts. This pattern used to hold true in Denmark but no longer seems to do so.

Alder and hazel (*Alnus* and *Corylus*)

April to May
In the past, the hazel pollen season in Norway, Sweden and Finland has been short, beginning in late April. With the milder winters of recent years, hazel has begun to release pollen in January and February around Oslo and elsewhere in the south. This has had a noticeable priming effect (see p41) on those with birch pollen sensitivity.

In Denmark, hazel pollinates from January or February. Northern Scandinavia has very low pollen counts for hazel.

The alder season has also been getting longer in recent years, due to warmer weather. The alder season begins earlier in Denmark, from mid-February or early March. Pollen counts are moderate in most areas, very low in the far north.

Oaks (*Quercus*)

May to June
Significant pollen counts are found in southeastern Sweden and Denmark only.

Ash trees (*Fraxinus*)

May
Only in the south of the region. Not a common cause of hayfever.

Elms (*Ulmus*)

March to May
Not considered a cause of hayfever elsewhere in Europe, but identified as an allergen in Denmark. Cross-reactions with birch seem to be involved.

Pines (Pinaceae)

May to July
Only Denmark is likely to have appreciable amounts of pollen in the air before mid-May.

Cypresses (Cupressaceae)

May to July
Low pollen counts in most areas, peaking in June. Not observed in Denmark, but junipers (which cross-react with cypresses) pollinate from March to June. This pollen is not believed to cause any hayfever in Scandinavia.

Bog myrtle or sweet gale (*Myrica gale*)

April to May
Seems to cross-react with birch pollen.

Mugwort and wormwoods (*Artemisia*)

July to September
Rarely begins pollination before mid-July. The peak is in August. Pollen counts are highest in Denmark and around the Oslo Fjord region, but low in central and northern Scandinavia. This is the third most common source of hayfever in Scandinavia.

Nettles (*Urtica*)

June to August
The season begins earlier in Denmark and continues into September. Pollen counts are very low in central and northern Scandinavia.

Docks and plantains (*Rumex* and *Plantago*)

June to August
Pollen counts are low in most areas, but dock pollen reaches moderate levels in central Scandinavia.

NORTHERN AND EASTERN EUROPE

This includes northern France, Belgium, Luxembourg, the Netherlands, Germany, Switzerland, Austria, Hungary, Czechoslovakia and Poland.

Grasses (Gramineae or Poaceae)

April to September
The most important allergenic pollen throughout this region. As well as wild and cultivated grasses, fields of rye contribute to the pollen count in Germany, Austria and eastern Europe.

The season is much shorter in the west and north of this region, ending in July. The Rouen area, for example, has very high grass pollen counts from April to

June. In Belgium and the Netherlands the grass pollen season is later, from mid-May to mid-July. In the west of Germany it runs from May to July. In central France, central Germany, Austria and eastern Europe the grass season is long, from May through to September, although counts are fairly low after mid-August. Hungary has a relatively short season, from May to mid-July. At high altitudes, the pollen season generally runs from June to July only.

Pollen counts are lower on the west coast of France and near the Brittany coast. They are also low in forest areas, notably the Black Forest, and in the high Alps. Particularly high in the upper Loire valley in June, and on the north German plain from June to early July. Reeds and sedges can provoke cross-reactions in those sensitive to grass pollen, and areas with many reeds, such as Lakes Balaton and Velencei in Hungary, can provoke severe symptoms; the pollination season is from April to early July.

Birches (*Betula*)

April to May
The season can begin earlier, during March, in eastern Europe. In western Germany it runs from mid-March to June, but with the peak in late April and early May. Mountainous areas generally begin one to three weeks later than nearby lowlands.

High pollen counts occur in Belgium, Luxembourg, Austria and parts of northern Germany, but not in France, except around Paris and to the east of Paris. A major allergen in the Netherlands and Belgium.

Alder, hornbeam and hazel (*Alnus, Carpinus* and *Corylus*)

February to May
Peak pollen production is in March and April. Hazel can begin pollinating in January. In the Netherlands, alder sensitivity is more common than birch sensitivity.

Oaks and beeches (*Quercus* and *Fagus*)

April to June
The pollen count peaks in May. Beech pollen is highest in eastern France. Oak pollen can be high in central Germany and the eastern lowlands of Austria.

Chestnut trees (*Castanea*)

June to July
Those sensitive to this pollen usually react to birch pollen as well. Chestnuts are common in France, particularly around Paris, but pollen counts are relatively low. Counts can be high in the south and east of Austria.

Plane trees (*Platanus*)

March to May
Widely planted on city streets. There is a high pollen count for planes in Paris, usually from late March, ending in early May; similarly in some Swiss and Austrian cities, from April to May. Not a particularly common cause of hayfever.

Ash trees (*Fraxinus*)

April to May
Not a particularly strong allergen, but those already allergic to olive pollen may be sensitive to it through a cross-reaction.

Cypresses (Cupressaceae)

February to May
The peak is in March and April. Not considered a cause of hayfever in this region, but might affect visitors sensitized elsewhere. Pollen counts are low in the north, higher in the south.

Yew (*Taxus*)

March to April
Causes some hayfever in northern Switzerland and northern Austria, but not elsewhere in this region nor in most other parts of the world.

Pines (Pinaceae)

April to July
The season is shorter in the north and in central and eastern Europe, from May to June only. In Switzerland it is longer, continuing into August. Pollen counts are especially high in the Black Forest. Not considered a cause of hayfever anywhere in this region, but might affect visitors sensitized elsewhere.

Mugwort and wormwoods (*Artemisia*)

July to September
The main pollen season is in August. An important allergen in Austria, Belgium and some parts of the Netherlands.

Plantains (*Plantago*)

May to September
A long flowering season, but pollen counts are never particularly high. The maximum levels occur in July. Fairly common as a cause of hayfever in Belgium and parts of Austria.

Pellitories (*Parietaria*)

May to September
The season starts later in the north, usually in June. Widespread in France, Czechoslovakia, Austria and Hungary, but only found in certain localities in the other countries making up this area. Abundant along the banks of the Danube.

Docks and sorrels (*Rumex*)

May to August
Pollen counts are generally low after the end of June, so sensitivity to docks and sorrels may be mistaken for grass-pollen hayfever. There is less pollen in the air in the north of the region. Docks are considered an important allergen in Poland.

Nettles (*Urtica*)

June to September
Very high pollen counts have been recorded in some areas (e.g. Belgium), yet this is not a common cause of hayfever. The season is earlier in central Germany and Austria, from mid-May to the end of August.

Ragweeds (*Ambrosia*)

August to September
Do not grow in significant numbers in western Europe, except in Switzerland (particularly around Basle) and in the east of Austria, from Vienna to the Hungarian border. May also be spreading into the upper Rhône valley from the Lyon area. In eastern Europe, ragweeds are an increasing problem (see p131).

Goosefoots and amaranths (Chenopodiaceae and Amaranthaceae)

May to October
The main pollen season is from June to September. Various species grow widely, but there is relatively little airborne pollen in most areas. Significant amounts have sometimes been found in northeastern France and eastern Europe. This pollen is not considered a common cause of hayfever in this region.

SPAIN AND PORTUGAL

Grasses (Gramineae or Poaceae)

April to June
Although the highest counts are in the spring and early summer, there can be some airborne pollen all year round in the warmest areas. Portugal has significant pollen counts from late March through to early September.
　On the Costa del Sol, the main season begins at the end of April. The rest of Andalusia and the Madrid area follow on in May. There are a great many variations due to the weather. Dry winters delay the season, wet ones bring it forward.
　In general, pollen counts inland are higher than those near the coast.

Olive trees (*Olea*)

May to June
There is considerable variation in the pollen count from one year to another. In Andalusia, for example, the average count is 25 times higher in some years than in others.
　The season begins much earlier in Portugal, from March onwards. It is early on the Costa del Sol and in the southwest, later in the northeast. In the warmest areas, the last week of May is the worst time for this pollen.
　Few olives are grown in the north; the main growing regions are Portugal, Andalusia, Catalonia and central Spain.

Cypresses (Cupressaceae)

January to March
Although the pollen peaks in early spring, there is some in the air almost all year. In

the south, the peak season usually starts in February.

Birches (*Betula*)

April
Only common in the mountainous areas of northern Spain. Where it does occur, birch is an important allergen.

Alders (*Alnus*)

February to March
Only common along riversides in the mountains. The pollen counts are usually low.

She-oaks or 'Australian pines' (*Casuarina*)

October to November
Pollen counts can be quite high wherever this tree has been planted. Whether it is an important allergen among local people is not clear, but it could affect sensitized visitors from Australia. The season is two or three weeks earlier on the Costa del Sol.

Plane trees (*Platanus*)

March, April or May
The season is short, only about a week. It occurs in March in the south, as late as June in the far northwest or the high mountains. A very common street tree, so pollen counts can be high.

Oaks (*Quercus*)

March to June
There are large oakwood areas which can produce high pollen counts. Not a particularly allergenic pollen.

Ash trees (*Fraxinus*)

February to May
Common along riversides, mainly in Castille, around Madrid, and in the north. Cross-reacts with olive pollen, so it may cause symptoms in those sensitized to olive.

Pines (*Pinaceae*)

March to July
A rare cause of hayfever in Spain.

Eucalyptus or gum trees (*Eucalyptus*)

May to June
Some pollen in the air all year round. Not a powerful allergen, and no cases of hayfever have so far been recorded in Spain, but there are a few well-documented cases in California, Hawaii and India.

Sunflower (*Helianthus*)

June to August
Although sunflowers pollinate from June to July, many people experience symptoms during the harvest period in August. The reason for this is unknown. Mainly grown in southern Spain. People living near sunflower fields may be sensitized.

Goosefoots and amaranths (Chenopodiaceae and Amaranthaceae)

May to September
Among the most important allergenic weeds in this region, mainly in the driest areas.

There may be some pollen in the air all year round, but the peak is in summer. In southern Spain, the peak comes in May and June. In central and northern Spain it is later, in July and August. The season is generally shorter in Portugal, running from July to August only.

Pellitories (*Parietaria*)

March to May, May to July
The season varies, depending on which species grow locally. Pellitories are not a common cause of hayfever here, whereas they are in other Mediterranean countries. It seems that the local pellitory species produce less pollen, and what they do produce is less allergenic. Pellitory hayfever is only common in Catalonia.

Nettles (*Urtica*)

May to July
Common weeds throughout the region, causing some hayfever.

Mugwort and wormwoods (*Artemisia*)

August to September
Very common in drier areas and in the

mountains of the south, southeast, east and centre of the Iberian peninsula.

Plantains (*Plantago*)

March to June
The season begins first on the Costa del Sol, later in Catalonia, and not until May in the centre and south. Relatively few people are allergic to this pollen.

THE CANARY ISLANDS

There is very little grass on some islands (e.g. Gomera) except in the small fields beside streams. Other islands may have more grass but it will flower early, in about April. The islands have a specialized native flora and are home to very few of the more troublesome hayfever plants. Along the coasts of the islands, particularly in the north, pollen counts are very low, because of the strong onshore winds. Tree heather (*Erica arborea*) grows on some islands, and has been implicated in hayfever elsewhere (e.g. Turkey). Olives (*Olea*) may be grown on some islands.

THE MEDITERRANEAN

Southern France, Italy, Greece and the Mediterranean islands. For northeastern Greece, the information for Turkey and the Balkans (see p288) may be more relevant.

Grasses (Gramineae or Poaceae)

April to September
The season is much shorter in Greece, from mid-April to June only. Throughout the region, grass pollen counts are much lower than in Britain or northern Europe, particularly in hot dry areas where they may be insufficient to provoke hayfever. Sicily and the Greek islands have low counts, as do the Bordeaux region, Calabria and the Adriatic coast of Italy.
   A few species of grass flower in winter in Greece and might cause problems in some areas.

Olive trees (*Olea*)

March to July
Peak pollination is in May and June. In southern France and southern Italy, the season starts later, in late April or early May.

Cypresses (Cupressaceae)

December to June
The season is earlier in Italy and Greece, and along the Mediterranean coast of France (December or January to May). It is later (February to June) in inland areas of southern France. Cypress hayfever is rising rapidly in southern France where many cypresses have been planted to protect crops and fruit trees from the wind.

Birches (*Betula*)

April to May
Pollen counts are generally low. Only significant in mountainous areas of France and northern Italy.

Alder and hazel (*Alnus* and *Corylus*)

January to May
The season begins in January only on the Mediterranean coast. Pollen counts can be quite high in northern and central Italy; elsewhere they are very low.

Pines (Pinaceae)

March to July
Pollen counts are not particularly high, yet there are isolated cases of pine allergy reported.

Oaks (*Quercus*)

April to June
Not a major source of hayfever.

Chestnuts (*Castanea*)

June to July
Only common in southern France and northern and central Italy, where they may cause some hayfever.

Mimosa (*Acacia*)

February to May
Only important in the area around Nice.

Poplars (*Populus*)

March to April
Grown for shade in some parts of Greece and may cause hayfever.

Paper mulberry (*Broussonetia papyrifera*)

April to May
Only grown in southeastern France; it can cause very severe symptoms, particularly in the eyes.

Pellitories (*Parietaria*)

March to July, September to November
This very long season, with a lull in midsummer, is typical of southern Italy only. In Sicily, there may be some pollen in the air all year round. In Greece, the hot dry climate keeps the season shorter, from April to June, with low levels continuing until September. In central and northern Italy, and in southern France, the season is from April to October, beginning later in the north.

Nettles (*Urtica*)

April to June
Some pollen in the air all year round.

Docks and sorrels (*Rumex*)

April to September
Moderate amounts are found in the air in southern France and northern Italy, but not elsewhere in this region.

Plantains (*Plantago*)

May to September
Pollen counts are negligible in Greece.

Mugwort and wormwoods (*Artemisia*)

August to October
Pollen counts are fairly low everywhere, especially in the far south.

Goosefoots and amaranths (Chenopodiaceae and Amaranthaceae)

May to October
'Russian thistle' is a common cause of hayfever in some areas.

Ragweeds (*Ambrosia*)

August to September
The season may start a little earlier in northern Italy, in mid-July. It continues into October in parts of Italy. Ragweed pollen is particularly abundant in the Rhône valley, around Lyon.

TURKEY AND THE BALKANS

Turkey, Bulgaria, Romania, and the countries of the former Yugoslavia. No data available for Albania.

Grasses (Gramineae and Poaceae)

May to September
Counts are highest in May and June for much of this region. The pollen count falls sharply at the end of June, and is fairly low by mid-July. Rye is grown in Croatia, adding to the pollen count. In southern Bulgaria the season may start earlier, at the end of April, but for northern Bulgaria the peak pollen season is in July.

Sedges and reeds, pollinating in April and May, may cross-react with grass pollen. Counts may be high near large lakes.

Birches (*Betula*)

April to May
Only common in Romania, Bulgaria and other parts of the Balkans, but the species of birch found in Turkey produces highly allergenic pollen.

Alder, hornbeam, hop-hornbeam and hazel (*Alnus, Carpinus, Ostrya* and *Corylus*)

February to May
The pollen counts for hazel can be fairly high in some areas. The hazel season in Turkey is largely over by April.

Olive trees (*Olea*)

May to June
Only significant in Turkey, mainly in coastal regions.

Poplars (*Populus*)

March to April
Considered an important allergen in the countries of the former Yugoslavia.

Ash trees (*Fraxinus*)

March to April
Pollen counts can be high in parts of Turkey and on the Adriatic coast.

Cypresses (Cupressaceae)

March to May
Pollen counts can be high in Turkey, but the season ends earlier, in April.

Pines (Pinaceae)

April to July
The season is shorter in Turkey, from May to June, but counts are very high.

Oaks, beeches and plane trees (*Quercus, Fagus* and *Platanus*)

April to May
Planes produce very high counts for a brief period in parts of Turkey.

Box elder or ash-leaved maple (*Acer negundo*)

March to May
A tree introduced from the USA which is found in parts of Turkey and produces highly allergenic pollen.

Tree heather (*Erica arborea*)

April to May, September to October
Produces highly allergenic pollen.

Plantains (*Plantago*)

May to August
Season does not start until June in Turkey. The pollen can be highly allergenic.

Goosefoots and amaranths (Chenopodiaceae and Amaranthaceae)

June to October
Peak pollen production is in August and September. An important source of allergenic pollen along the Bulgarian coast.

Pellitories (*Parietaria*)

May to August
Pollen counts are not particularly high, except on the Romanian plains, along the Adriatic coast and in parts of Croatia.

Mugwort and wormwoods (*Artemisia*)

July to September
Common allergens in Romania and Bulgaria, not particularly important elsewhere.

Docks and sorrels (*Rumex*)

April to June
Pollen counts are generally low.

Nettles (*Urtica*)

March to August
Not a particularly important allergen. Counts can be high in Bulgaria.

Ragweeds (*Ambrosia*)

August to September
Recorded in Bulgaria, along the Adriatic coast and in much of Croatia, where the pollen count is steadily rising.

THE FORMER USSR

In Russia (west of the Urals), Bielarus, the Ukraine and the Caucasus region, the pollen seasons are similar to those of eastern Europe (see pp283–5). Ragweeds (*Ambrosia*) are a major allergen in large parts of this area, often the most common cause of hayfever. Rye (*Secale*) grown as a crop, boosts the grass pollen count in early summer. Birch (*Betula*), alder (*Alnus*), hazel (*Corylus*), wormwood (*Artemisia*), plantains (*Plantago*) and goosefoots (Chenopodiaceae) are other notable allergens. Sunflowers (*Helianthus*) cause hayfever in some localities.

Information is sparse for other countries in this region. Ragweed (*Ambrosia*) grows in Georgia, and probably in several other states.

THE MIDDLE EAST

In most of the area, desert conditions prevail and pollen counts are very low, especially from July to January. What pollen there is becomes airborne in April. Where there are extensive tree plantations, as in Saudi Arabia, the pollen may cause hayfever. Grass pollen is found in Israel, Lebanon, and the western regions of Jordan and Syria. The season runs from March to May, continuing into June in parts of Israel. The same regions have olive (*Olea*) pollen in May and June and some mugwort (*Artemisia*) from August to October. Goosefoots

(Chenopodiaceae) are widespread on dry soils, particularly 'Russian thistle' (*Salsola kali*) which is a common source of symptoms in parts of Iran. Cypresses (Cupressaceae) pollinate in the winter, continuing into February, and are an increasing cause of hayfever. Rural areas in Israel growing irrigated crops produce very high pollen counts (see p52) and hayfever is a serious problem. Australian she-oaks (*Casuarina*) and wattles (*Acacia*) are planted for shelter in places and have been implicated in hayfever.

INDIA AND PAKISTAN

During the monsoon rains, the air is practically free from pollen. The period immediately afterwards sees very high pollen counts for most plants, including grasses. This continues for about two months, then the grass pollen count declines for about two months, followed by a period with low or moderate pollen counts. This is a very generalized picture and exact dates cannot be given for every area. The monsoon seasons vary from north to south and within particular regions, so the grass pollen season will also be variable. Try to find out the timing of the rainy season in the area you plan to visit, and avoid the months immediately after this. For most of the sub-continent, excluding the far south, the period from February to April will have the lowest pollen counts.

There are many other plants that cause hayfever in India, such as mesquite (*Prosopis*) and American feverfew (*Parthenium*).

JAPAN

Grasses (Gramineae or Poaceae)

April to June

About 30 per cent of hayfever sufferers react to grasses. Many of these people are also sensitive to Japanese red cedar.

Although grass pollen can continue into September, the pollen counts are low after June. The season begins later in the north and at higher altitudes.

Highest pollen counts are in the central areas such as Matsukawa where there are extensive apple orchards.

Japanese red cedar or 'sugi' (*Cryptomeria japonica*)

February to April

More than 90 per cent of patients with hayfever in Japan are allergic to Japanese red cedar. Anyone travelling to Japan from abroad is unlikely to be affected unless they are already allergic to cypress (Cupressaceae) pollen: there is considerable cross-reactivity between these pollens. Reactions to Japanese red cedar seem to be considerably worse in towns or along roads with serious air pollution.

The main pollination period for Tokyo and surrounding areas is in February and March. The season begins later further north, and at higher altitudes. In the district of Nikko-Imaichi, for example, 120 km (75 miles) north of Tokyo and 800 metres (2600 feet) above sea level, the season is in March and April.

The tree is native to the northern part of Honshu – the main island. It grows in forests between 220 and 400 metres (730 and 1320 feet) above sea level, sometimes alone, sometimes mixed with cypresses. Elsewhere it is now grown in plantations for timber. A very beautiful conifer, with glossy green foliage, it is also widely grown in gardens, palaces and sanctuaries, providing a source of pollen within towns.

The amount of pollen produced varies enormously from year to year. Patients who are not particularly sensitive may be free from symptoms in low-pollen years.

Cypresses (Cupressaceae)

March to April

Cypresses grow wild, particularly in the mountains. They are also cultivated widely in gardens, and are grown as *bonsai*, or miniature trees. Since *bonsai* trees are brought indoors for special occasions, cypress pollen can be liberated in the home itself.

Those sensitive to cypresses may be allergic to Japanese red cedar as well.

The season usually ends in early April, but sometimes continues to late April. The amount of pollen produced varies greatly from one year to another.

Birches (*Betula*)

February to May

The season does not usually begin until

late February. Pollen production is prolific and the pollen spreads widely, but a relatively small proportion of hayfever sufferers are affected.

Birches grow mostly in mountain valleys in light woodland. They also border coniferous forests along the tree line at high altitudes. Some are planted for ornamental purposes.

Alders (*Alnus*)

March to April
Alders have recently been identified as a cause of hayfever in Japan. A large number of cases of alder hayfever are found close to the alder plantations that exist in some areas. Cross-reactions between birches and alders are known to occur.

Ragweed (*Ambrosia*)

July to August
The season does not usually begin until late July. This highly allergenic weed was introduced from America about a hundred years ago and is now widespread in open habitats.

Mugwort (*Artemisia*)

July to September
This pollen does not spread widely, so it only causes localized problems, in areas where mugwort grows.

Hops (*Humulus*)

July to August
Localized in lowland areas, so a relatively rare cause of hayfever. Hops and hemp (cannabis) belong to the same plant family, and there are occasional reports of hayfever reactions to their pollen from various parts of the world.

Goosefoots, plantains and nettles (Chenopodiaceae, *Plantago* and *Urtica*)

August to September
Widespread weeds of open habitats, but the pollen does not spread far. Allergy to these pollens is relatively rare in Japan, but they could cause problems for visitors from abroad.

HAWAII

Grass pollen can be in the air for most of the year, with the exception of late December. Tree pollens, of various native and introduced species, are airborne from January until late April. Japanese red cedar (*Cryptomeria*) is planted for landscaping and windbreaks. Gum trees (*Eucalyptus*) seem to cause hayfever quite commonly here, unlike other parts of the world. The weed season is from mid-May to December. There are marked regional differences in pollen counts.

APPENDIX 2
Particles, droplets and dust – the range of sizes

(A micron is a thousandth of a millimetre.)

Type of particle	Size (diameter) of particle
Absidia spores	2–4 microns
Alder pollen	22–34 microns
Alternaria spores	4–10 microns, some larger
Amaranth pollen	20–40 microns
Arthrinium spores	4–10 microns
Ash pollen	18–27 microns
Aspergillus spores	2–4 microns, some smaller than 2 microns
Aspergillus tereus	less than 2 microns
Aureobasidium spores	2–10 microns
Australian white cypress pine	20–24 microns
Bacteria	0.1 micron–5 microns
Bald 'cypress' pollen	28–36 microns
Birch pollen	18–28 microns
Bird allergens	see 'Feather allergens'
Cat allergen	less than 2.5 microns (perhaps as low as 0.05 micron) up to 20 microns or more
Cladosporium spores	4–10 microns
Coal dust	1–100 microns
Coniophora cerebella spores	14 microns x 9 microns
Cryptostroma spores	2–4 microns
Cypress pollen	19–38 microns
Diesel exhaust particulates	1–10 microns, most are 2.5 microns or less
Dock pollen	21–27 microns
Dog allergen	no figures available
Dry rot spores	4–10 microns
Epicoccum spores	over 10 microns
Feather allergens	most are 1 micron
Flour	1–90 microns
Fog and mist	2–100 microns
Goosefoot pollen	20–30 microns
Graphium spores	2–10 microns
Grass pollen	25–37 microns

Greasy particles found in domestic air	0.01 micron–5 microns
Hazel pollen	18–23 microns
Horsetail (*Equisetum*) spores	38–56 microns
House-dust mites	200–300 microns
House-dust mite droppings	4–20 microns
House-dust mite droppings – fragmented	0.5 micron-3 microns
Japanese red cedar pollen	24–32 microns
Micropolyspora faeni spores	less than 2 microns
Mould spores	less than 2 microns to over 10 microns (see individual entries if you know which mould is your allergen)
Mucor spores	2–10 microns
Nocardia asteroides spores	less than 2 microns
Mugwort pollen	18–24 microns
Olive pollen	17-28 microns
Paxillus panuoides spores	4–5 microns
Pellitory pollen	14–19 microns
Penicillium spores	mostly 2–4 microns, some larger
Pine pollen	60–85 microns, but air bladders keep it airborne despite its large size
Plane pollen	18–25 microns
Plantain pollen	16–36 microns
Pollen	5–200 microns, although the main allergenic pollens fall in the range 10–40 microns, with the majority between 20 and 35 microns (see individual entries if you know which pollen is your allergen)
Pollen fragments* (see next page)	0.5 micron upwards
Privet pollen	28–38 microns
Puccinia spores	over 10 microns
Ragweed pollen	19–20 microns

Rat urinary proteins	associated with particles of 5–10 microns
Redwood pollen	22–25 microns
Smog	0.01 micron–2 microns
Smoke from cigarettes	see 'Tobacco smoke particles'
Smoke from coal fires and boilers	0.01 micron–4 microns
Smoke from oil-burning boilers, etc.	0.04 micron–1 micron
Sporobolomyces spores	2–10 microns
Thermoactinomyces spores	less than 2 microns
Tobacco smoke particles	0.01 micron–1 micron
Ustilago spores	4–10 microns
Viruses	0.02–0.3 micron
Wet rot spores	see *Coniophora cerebella* spores and *Paxillus panuoides* spores

* Covers all smaller-than-pollen-grain particles carrying pollen allergens. This includes both fragmented pollen grains, and very small particles containing pollen-type allergens that are released by the plant at the same time as the pollen. These are known to exist for ragweed, some grasses, Japanese red cedar and Australian white cypress pine. They may exist for other plants, but this has not been widely investigated.

APPENDIX 3
Useful products

One of the problems facing allergy sufferers is that the trade in protective goods is not well regulated. To quote just one example, there is a small aerosol spray containing herbal extracts, manufactured in the USA and sold in some shops in Britain which claims to 'safely clear the air of smoke and pollen'. The claim is absurd, but there is apparently nothing to prevent this spray being sold. Fortunately, most manufacturers' claims are not as misleading as this, but one still needs to be wary of believing everything that is claimed about certain air filters, for example, or some of the anti-pollution masks. The details given here are primarily intended to make potential buyers more informed about the goods available, and better able to choose the right product.

The names of suppliers are given here. For their addresses please turn to the list in *Appendix 4* (p311).

While we have made every effort to ensure that the details and prices given here are correct, we cannot take any responsibility for errors or omissions. Nor have we carried out any independent testing of the products. Purchasers should check all details carefully before buying any product.

VAT exemption

In Britain allergy sufferers with asthma, perennial rhinitis or eczema do not have to pay VAT on certain goods that can alleviate their medical condition. This applies to the specialized vacuum cleaners for dust-mite allergy, anti-mite sprays and mite-proof covers for mattresses, duvets and pillows. It may also apply to certain other products – ask the supplier. You need to fill in a VAT exemption form, which is included in the order form sent to you by the company selling the goods. Make sure that you are buying from a company that operates this scheme, otherwise you will be paying VAT unnecessarily.

This scheme does not operate throughout the EC, but there may be reductions in VAT in other countries.

FACE MASKS

Face masks, which filter air going into the nose and mouth, can be helpful in certain situations, where you are exposed to a high level of allergen for a short period. The mask must fit tightly against your nose and face, forming a seal at all the edges. A beard or moustache may prevent a good seal being formed.

If you experience any difficulty in breathing, you should remove the mask immediately.

Occasions when masks can be useful

You might want to wear a mask at certain times of year, or in certain places, to protect against various items in the air, as follows.

Natural allergens and irritants in outdoor air
- pollen
- pollen fragments
- volatile chemicals produced by plants (occasionally a source of trouble if they act as irritants)
- mould spores in the air
- mould spores being released in large amounts, e.g. from a compost heap, rotting wood, or crop plants during harvesting
- other allergens, such as insect particles (rare causes of allergy)

Pollutants in outdoor air that might aggravate hayfever symptoms, or trigger an asthma attack
- sulphur dioxide (from factories and power stations)
- acidic droplets in the air (from factories and power stations)
- ozone (from sunlight + vehicle exhaust)
- nitrogen oxides (from vehicle exhaust)
- diesel particles (from buses, lorries and other diesel engines)
- volatile hydrocarbon molecules (from petrol etc.)

Natural allergens in indoor air
- pollen stirred up during ordinary housework
- pollen coming into the house when the windows are open
- mould spores stirred up during ordinary housework
- mould spores coming into the house when the windows are open
- mould spores being released in large amounts by renovation work, redecorating or a major clean-up operation in a damp (or previously damp) house
- mould spores being released in large amounts from stored hay, bird droppings or bird nesting material, mushroom compost or rotten timbers
- house-dust mite droppings stirred up during ordinary housework
- house-dust mite droppings stirred up during a major clean-up operation, replacement of a carpet, or removal of an old sofa, mattress, etc.
- cat, dog or feather allergens stirred up during ordinary housework
- cat, dog or feather allergens stirred up during a major cleaning operation, replacement of a carpet, or removal of an old sofa, armchair, etc.
- other allergens (e.g. insect particles) stirred up during a major cleaning operation
- animal allergens found in urine (laboratory workers only)
- wood dust or other allergens encountered at work

Pollutants in indoor air that might irritate the airways
- paint fumes during decorating
- solvent fumes following protective wood treatment

Finding the right mask for the job

There are two basic types of mask: those that have a dust filter only, and those that combine a dust filter with an activated carbon filter. (Powered respirator helmets, used for special applications, are dealt with on p297.)

Activated carbon masks

Activated carbon masks filter out certain gases and volatile chemicals (see p120) which cannot be removed by dust masks because they are not particles. They are used, primarily, to protect against synthetic pollutants, but should also take out natural volatile substances produced by plants.

The activated carbon is made by heating coal or wood to very high temperatures (when made from wood it is sometimes called **activated charcoal**). Heating to a high temperature turns carbon into highly porous material, rather like a hard sponge. The surface of the carbon acts like a 'molecular magnet' – it holds a variety of airborne chemicals (see below) by forming weak chemical bonds with them. As the activated carbon is riddled with holes, there is a large surface area which can interact with chemicals in the air.

To make face masks, a thin pad of fabric, or a piece of foam rubber, is impregnated with particles of activated carbon.

The ability of activated carbon to attract and hold chemicals will decline with use because the surfaces become coated with the chemicals already filtered from the air. According to some manufacturers, its powers can be regenerated by washing with detergent, which they claim removes the chemicals that are bound to the carbon. Other manufacturers dispute this claim. Replacement carbon filters are sold for some of the masks.

Activated carbon is used in all the anti-pollution masks currently sold in Britain. As explained in the next section, these are not covered by any compulsory standards. Some have been independently tested, as described below, and one complies with standards for particle (dust) removal, but not to any for the removal of gas or volatile substances, since there are no relevant standards.

Activated carbon is also used in certain masks for industrial use, which do have to conform to standards. One of these could be used to protect against pollutants.

Activated carbon will take out various chemicals from the air, including:

- sulphur dioxide (from factories and power stations)
- acidic droplets in the air (from factories and power stations)
- ozone (from sunlight + vehicle exhaust)
- volatile hydrocarbon molecules (from petrol etc.)
- volatile substances from plants (e.g. oil-seed rape)
- solvent vapour from paint
- solvent vapour following protective wood treatment

Some anti-pollution masks take out nitrogen oxides as well. Activated carbon alone cannot take out these gases, but the carbon can be treated so that some nitrogen dioxide is absorbed.

Very few masks contain a pad of activated carbon material alone, but a few do. Although the activated carbon may take out some dust particles, it is not designed for this purpose, so it will have limited action against pollen or diesel particulates, for example. There is also a strong possibility that some activated carbon particles will become detached from the fabric or foam which carries them, and thus be inhaled. Since activated carbon can act as an IgE-specific adjuvant (see p45) in just the same way as diesel particulates, inhaling carbon particles is not a good idea. Any mask where the activated carbon pad is directly against the nose and mouth could represent a hazard, and should therefore be avoided. There should be a dust filter between the activated carbon material and the face.

Dust masks

Dust masks will take out particles from the air, but it is crucial to know the smallest size removed; the simplest dust masks remove only fairly large particles. A claim that a dust mask or anti-pollution mask removes '95 per cent of particulates' is meaningless unless the size of those particulates is given.

Dust masks that are manufactured and sold for the protection of workers have to meet certain standards based on the smallest particle size they will filter out efficiently. (These are technically known as **dust respirators**.)

Masks sold *only* for protection from traffic pollutants are not governed by any compulsory standards in Britain at the time this book went to press, but this situation may change in the future. If there are no standards, it may be difficult to discover what particle size the anti-pollution mask removes (indeed, the manufacturer may not know). One of the anti-pollution masks, made by 3M, is based on dust masks designed for industrial use, and complies with the standards applied to them.

Standards for dust masks

The standards applied in Britain to industrial dust masks (respirators) are as follows. (In all cases, particles smaller than 0.5 micron will also be removed, but with less efficiency.)

Health and Safety Executive Standards

EN149 FFP 3SL Filters out particles of 0.5 micron and above with an efficiency of 98 per cent. Also filters out mist droplets with an efficiency of 98 per cent.

EN 149 FFP2S Filters out particles of 0.5 micron and above with an efficiency of 92 per cent. Also filters out mist droplets with an efficiency of 96 per cent.

EN 149 FFP1 Filters out particles of 0.5 micron and above with an efficiency of 78 per cent. Filters out mist droplets with an efficiency of 78 per cent.

British Standards

These are no longer in use, but you may see them quoted on products that were first marketed some time ago.

BS 6016/2 Filters out particles of 0.5 micron and above with an efficiency of over 95 per cent.

BS 6016/1 Filters out particles of 0.5 micron and above with an efficiency of over 90 per cent.

Nuisance Dust masks

Nuisance Dust masks only filter out particles larger than 5 microns. There are no compulsory standards set for the efficiency with which they remove these particles. The manufacturers are allowed to state that such masks filter out pollen, and of course they do. However, fragments of pollen grains, and fine dust from plants containing the same allergens as pollen, can be smaller than 5 microns in size. Some plants are known to produce these (see p23), and they may exist for other plants as well. At least some of these particles would get through a Nuisance Dust mask.

The dust masks sold in chemists' shops (e.g. Boots) are designed only for Nuisance Dusts. Thus, they will not give full protection against pollen fragments or small particles of dust-mite allergens made airborne during vacuum cleaning (see p185), despite the claim on the packet that they are 'suitable for those sensitive to dust'.

You should check the size of the particles that you need protection from, using Appendix 2 (see p292). If the

particles are larger than 5 microns, a Nuisance Dust mask will be adequate. If some or all of the particles are smaller than 5 microns, you may need a mask that complies to standards. However, since Nuisance Dust masks are cheap and readily available, it is worth trying them to see if they reduce your symptoms.

Manufacturers and suppliers

Allergy Aid Centre, Australia

Produces a respirator that protects against dust, mists and some volatile substances.

Arco

Sell occupational masks made by 3M. Can be bought in Arco retail stores in some parts of Britain; also available mail order.

British Lung Foundation

Sells an anti-pollution mask produced by 3M (see p297). Available by mail order.

R.J. Chicken

Distribute 3M anti-pollution masks to cycle shops. Cannot sell directly to the public, but masks can be ordered through any cycle shop.

Greenscreen

Produce and sell anti-pollution masks, including one incorporated into a scarf. The Uno model, widely available in cycle shops, contains an activated carbon pad sandwiched between two foam dust masks. The other models, which must be ordered by mail, have a dust filter with an electrostatic charge for better filtration of small particles. Manufacturer cannot give size for particles removed. Independently tested by a research laboratory in the USA and another in Mexico. Reduces sulphur dioxide by 60 per cent, nitrogen dioxide by 50 per cent, ozone by 84 per cent.

Martindale

Produce and sell Nuisance Dust masks and occupational dust masks complying to standards. Also produce and sell occupational masks for both dusts and gases complying to standards (suitable model for use against pollutants: Flatmate Gas). All masks available by mail order; Nuisance Dust masks sold in Boots the Chemists.

Respro

Produce and sell anti-pollution masks.

Available in some cycle shops; can also be bought by mail order.

3M

Produce occupational dust masks complying to standards, and Nuisance Dust masks. Both sold through Arco and other retail outlets; call freephone 0800 212490 for your nearest store. Produce an anti-pollution mask based on industrial masks. This is sold through the British Lung Foundation, Allerayde and some cycle shops. Unlike other anti-pollution masks, this complies with EN 149 FFP1, so it will take out 0.5 micron particles with an efficiency of 78 per cent. It also contains activated carbon which will remove ozone, sulphur dioxide, acid droplets and volatile organic compounds, but is not designed to protect against nitrogen oxides.

Approximate costs

Nuisance Dust masks cost about £1–£2.

Occupational dust masks, complying to standards, cost between £1 and £4.

The inclusion of activated carbon makes anti-pollution masks more expensive. The 3M anti-pollution mask costs about £5 and is available in packs of two. The filters are not replaceable. The simplest Greenscreen anti-pollution mask costs about £4, plus about £2 for five refill carbon filters. Masks incorporated into scarves tend to cost more, about £10. The Flatmate Gas filter from Martindale costs £3–£4.

POWERED RESPIRATORS

These are used mainly by laboratory workers who are exposed to high levels of allergen from mice or rats (see p216). They may also be of value to farm workers or plant breeders with hayfever. Air is filtered by a battery-powered unit strapped to the waist (see p126).

Manufacturers and suppliers

Arco
Sell Racal 'airstream' respirators, which offer a good range of helmets.

Martindale
Sell a wide range of models, some with ultra-lightweight hoods or helmets.

Protector Safety, Australia
Sell Racal 'airstream' respirators, which offer a good range of helmets.

Approximate costs

Powered respirators cost £150–£190, plus the cost of the filters.

PROTECTIVE EYEWEAR

Plastic goggles are widely available in do-it-yourself shops, and are very cheap. You can also add your own shields to an existing pair of glasses or sunglasses (see p123).

More sophisticated protective eyewear, designed to look like ordinary glasses, is now available. Some designs are very attractive indeed, and can be supplied with plain or prescription lenses, tinted or untinted.

Choose a pair that gives as much coverage as possible at the side and above the lens. A few designs (such as the Deflector XR10 from ILES Opticals) also give coverage below the lens.

Manufacturers and suppliers

Some companies manufacturing safety spectacles deal with the public through opticians, rather than directly, even if the glasses are fitted with plain lenses (known as plano lenses in the trade) for those with good eyesight. Some opticians stock a few types of protective spectacles which you can look at, but they rarely have a wide range. Colour catalogues are available, however, and the optician can obtain these so that you can see the designs for yourself. The optician should also be able to order a frame that you like the look of, and either adjust it to fit you, or return it to the manufacturer if you are not happy with it. Be prepared to shop around and find an optician who will order two or more catalogues for you to look at.

Companies dealing in protective wear (e.g. Arco, Iles Opticals) also supply protective glasses in excellent designs. They feature these in their catalogues, which can be sent free of charge to anyone, so that you can see what is available. Some of these companies deal only through opticians, while others will sell the glasses direct to the public, if fitted with plano lenses. Should you need corrective lenses, these companies can have your prescription made up and fitted into the chosen frame.

Tinted lenses are available in some of the models.

Arco
Sell a wide range of protective spectacles made by various other companies. Will send a free colour catalogue on request, and can supply the spectacles mail order with plano lenses, or via an optician with prescription lenses. Their spectacles (with plano lenses) are also available in Arco stores (see p311).

Iles Opticals
Produce a good range of protective eyewear, of which the Hy-Line and the Deflector XR range give good all-round coverage. Will send a free colour catalogue, and a price list. Spectacles with plano lenses are available in retail outlets around the country; ask about your nearest store. If corrective lenses are needed, can supply the spectacles through an optician.

Medivac
Sell protective eyewear mail order.

Norville Optical Company
Produce a range of safety spectacles, some with top-and-sides coverage. Catalogues and spectacles can only be ordered by opticians.

Approximate costs

Plastic safety goggles cost £2–£3.

Safety spectacles with plano lenses cost £3–£12. For prescription lenses add £20–£30, more for bifocals.

AIR FILTERS AND CLEANERS

A research paper published by a team of scientists in the USA concluded that the 'use of room air-cleaning devices in the absence of other forms of environmental control is not reasonable'. However, they did find that the air cleaners could be useful in certain circumstances, if combined with other measures. These measures are described in the main text of this book, in relation to pollen, dust mites, mould spores, cat allergens and other items in the air.

With the exception of HEPA filters (see below), there are no compulsory standards governing air cleaning devices in Britain. Making sense of the sales literature on different brands of air filters and assessing their relative merits is far from easy. The information given below is intended to help you understand the claims made and compare one filter with another.

The small, table-top filters sold in electrical shops which claim to 'remove pollen' are most unlikely to be powerful enough to make any impact on the air in an average room. Any filter that is on sale without technical information on air throughput (see p300) and filtration efficiency should be rejected. With any air filter or cleaner you need to ask some pertinent questions of the supplier or manufacturer, and try out the device at home (see p302) before you buy.

How air filters and cleaners work

As with masks (see pp294–5), an air filter may remove either particles, or gases and volatile chemicals, or both. Most deal with both.

The removal of gases and volatile chemicals relies on **activated carbon**, as in masks. See p295 for further details on how activated carbon works.

In the case of particles, there are two basic approaches to removing them. One is to use a fibrous filter that takes them out by a sieving action; **HEPA filters** work in this way and offer the maximum efficiency among sieving filters. The other approach is to give the particles an electrical charge and then attract them to a plate that carries the opposite charge; devices employing this method are called **electrostatic precipitators, electronic air cleaners** or **electrostatic air cleaners**.

A hybrid method also exists, using a fibrous filter in which the fibres carry an electrical charge. The particles in the air apparently have sufficient natural charge to attract them to the fibres of the filter, and this supplements the sieve-like effect of the filter. These are known variously as **charged media filters, precharged electrostatic filters, electrostatic microfilters** or **electrets**.

HEPA filters
High Efficiency Particulate Air (HEPA) filters must remove particles of 0.3 micron

diameter with an efficiency of at least 99.97 per cent – a stringent requirement indeed. With any high quality filter, the 0.3 micron particle is the one that is most difficult to filter from air. Smaller particles, paradoxically, are caught more easily, due to the complexities of air movement through a filter. Thus, 99.97 per cent is the minimum efficiency, and both larger and smaller particles will be trapped with greater efficiencies.

HEPA filters are made of glass fibres less than a micron wide, embedded in a matrix of slightly larger fibres. They were developed during World War II by the Atomic Energy Commission in the USA to remove radioactive dust from waste gases. Today, HEPA filters are used in a variety of situations, including operating theatres in hospitals.

Once in use, the efficiency of a HEPA filter actually increases because the particles caught reduce the size of the channels through which other particles can flow. However, there is a downside to this: the **air throughput** or **airflow** (the amount of air processed each minute) declines because of the increased resistance. The specification for HEPA filters stipulates that this should not drop more than a certain amount.

These filters have a very long life – at least a year, and sometimes as much as five years. The filter is replaced when it is so full of particles that the air throughput drops considerably.

Other sieve-like filters

Some air filters use sieve-like filters that are not up to HEPA standard, but are still good enough to help those with allergies. (These are sometimes referred to as **panel filters, extended surface filters**, or '**HEPA-type filters'**.) If there are no figures given in the sales literature supplied, you should ask for the filtration efficiency at 0.3 micron or 0.5 micron.

Very simple sieve-like filters are used in small, table-top air filters of the kind sold in electrical shops. They are unlikely to state their filtering efficiency, but tests have shown that it is about 75 per cent at 20 microns – the size of pollen grains. This filtration rate might help some hayfever sufferers, but the fans in these machines are too weak to achieve the air throughput needed for cleaning the air in a normal room.

Electrostatic precipitators

These have an electrode which discharges ions into the incoming air, thus giving the particles an electrical charge. A fan draws the air towards collecting plates, which carry the opposite electrical charge. The charged particles are attracted towards the plates and stick to them.

When first running, electrostatic precipitators have a very high efficiency, even for very small particles. Tobacco smoke particles, for example, will be removed with 80–90 per cent efficiency. However, within a few days the efficiency begins to drop because the particles already deposited on the plates interfere with their ability to attract and hold more particles. The plates therefore have to be cleaned regularly to maintain the filtration effect.

If considering an electrostatic precipitator, you should ask how often the plates need to cleaned, and how much their efficiency drops in the interval between cleaning. Also find out how difficult it is to remove the plates, and how much scrubbing is needed to get them clean.

Electrostatic precipitators inevitably produce small amounts of ozone because they ionize the oxygen in the air. Ozone can cause irritation of the airways (see p70), but with newer devices this is said not to be a problem because the amount produced is very small. However, should you experience any irritation, or find that you are coughing more than usual, ozone may be the explanation. Experiment with not using the filter for a while and see if your symptoms change.

Charged media filters

Also known by a variety of other names (see p298), these filters are relatively new and have not yet been tested by researchers looking at their effects on allergy patients. According to one manufacturer in Australia (Aironic) the efficiency of their filtration medium is 99 per cent at 1 micron and 93 per cent at 0.3 micron. While not as good as a HEPA filter, this efficiency may be sufficient for many allergy sufferers. The medium does not have to be as dense as a HEPA filter because a particle that is smaller than the channels running through the charged medium can still be caught by means of electrostatic attraction. The filter, being less dense, does not create as much air resistance as a HEPA filter, so air throughput is proportionately higher. In general, these devices are less expensive than HEPA filters, but the filter medium has to be replaced more often.

Air ionizers

Air ionizers have an effect very similar to that of an electrostatic precipitator, except that walls and other surfaces in the home act as the collecting plates. Their effects as air cleaners are discussed on p304.

Which type of device is best?

If you want your filter to remove irritant gases and volatile chemicals from the air, or to eliminate bad smells, you need to buy one with an activated carbon filter as well as a particle filter.

For particle filtration most researchers favour HEPA filters over electrostatic precipitators because their efficiency tends to increase with use, rather than declining, and less maintenance is involved. An electrostatic precipitator also has the disadvantage that, if an electrical fault develops which prevents the collecting plates from becoming charged, the filter stops working entirely, yet the fan can still be running, so the machine seems to be functioning. Charged media filters do not have this drawback as the charge is intrinsic to the fibres of the filter. They are also easier to maintain. This type of filter may come to rival HEPA filters in the future, but still needs to be tested more fully.

Ensuring the filter is up to the job

Once you have established that the filter will efficiently take out particles of the size required (see p299), there is another important measurement to look at: **air throughput** or **airflow**. This may be stated in cubic metres per minute (cmm), cubic metres per hour (cmh) or cubic feet per minute (cfm). If you are trying to make sense of brochures and leaflets on air filters obtained from manufacturers, look out for these abbreviations. Occasionally, air throughput is stated in yet another way: litres per second. Table 3 gives conversions between these three different units, allowing you to compare the throughput of different brands of air filter.

Work out the minimum air throughput that you need as follows. Measure the

length, breadth and height of the room in which you want to use the filter. If several rooms are to be treated and you therefore want to buy a portable filter for moving around the house, measure the largest of the rooms. (Remember to consider ceiling height in assessing which is the largest.)

Multiply the three figures:
length x breadth x ceiling height.
This gives the volume of air in a room. For example, a room that is 5 metres long by 6 metres wide, with a ceiling height of 3 metres, will have an air volume of 90 cubic metres.

Divide the air volume in the room by the 'air throughput' of a filter, and you can discover how often that filter will clean all the air in the room.

For example, if you buy a filter with an air throughput of 1.5 cubic metres per minute (cmm), it will take 90 divided by 1.5 to process all the air in the room – that is, 60 minutes – so the air in the room will be cleaned every hour. This is considered the absolute minimum rate, and is not ideal. (Far higher rates of air exchange are achieved in an old-fashioned house without draught-proofing for example.) The recommended rate is to clean the air in a room four times an hour. Thus a filter

---

TABLE 3
Air throughput conversions

The air throughput figures given here are typical values for the widely available brands of air filters and cleaners.

cubic metres per minute (cmm)	cubic metres per hour (cmh)	cubic feet per minute (cfm)	litres per second
0.67	40	23.7	11
1.0	60	35	16
1.5	90	53	25
2.5	150	88	42
2.8	168	99	47
3.3	200	118	55
4.3	255	150	71
5.0	300	175	80
5.9	349	208	97
6.6	400	236	110
8.5	510	302	142
16.6	1000	600	278
21.7	1300	760	360
34	2050	1200	570

with an air throughput of 6 cmm is needed for a room of 90 cubic metres. (However the air in the room will not be completely cleared of particles every 15 minutes because there is bound to be some mixing between cleaned and dirty air.)

If buying a HEPA filter, choose one with an air throughput figure slightly above that required, since this tends to drop as the filter booomoo dirty.

Some manufacturers and suppliers give a figure for the size of room to which an air filter is suited, rather than revealing the air throughput. They may refer to this as the capacity of the filter. Ask how this room size figure is calculated – that is, how many air changes per hour the filter gives in a room of that size.

Another figure that may be given is the clean air delivery rate. This is a measure of how much the rate of removal of particles by the air cleaner exceeds that occurring due to natural settling of particles (see p202).

Allergen disturbance by fans

All the filters rely on a fan to move air through them, and the fans themselves create a disturbance in the air. The more powerful the fan, the more the air is disturbed. If there is a large reservoir of allergen particles on the floor or on other surfaces, the air movements created by the fan will make some of these particles airborne, partially offsetting the effects of the air filter. This is particularly likely with small particles such as those produced by cats. To get the best effects from your filter, therefore, you need to reduce the amount of allergen in the carpets and furniture by thorough cleaning measures (see p207 for those needed for cat allergens).

If it is difficult to reduce the reservoir of allergens, there are other measures you can take. Placing the filter off the floor will reduce the amount of allergen disturbed from the carpet. Two filters running simultaneously, each with an air throughput of, say, 2.5 cmm will have the same cleaning effect on the air as one filter with a throughput of 5 cmm, but will not cause as much disturbance of allergens because the fans are less powerful.

Other features

Several air filters and cleaners have an additional feature of some kind.

Dehumidifier

If you are sensitive to both pollens and house-dust mite, or pollens and mould spores, a combined air filter and dehumidifier may well be your best choice, since it will allow you to keep the windows closed without suffering the consequences in condensation and damp. For more details on dehumidifiers, including those that also filter the air, see p306.

Humidifier

Anything that increases the humidity of the air is not recommended for most houses (see p201).

Air ionizer

When ionizers are added to air filters or cleaners, they may improve their air-cleaning performance to some extent. In the case of air filters with a low air throughput, this may be valuable. However, this is not the reason for adding them to high powered filtering devices. In such cases, they are added because ions are claimed to have a direct benefit on health. These claims are considered in more detail on p305.

Fragrance diffuser

These are not recommended for anyone with asthma or rhinitis, as continuous exposure to the fragrance may irritate the airways. The use of the fragrance diffuser is usually optional, even if one is fitted.

Questions to ask about air filters and cleaners

- Does it contain an activated carbon filter?
- What type of system is used for removing particles from the air?
- With what efficiency are particles of 0.3 micron or 0.5 micron removed?
- What is the air throughput when operating at its highest speed?
- Is the device designed to be portable?
- Is the device available for a free trial period, or on a money-back basis, or

for hire so that its effectiveness can be assessed before buying?
- What are the running costs in terms of electricity used?

For electrostatic precipitators
- How often do the plates need cleaning, and how difficult are they to clean?
- With what efficiency are particles removed a month after cleaning? And after two months?

For all other types of air filter
- How often do the filters need replacing, and how much do they cost?

Manufacturers and suppliers

Aironic, Australia
Produce and sell a range of air filters. These use charged media filters, combined with an activated carbon filter in some models. *Air throughputs*: 302 – 540 cfm. Sold directly by mail and through the Allergy Aid Centre.

Allerayde
Sell an air filter produced in the USA, the Enviracaire, adapted for British electricity supplies. This includes a HEPA filter and activated carbon filter. It is the only filter to have been directly tested for its benefits to allergy sufferers and shown to reduce symptoms in certain contexts. *Air throughput*: 350 cfm. The filter can be supplied for a trial period of a few weeks to assess its usefulness.

Allergy Aid Centre, Australia
Sells the Aironic air filter (see above) by mail order.

Beta Plus
Sell a range of air filters and cleaners (also air conditioners, ionizers and dehumidifiers). Some are electrostatic precipitators, while others use activated carbon and a charged media filter. *Air throughputs*: a wide range is available, including some high-powered filters suitable for offices and bars. All products may be hired so that their effectiveness can be judged before purchase; the hire fee for two weeks is deductible from the price.

Beta Plus also sell an air filter designed for use in cars (see p304).

Products can be seen at their showroom in London, or ordered by mail.

The Healthy House
Produces and sells its own air cleaner. This contains six different filters, including a HEPA filter and two activated carbon filters. The unit is designed for allergy sufferers, and for those sensitive to pollutants . *Air throughput*: 159 cfm. The air cleaner can be returned for a refund within fourteen days of purchase if you are not satisfied with its effectiveness; a charge of about £18 will be made for replacing one of the filters.

This company also sell filters for use with cars (see p304).

Medivac
Produces and sells the Enviro-dry, which combines a charged medium filter with a powerful dehumidifier (see p306).

Also sells a small table-top filter which includes an ionizer. *Air throughput*: 40 cmh. All products can be returned within fourteen days for a refund if you are not satisfied with their usefulness. Sold by mail order, and can be ordered in chemists' shops from mid-1993.

Mountain Breeze
Produce ionizers with a filter system attached (see p305). *Air throughputs*: 40– 60 cmh. Sold by mail order, also through Beta Plus and in Boots the Chemists.

Rentokil
Produce and sell air filters for commercial use.

Approximate costs

Low-powered air filters combined with an ionizer are relatively cheap, £70–£100.

With other filters always assess the price in relation to the air throughput figure. If you divide the air throughput (in cfm) by the price (in £, excluding VAT) you will get a figure between 0.25 and 1.5. The higher the figure, the better value the machine, although you should also consider whether it offers the best type of filtration method for particles, and whether an activated carbon filter is included.

For example, the Enviracaire device has a maximum air throughput of 350 cfm and costs £225 excluding VAT. This gives a figure of 1.5 by the calculation method described above.

The device includes a HEPA filter and an activated carbon filter, and therefore offers excellent filtration efficiency. On the down side, the cost of replacement HEPA filters is quite high (£70 each). However, the filters only need replacing every 5–7 years, so the cost is actually about £10–£15 per year.

Electrostatic precipitators are generally more expensive to buy than other types at the outset (about twice the price), but replacement filters are not needed.

For people with certain conditions (see p293) VAT exemption is available on some filters, including the Enviracaire filter and The Healthy House filter.

AIR CONDITIONERS

As well as cooling the air, these will take out over 90 per cent of the pollen grains (see p116). The air also becomes drier, which helps to decrease the number of house-dust mites.

Suppliers

Beta Plus
Stock a wide range of mobile air-conditioning units produced by different manufacturers.

Approximate costs

Prices start at £760, including VAT.

FILTRATION UNITS FOR EXISTING AIR CONDITIONING SYSTEMS

These are available, but research has shown that air conditioning itself reduces the pollen count in the air considerably, and that adding a filter produces only a small improvement (see p116).

Suppliers

Beta Plus

FILTERS FOR EXISTING HEATING DUCTS OR VENTILATION SYSTEMS

Some modern buildings have central heating systems that provide warm air by running it through air ducts. These can be fitted with filters that effectively reduce the pollen and mould spore counts in the air. Filters are also useful in the ventilation systems of large office blocks, where the air travels in through air ducts. These will probably have some type of filter already, but the filtration performance can usually be improved.

Suppliers

Beta Plus

Healthy Buildings International

Rentokil

FILTERS AND IONIZERS FOR CARS

There are relatively few products available, and none have been independently tested, so it is difficult to say how much help they might give.

Any filtration or ionization system within a car will work only if the windows are closed. There is little doubt that a car with built-in air conditioning will provide a cooler and more comfortable solution to the problem of pollen when driving.

Removal of pollen

A dust filter will remove pollen within the car as long as the air throughput (see p300) is adequate to change the air in the car four times an hour or more.

An air ionizer should also remove some pollen grains from the air in the car. As with domestic ionizers, a direct benefit from the ions on the well-being of driver and passengers is claimed, but this is a matter of debate (see p305). The effects of ionizers in cleaning the air are apparent in the home (see p304) but how effective they are within a car is unknown. Car ionizers plug into the cigarette lighter socket.

Dust filters that are taped over the air intake on the vehicle will take out pollen entering the car by this route. However, the pollen that was in the car to begin with will remain. To what extent this settles from the air when the car is in motion with windows closed is unknown.

A *combination* of dust filters taped over the air intake, and an ionizer or filter within the car, may be the most effective way of reducing the pollen and pollution load. It does not, however, solve the problem of heat building up within the car.

Removal of pollutants from traffic

To remove gases and petrol fumes, activated carbon (see p294) is required.

Diesel particles require a dust filter (see p299), preferably one that can deal with particles smaller than a micron. They might also be removed by an air ionizer.

Manufacturers and suppliers

Aironic, Australia
Produce and sell an ionizer for use in cars. Sold directly, or through the Allergy Aid Centre.

Beta Plus
Sell an air cleaning device for cars made by National Safety Associates, the only one currently on sale. No details available on filtration method or air throughput. Also sell the Mountain Breeze car ionizer.

The Healthy House
Sell filter pads, known as Breathe Easy filters, designed to fit over the air intake on a car. They contain activated charcoal and an electrostatically charged dust filter, and will reduce the pollutants and pollen coming into the vehicle. The Breathe Easy is unaffected by water and car washes. It is large enough to fit most makes of car. Also sell the Mountain Breeze car ionizer.

Mountain Breeze
Produce and sell an ionizer for in-car use. Available directly by mail order; also sold through Beta Plus, The Healthy House and Boots the Chemists.

Approximate costs

The air-cleaning device available from Beta Plus costs about £95 excluding VAT.

Breathe Easy filters cost £15 each. A new filter is needed every three to four months.

The car ionizer from Mountain Breeze costs £30 excluding VAT.

AIR IONIZERS

These produce a stream of negative ions by applying a high negative voltage to a set of needles. Electrons leave the tip of each needle and combine with oxygen molecules in the air, forming negatively charged ions. Particles of pollen, dust or smoke are attracted to the negatively charged oxygen molecules and cluster around them. The particles acquire the negative charge, which attracts them to positively charged surfaces such as walls, furniture and television screens. In this way, the particles are removed from the air far more quickly than if they just settled naturally.

The cleaning effect of ionizers is beyond dispute: the dirt that accumulates on the wall behind them is testimony to their effectiveness. They are, in fact, like electrostatic precipitators, but instead of having collecting plates, they use the walls and other surfaces. Unlike electrostatic precipitators, however, they have no fan, so air is not circulated around the room. This means that the cleaning power tends to decline as you move further away from the ionizer, but this can be overcome by having two or more ionizers operating in the room.

Coping with the mess created by an ionizer is something that has concerned many purchasers, particularly those using the device to combat cigarette smoke. A sticky brown deposit collects close to the ionizer, and can be very difficult to clean off. Some users have found that taping a large piece of paper to the wall behind the ionizer is the solution, or hanging a curtain behind it, which can be washed regularly.

A few of the newer ionizer models now incorporate a 'Faraday cage' and a charged medium filter, which help to reduce the amount of dirt deposited.

Despite the drawbacks, an ionizer may be a good solution to allergen-loaded air in certain circumstances. Ionizers are inexpensive to buy and very cheap to run since they use hardly any electricity. They are also quieter than air filters and cleaners. For an elderly person, or someone on a low income, where keeping the decor looking nice is not the top priority, an ionizer could be useful in cleaning the air. Unlike an air filter or cleaner, an ionizer will not disturb settled allergens from the carpet and other surfaces (see p301) because it has no fan.

Ozone is produced in small amounts by ionizers, but the levels are within government safety limits. Should you experience any irritation of the airways, however, or an increase in coughing, this could be due to ozone. Try moving the ionizer further away from you, if it is very close to your bed or armchair. If the symptoms persist, stop using the ionizer.

Other benefits claimed for ionizers

Ionizers were originally developed as a result of observations on 'winds of ill repute' – hot dry winds that blow regularly in certain parts of the world and are said to cause irritability and malaise. It was found that these winds were short on negative ions, but rich in positive ions. Close to the sea and on mountains there are more negative ions, and the well-being that people experience in these places has been attributed to the ions. Needless to say, there are a great many other reasons why people may feel good at the seaside or on a mountain-top, and the ill effects of hot dry winds could also be caused in a variety of ways.

Some scientific studies have been carried out with ionizers to test these claims, and one reported that office workers felt more alert with an ionizer running. This could be due to breathing cleaner air, however. Effects on well-being are certainly not universal, and many people who have tried ionizers report no difference in their mood or health. It is possible that individuals vary in their response, just as static electricity affects some people far more than others.

The claim that ionizers can have a direct effect on allergy symptoms has been made repeatedly. One hayfever sufferer has informed us that by allowing the ions to stream over his eyes and nose for a few minutes, he can greatly reduce his hayfever symptoms. How this might work is difficult to see, and most doctors are profoundly sceptical about such claims. Indeed, the ozone produced by ionizers (see p304) could make some symptoms worse.

In brief, we would suggest that ionizers can be useful as air-cleaning devices, in certain situations, but that the other claims made for them are unproven and need scientific investigation.

Choosing an ionizer

The most important figure to be quoted for an ionizer is the cleaning range. Most achieve 6 metres (20 feet), but some can manage more on a higher setting, up to 9 metres (30 feet) on the maximum setting.

The ion concentration at a given distance from the ionizer is often quoted. This should be over 100,000 ions per cubic centimetre (cc) at 1 metre (3.3 feet) away, and over 1,000 ions per cubic centimetre at 5 metres (16.5 feet) away.

Is the ionizer working?

A survey by the consumer magazine *Which?* (March 1992) found that some of the ionizers tested produced no ions at all. If there is no dirt deposited on surfaces near the ionizer, then it is probably not working.

The effects of the ionizer in cleaning the air will also be much reduced by objects being placed too close to it, particularly television sets. The ionizer should be positioned at the very front of a shelf, or the front edge of any other surface, as long as it is not metallic. The needles should be cleaned with a matchstick every three to four weeks.

Manufacturers and suppliers

Aironic, Australia
Produce and sell straightforward ionizers, and ionizers combined with an air filter (see p302). Sold directly, or through the Allergy Aid Centre.

Beta Plus
Sell a range of ionizers made by different manufacturers.

The Healthy House
Sell the Pifco ionizer and other brands.

Medivac
Sell an ionizer with a 'Faraday cage', which also incorporates an air filter (see p302). Also sell a much simpler ionizer.

Mountain Breeze
Produce and sell straightforward ionizers, and ionizers combined with air filters (see p302). Available directly from them by mail order, also from Beta Plus or The Healthy House; sold in Boots the Chemists.

Pifco
Produce the ionizer that was chosen as 'best buy' by *Which?* magazine. Can be bought by mail order from The Healthy House, or ring Pifco on 061-681 8321 to find out about local stockists.

Approximate costs

Straightforward ionizers cost £20–£40. Running costs are very low – less than £3 per year. Ionizers with air filters included cost £70–£100.

DEHUMIDIFIERS

Dehumidifiers are useful for anyone with allergy to mould spores or house-dust mites. To be effective, a dehumidifier must reduce the relative humidity of the air to 45 per cent, which is the target for most ordinary dehumidifiers.

One model, the Banamite Enviro-dry Dehumidifier, reduces the relative humidity further, to 25 per cent. In these very dry conditions, the dust-mite population is greatly reduced. It is best to use this device when the room is unoccupied (for example, in a bedroom during the daytime). The door should be closed for maximum effect. At bedtime turn the dehumidifier off and leave the door to the room open for 30 minutes. This will restore the humidity to a normal level, making it comfortable for human occupants.

All dehumidifiers work by cooling the air, using the same technology as a refrigerator. Water condenses out of the air as it is cooled, and is collected in a tank from which it cannot evaporate again. The dry, cool air is blown out of the device and is heated up by contact with the warmer air in the room.

Choosing a dehumidifier

Dehumidifiers are rated according to the amount of water they can remove from the air in a 24-hour period, but these figures cannot be compared unless the temperature and humidity of the air are quoted; the amount of water removed varies as these figures vary. Ask for the removal rate at 21°C (70°F) and 70 per cent relative humidity, as these are fairly typical conditions.

Ideally, a dehumidifier should have an in-built control which regulates it according to the humidity of the air, switching the device off when the air gets sufficiently dry.

Check how large the water tank is in relation to the amount of water the device can remove each day. It should be large enough to allow you to empty the tank

just once a day. Good machines have an automatic cut-out to turn the device off when the tank is almost full. The next best option is a warning light which tells you when the tank is nearly full.

Manufacturers and suppliers

Electrical stores, such as Currys, sell dehumidifiers, but these are relatively low-powered machines.

Beta Plus
Sell a good range of dehumidifiers that will reduce the relative humidity to 45 per cent. They also sell an inexpensive meter that will measure the humidity in your home. All their products can be hired before purchase to see if they are effective.

Specialized dehumidifiers for use after building work (see p199) are also available for purchase or hire.

The Healthy House
Sell one type of dehumidifier by mail order.

Medivac
Produce and sell the Banamite Enviro-dry Dehumidifier. This also incorporates an electrostatic microfilter to remove particles such as house-dust mite droppings, mould spores and pollen from the air. If the water tank becomes full, the dehumidifier cuts out to prevent an overflow, and an indicator light warns that it has cut out.

Approximate costs

About £200–£300 for a device that will dry out a two- or three-bedroom house. The Banamite Enviro-dry Dehumidifier costs about £400, but offers more than an ordinary dehumidifier, and incorporates an air filter.

BEDDING AND MATTRESS COVERS

An allergen-proof cover for the mattress is the single most valuable preventive measure in dust-mite allergy. You should, if possible, kill the mites already in the mattress first (see p179). Putting allergen-proof covers on to the duvet and pillows will further reduce exposure to the mite allergen. Alternatively, you can replace duvets and pillows with ones that can be laundered regularly at 60°C. The most widely used are microporous covers, made from a special material that lets water vapour through. There are also covers made of heavy duty PVC. These are a little cheaper than the microporous covers, but may make you feel hot and sweaty in bed.

One rather unusual product offered for sale is a 'herbal allergy pillow' which contains cedarwood chippings and 'other powerful anti-allergy herbs'. The cedar chippings are said to deter dust mites from entering the pillow. The product is not cheap (£19) and a good microporous pillow cover could be bought for half this price. We would not recommend anyone with rhinitis or asthma to expose themselves to a strong smell such as cedarwood every night. Allergies to wood dust sometimes occur (see p216) and are a potential risk with this product.

Manufacturers and suppliers

The companies listed here should be able to offer VAT exemption, but enquire before buying. Some can also give interest-free credit for up to twelve months. Most of those using microporous material will send a small sample of it, on request.

Allerayde
Sell mattress covers, pillow covers and duvet covers made in the USA. These are made of a microporous material that has cotton polyester on the outside, vinyl on the inside. Custom-made covers can be ordered for unusual mattresses.

Allergy Aid Centre, Australia
Sell allergen-proof covers for mattresses, pillows and doonahs.

Allergy Relief Products
Produce and sell mattress covers, duvet covers and pillow cases. These are welded at the seams, rather than sewn, to minimize the escape of allergens. When in place, they are sealed with adhesive tape, rather than closed with a zipper, again minimizing the escape routes for allergen particles. A spare roll of the tape is provided.

The Healthy House
Sell mattress covers, duvet covers and pillowcases made of microporous materials. Can make unusual sizes to order.

Intervent
The Intervent range of mattress covers, duvet covers and pillowcases are made from a microporous material. They are manufactured by Slumberland, and sold exclusively in Boots the Chemists.

The Linen Cupboard
Sell heavy-duty PVC mattress covers. These can be custom made for unusual mattresses. Also sell dust-proof pillowcases.

Medivac
Produce and sell a mattress cover of microporous material, which covers the top and sides of the mattress like a fitted sheet. This may be of value to some allergy sufferers, but will obviously not contain the mite allergens as thoroughly as a cover that entirely encloses the mattress.

Medivac also produce and sell a duvet made of two separable layers. The layers can be washed separately in an ordinary washing machine at 60°C. Pillows made of the same material (soft terry towelling) can likewise be washed at this high temperature, sufficient to kill the mites. It is recommended that pillows and duvet be washed every three months.

All Medivac products are available in chemists' shops from mid-1993, as well as directly, by mail order.

Slumberland
Make the Intervent range of covers, sold in Boots the Chemists.

Also sell new mattresses which are 'sealed in' with a microporous cover during manufacture. This type of cover is available with any of their mattresses. Enquire at stores selling Slumberland beds.

Approximate costs

There are large variations here, and it is worth shopping around: pillowcases £8–£25, single duvet covers £17–£120, double duvet covers £25–£150, kingsize duvet covers £27–£170, single mattress covers £28–£110, double mattress covers £36–£140, kingsize mattress covers £42–£160.

The cheapest prices at the time this book went to press were those of Allergy Relief Products and The Healthy House. Some brands are suitable for washing, but with others this is not recommended. You should ask the suppliers how long their products are estimated to last, and if they are guaranteed. Some companies offer a discount if you buy a full bed set.

The washable duvets from Medivac cost £140 for a single, £186 for a double, £206 for a kingsize. Washable pillows cost £28 each.

VACUUM CLEANERS

High-retention vacuum cleaners are useful to some people with dust-mite allergy, although bedding covers (see p306) are considered a more important measure. These vacuum cleaners may also be valuable to people with cat allergy and, perhaps, to those with hayfever if they are being affected by pollen fragments (see p118). The crucial test is whether you suffer increased symptoms during vacuum cleaning, or after someone else has vacuum cleaned the house.

Ordinary vacuum cleaners release allergenic dust particles into the air during cleaning (see p185). The amount and size of the particles emitted varies considerably from one manufacturer to another, but all let out enough to affect someone who is highly sensitized to dust-mite allergen.

Specialized vacuum cleaners, designed for those with dust-mite allergy, should retain over 99 per cent of particles at 0.3 micron. Several models are now available which achieve this, and others that achieve good filtration at 0.6 micron, which can be sufficient for some people.

These machines are considerably more expensive than a normal vacuum cleaner because they have to be made to much higher specifications, and the motor has to be more powerful to overcome the air resistance created by the high quality filter (usually a HEPA filter, see p298) over the exhaust.

Several companies producing standard vacuum cleaners have now begun to make claims about the dust retaining power of their machines in an attempt to attract allergy sufferers. A claim of the type 'Retains 99.9 per cent of dust' is valueless unless the particle size to which the claim relates is given. It may well be relevant only for particles more than a micron in size, in which case smaller allergenic particles will be emitted.

In view of the cost of specialized vacuum cleaners, a filter pad which can be taped over the exhaust of a conventional vacuum cleaner is now sold as a 'second best' solution. This has been tested scientifically and shown to remove 99.3 per cent of particles down to 0.5 micron in size from exhaust air. However, it will not stop dust particles being emitted from poorly fitting joints in the machine, or from the space around the switch, unless you cover these as well.

One company offers a wet vacuuming system with a special anti-mite shampoo. Although good results are claimed for this treatment, one study showed that it was no better than intensive dry vacuum cleaning. Another found that there was an increase in mite populations in the carpet after the treatment, probably because of the increase in humidity and the selective removal of other mites which normally prey on *Dermatophagoides*. The general conclusion is that wet vacuuming cannot be recommended at present.

Manufacturers and suppliers

All the suppliers listed here offer VAT exemption and a free trial period for vacuum cleaners. Nilfisk and Medivac offer twelve months interest-free credit.

Allerayde
Sell Vacu-Filt exhaust filters for conventional vacuum cleaners. Also sell the Nilfisk vacuum cleaner.

BVC bivac
Sell a vacuum cleaner that retains 99.997 per cent of particles at 0.6 micron.

Medivac
Sell a vacuum cleaner that contains a HEPA filter. Retains 99.97 per cent of particles at 0.3 micron. Has been independently tested with good results. Also sell an electronic dust monitor which shows when an area of carpet is clean.

Nilfisk
Sell the Allergy Vac vacuum cleaner which contains a HEPA filter. Retains 99.997 per cent of particles at 0.3 micron. Has been independently tested with good results.

Approximate costs

Vacuum cleaner prices start from £260 excluding VAT. Check exactly what is included in the price.

Attachments for special purposes, such as vacuuming dogs, start from about £20. Replacement HEPA filters are needed for some machines, and you should ask about the costs of these and how often replacement is needed. Also check the cost of the disposable paper bags.

Vacu-Filt costs £20 including VAT for a pack of three sheets. You cut out a piece of the right size for your vacuum cleaner exhaust, and each sheet gives two or three pieces. The filter lasts three to four months, so a single pack lasts from eighteen months to three years. Be sure to change the filter when it is dirty, as it will begin to slow down the motor on the vacuum cleaner, which could lead to overheating.

DUSTERS

There is only one brand on the market at present, the Guardsman One-Wipe. It consists of a cloth with an electrostatic charge, similar to that of a charged media filter (see p299). This attracts and holds the dust so that very little becomes airborne during dusting. (A similar effect can be obtained by wet dusting, but the electrostatic cloth is less bother.) The duster can be washed and will not lose its charge until it has been through the wash about twenty times. Thereafter, it can be used as an ordinary polishing cloth.

Supplier and cost

The Guardsman One-Wipe is available from Allerayde and costs £3.

ACARICIDE TREATMENTS

The pros and cons of using acaricides are discussed on p184 and p189. They must be followed by very thorough vacuuming, preferably with a vacuum cleaner that has a filter attached or with a specialized vacuum cleaner (see p308). The allergy sufferer should be out of the room throughout the process, and should remain out for some hours afterwards because there will be considerable disturbance of the allergen from moving furniture, and by vacuum cleaning if the cleaner exhaust is not filtered. Should the allergy sufferer have to do the job in person, a good quality dust mask should be worn (see p295).

According to the National Asthma Campaign, some asthma sufferers experience symptoms from the sprays themselves.

VAT exemption is available on the do-it-yourself sprays. If you prefer to get the spraying done by a contractor, this is also possible (see below).

Another type of spray, containing a fungicide, natamycin, has sometimes been used in an attempt to control dust mites. The theory is that without the moulds (fungi) that break down skin particles for them, dust mites will starve. In practice, these sprays did not have much effect on the mites.

Suppliers

Crawford Pharmaceuticals

Produce and sell the Acarosan range, which includes foam in a spray can (used for mattresses and upholstery), and a moist powder (used for carpets). Both are designed to minimize the amount inhaled. The active ingredient is benzyl benzoate. Can be bought directly by mail order.

Rentokil

This company will spray the house for you, using permethrin, which is also an insecticide, and therefore effective against woodworm and any insect pests in the house.

Searle

Produce and sell the Actomite spray, supplied in an aerosol. The active ingredients are two synthetic pyrethroids, bioallethrin and S-bioallethrin. Can be bought in Boots the Chemists and other chemists' shops.

Approximate costs

The costs, taken over a whole year, are roughly the same for the two do-it-yourself treatments available: about £70–£80.

The amount of Acarosan needed to treat an average living room and bedroom (two cans of foam and two cartons of moist powder) would cost about £35 excluding VAT. The treatment has to be repeated twice a year. A can of Actomite spray costs about £10 excluding VAT, and is sufficient for a single room. The treatment has to be repeated four times a year.

The Rentokil treatment would cost about £90. You would have to carry out the subsequent vacuum cleaning yourself.

LIQUID NITROGEN TREATMENT

This kills dust mites and leaves no residue at all (see p184). The company follows up the treatment with a very thorough vacuum cleaning of the house.

Supplier and costs

The main supplier in Britain at present is Nitroboost. They have contractors who can provide the treatment anywhere in Britain or Northern Ireland. Nitroboost can treat a single bedroom for £80, a double bedroom or living room for £95, and a whole house for £200. A maintenance contract, providing two treatments per year, is available.

TANNIC ACID SPRAYS

These are sprays that denature (see p182) the dust-mite allergen and are probably effective against other allergens too. As well as denaturing the allergen, the tannic acid makes it less sticky so that it is taken up more readily by a vacuum cleaner. The tannic acid spray itself dries to a powder within about three hours. This powder can likewise be removed by thorough vacuum cleaning.

By destroying the reservoir of allergen in carpets and upholstery, the tannic acid spray has an effect that lasts for two to three months, even though the mites themselves are still alive and the tannic acid does not have any ongoing effect on the allergens they produce. It takes two or three months for the allergen reservoir to build up to appreciable levels once more.

VAT exemption is available on this product.

Manufacturers and suppliers

Allerayde

Allergy Aid Centre, Australia

The Healthy House

Medivac

Approximate costs

The amount needed to treat a whole house costs about £50 excluding VAT.

DUST MITE TEST KITS

There is only one currently available, the Acarex test. The test procedure itself is quite simple to carry out, but getting a good sample of dust involves using a clean vacuum cleaner bag, vacuuming carefully, emptying the bag out on to paper, and tapping the paper to separate out the fine dust. *This must not be done by anyone sensitive to dust mite.*

The test measures the amount of guanine in the dust. This is the waste product produced by the 'kidneys' of mites and spiders. Studies show that mites are the main source of guanine in houses, the contribution made by spiders being negligible. The guanine is not itself allergenic, but it gives a good idea of how many mites and how much mite allergen are present.

Supplier and costs

Crawford Pharmaceuticals make the Acarex test and sell it directly, by post. The test kit costs £10 and will do ten separate tests.

SPRAYS AND SOLUTIONS FOR MOULD

There is a solution available for cleaning moulds from bathroom tiles, vinyl baths and bathmats, refuse bins and surfaces being prepared for painting. It contains a form of bleach and has a fairly strong smell, but is more effective in removing black mould than domestic bleach.

A spray that prevents mildew regrowth on curtains, carpets and shower curtains, as well as hard surfaces such as tiles and wood, is also sold. This contains a fungicide.

Supplier and costs

Both products are sold by Allerayde. The Mildew Remover costs £8 per bottle; the Mildew Stop aerosol costs £7.

INDOOR POLLUTION AND 'SICK BUILDING SYNDROME'

Two companies now offer consultancy and treatment services for offices that are afflicted by 'Sick Building Syndrome'. They are Rentokil W & V Consultancy Services, and Healthy Buildings International.

For indoor pollution, the best treatment is to eliminate the sources of pollutants (see p321). If formaldehyde is suspected as a problem, there is a formaldehyde monitoring badge, made by 3M, which can show how much formaldehyde you are exposed to every day.

APPENDIX 4
Manufacturers and suppliers

Aironic Pty Ltd
79 Mars Road
PO Box 216
Lane Cove
New South Wales 2066
Australia
Tel (02) 428 1334/ 428 4083
Fax (02) 427 7949

Allerayde
21 North End
Farndon
Newark
Notts NG24 3SX
Tel/Fax 0636 72636

Allergy Aid Centre
1st Floor
Pran Central
325 Chapel Street
Prahran
Victoria 3181
Australia
Tel (03) 529 7348

Allergy Relief Products Ltd
39 Spring Crescent
Portswood
Southampton
Hants SO2 1FZ
Tel 0703 586709
Fax 0703 676226

Arco Ltd
PO Box 21
Waverley Street
Hull
Humberside HU1 2SJ
Tel 0482 27678
Fax 0482 218536

This company has stores in Aberdeen, Linlithgoe, Lothian, Glasgow, Irvine, Blaydon-on-Tyne, Stockton-on-Tees, Hull, Ossett, Stockport, Ellesmere Port, Nottingham, West Bromwich, Bury St Edmunds, Bristol, Orpington and Eastleigh.

There is also a catalogue which can be sent free, and products can be bought by mail order.

Atom Imports Pty Ltd
Ashmore Estate
1A Coulson Street
Erskinville
PO Box 123
Alexandria 2015
Australia

Beta Plus Ltd
177 Haydons Road
London SW19 8TB
Tel 081-543 1142
Fax 081-543 4317

British Lung Foundation
8 Peterborough Mews
London SW6 3BL
Tel 071-371 7704

BVC bivac
Harbour Road
Gosport
Hants PO12 1BG
Tel 0705 584281

R.J. Chicken and Sons Ltd
Bisley Works
Landpark Lane
Kensworth
Dunstable
Beds LU6 2PP
Tel 0582 873329
Fax 0582 873583

Crawford Pharmaceuticals
71A High Street
Stony Stratford
Milton Keynes
Herts MK11 1BA
Tel 0908 262346
Fax 0908 567730

Greenscreen International Ltd
The Windsor Centre
2/18 Britannia Row
London N1 8QH
Tel 071-226 9282
Fax 071-226 9274

Healthy Buildings International Ltd
Wyvols Court
Swallowfield
Berks RG7 1PY
Tel 0734 880248
Fax 0734 880360

Healthy Buildings International
Townhouse 18
Greenwich Square
130-134 Pacific Highway
St Leonards
New South Wales 2065
Australia
Tel (02) 901 3933
Fax (02) 901 3939

The Healthy House
Cold Harbour
Ruscombe
Stroud
Glos GL6 4DA
Tel 0453 752216

Iles Opticals Ltd
Kingsley Works
Walmgate Road
Perivale
Greenford
Middlesex UB6 7LG
Tel 081-998 6600
Fax 081-991 5691

The Linen Cupboard
21-22 Great Castle Street
London W1
Tel 071-629 4062

Martindale Protection Ltd
Neasden Lane
London NW10 1RN
Tel 081-450 8561
Fax 081-450 4794

Medivac plc
Bollin House
Riverside Works
Manchester Road
Wilmslow
Cheshire SK9 1BE
Tel 0625 539401
Fax 0625 539507

Mountain Breeze Ltd
6 Priorswood Place
Skelmersdale
Lancs WN8 9QB
Tel 0695 21155

Nilfisk Ltd
Newmarket Road
Bury St Edmunds
Suffolk IP33 3SR
Tel 0800 252296

Nitroboost Ltd
395A Hardgate
Aberdeen AB1 6BW
Tel 0224 574705

Norville Optical Company Ltd
Magdala Road
Gloucester GL1 4DG
Tel 0452 528686
Fax 0452 300551/411094

Protector Safety Pty Ltd
17 Main Road
Wivenhoe
Burnie
Tasmania 7320
Australia
Fax: 004 31 6944

Rentokil Ltd
(Head Office)
Felcourt
East Grinstead
West Sussex RH19 2JY
Tel 0342 833022
Fax 0342 326229

Rentokil W & V Consultancy Service
Cheviot House
71 Castle Street
Salisbury
Wilts SP1 3SP
Tel 0722 335153

Rentokil Ltd
Auckland
New Zealand
Tel (9) 640079
Fax (9) 666977

Rentokil Pty Ltd
Sydney
Australia
Tel (02) 958 0277
Fax (02) 958 0776

Respro
Renaissance Design N.P.D. Ltd
28 South Island Place
London SW9 0DX
Tel 071-587 3663
Fax 071-587 0397

Searle Consumer Products
(Medical Information Department)
G.D. Searle & Co. Ltd.
Freepost
PO Box 53
Lane End Road
High Wycombe
Bucks HP12 3BR
Tel 0494 21124

Slumberland Medicare Ltd
Bee Mill
Shaw Rd
Royton
Oldham
Lancs OL2 6EH
Tel 061-628 5293

3M United Kingdom plc
(Occupational Health and Environmental
  Safety Group)
3M House
PO Box 1
Market Place
Bracknell
Berks RG12 1JU
Tel 0344 858000
Freephone 0800 212490

APPENDIX 5
Medicinal drugs

This appendix covers the drugs commonly used in hayfever and asthma.

Drugs are referred to in two ways – by their proper (generic) name, and by the trade names given them by manufacturers. The same drug may be marketed under a number of different trade names if it is produced by different manufacturers. Some medicines contain a mixture of two or more drugs. Drugs are described here under their generic names, which are given in italics, e.g. *salbutamol*. The trade names are shown with a capital letter e.g. Ventolin.

This list of drugs is reasonably comprehensive, but new drugs are introduced all the time, so a medicine you are prescribed may not be mentioned here if it is fairly new on the market.

How to use the lists

Beside each drug is a code number, which shows what type of drug it is. These are the code numbers:

1 Mast-cell stabilizers (see p87)
2 Antihistamines (see p89)
3 Sympathomimetic nose sprays and drops (see p96)
2/3 Antihistamine and sympathomimetic combined in tablet or liquid form (see p98)
4 Corticosteroids (see p100)
5 Bronchodilators (see p106)
5A ß2 adrenoceptor agonists (see p106)
5B Xanthines (see p107)
5C Anti-cholinergics (see p107)
5D Others (see p108)

Generic names

acrivastine 2
adrenaline 5D
alclometasone 4
aminophylline 5B
antazoline 2
astemizole 2
atropine 5B (also see pp230–31)
azatadine 2
azelastine 2
beclomethasone 4
betamethasone 4
brompheniramine 2, 2/3
budesonide 4

butethamate 5C
cetirizine 2
chlorpheniramine 2, 2/3
choline theophyllinate 5B
clemastine 2, 2/3
clobetasol 4
clobetasone 4
cyproheptadine 2
desonide 4
desoxymethasone 4
dexamethasone 4
diflucortolone 4
dimethindene 2
diphenylpyraline 2, 2/3
ephedrine 3, 2/3, 5D
fenoterol 5A
fluclorolone 4
flunisolide 4
fluocinolone 4
fluocortolone 4
fluorometholone 4
flurandrenolone 4
fluticasone 4
halcinonide 4
hydrocortisone 4
hydroxyzine 2
ipratropium 5C (also see pp230–31)
isoetharine 5A
isoprenaline 5A
ketotifen 2
levocabastine 2
lodoxamide 1
loratadine 2
mebhydrolin 2
mequitazine 2
methylprednisolone 4
nedocromil sodium 1
orciprenaline 5A
oxatomide 2
oxitropium 5C
oxymetozoline 3
phenindamine 2
pheniramine 2, 2/3
phenylephrine 3, 2/3, 5D
phenylpropanolamine 2/3
pirbuterol 5A
prednisolone 4
promethazine 2
pseudoephedrine 3, 2/3
reproterol 5A
rimiterol 5A
salbutamol 5A
salmeterol 5A
sodium-cromoglycate 1
terbutaline 5A
terfenadine 2
theophylline 5B
triamcinolone 4
trimeprazine 2

triprolidine 2, 2/3
xylometazoline 3

Trade names
Actidil 2
Actifed 2/3
Aerobec Autohaler 4
Aerolin Auto 5A
Afrazine 3
Aller-eze 2
Aller-eze Plus 2/3
Alomide 1
Alupent 5A
Asmaven 5A
Atarax 2
Atrovent 5C
Becloforte 4
Beconase 4
Becodisks 4
Becotide 4
Berotec 5A
Betnesol 4
Biophylline 5B
Boots Antihistamine Tablets 2
Bricanyl 5A
Bronchilator 5A
Bronchodil 5A
Brovon 5C
CAM 5C
Choledyl 5B
Clarityn 2
Congesteze 2/3
Contac 400 2/3
Cromogen 1
Cromolyn 1
Daneral 2
Dexa-Rhinaspray 4
Dimotane 2
Dimotane Plus 2/3
Dimotapp 2/3
Dristan Decongestant Spray 3
Dristan Decongestant Tablets 2/3
Eskornade Spansules 2/3
Eumovate 4
Exirel 5A
Fabahistin 2
Fenostil Retard 2
Fenox 3
Flixonase 4
FML 4
Franol 5B
Galpseud Plus 2/3
Haymine 2/3
Hismanal 2
Histryl Spansule 2
Intal, Intal Compound 1
Labophylline 5B
Lasma 5B
Maxidex 4

Maxivent 5A
Medihaler-Duo 5A
Medihaler-Iso 5A
Minims 4
Monovent 5A
Nalcrom 1
Nuelin 5B
Opticrom 1
Optimine 2
Otrivine-Antistin 2, 3
Otrivine 3
Oxivent 5C
Pecram 5B
Periactin 2
Phenergan 2
Phyllocontin Continus 5B
Piriton 2
Pollon-eze 2
Pred Forte 4
Predsol 4
Primalan 2
Pro-Actidil 2
Pro-Vent 5B
Pulmadil 5A
Pulmicort 4
Resiston One 1, 3
Rhinocort 4
Rhinolast 2
Rimasal 5A
Rynacrom, Rynacrom Compound 1
Sabidal 5B
Salbulin 5A
Salbuvent 5A
Seldane 2
Semprex 2
Serevent 5A
Slo-Phyllin 5B
Sudafed Plus 2/3
Syntaris 4
Tavegil 2
Tedral 5B
Theo-Dur 5B
Theodrox 5B
Uniphyllin Continus 5B
Thephorin 2
Tilade 1
Tinset 2
Triludan 2
Triominic Tablets 2/3
Vallergan 2
Vasocon-A 2, 3
Ventide 5A
Ventodisks 5A
Ventolin 5A
Vibrocil 2/3 (+ an antibiotic)
Vista-Methasone 4
Volmax 5A
Zaditen 2
Zirtek 2

APPENDIX 6
Getting additional help

POLLEN COUNTS AND FORECASTS

In the UK there are several telephone numbers offering information about pollen. A good telephone service should give pollen counts (from the previous day), pollen forecasts for the coming day, and the general outlook for the next three days. The best services cover different types of pollen separately and give counts for mould spores. Most run from May 1st to mid-August.

- Clarityline, a country-wide service, is available on freephone 0800 556610, starting mid-May
- Counts for London can be obtained from Pollon-Eze on: 071-753 7066
- Counts for different regions can be obtained from the Seldane Pollen Line on:

  0891 666451 – Scotland
  0891 666452 – Northern Ireland
  0891 666453 – Northern England
  0891 666454 – Wales
  0891 666455 – The Midlands
  0891 666456 – East Anglia
  0891 666457 – South and Southwest England
  0891 666458 – London

Calls to the Seldane Pollen Line cost 36 pence per minute cheap rate, 48 pence per minute at all other times.

- Boots the Chemists are offering a free telephone service. Cards with the telephone numbers are available in Boots stores.

POLLEN ADVICE SERVICES

Aerobiologists studying pollen can be of assistance when you are planning holidays. Check the information in Appendix 1 first. If this is not sufficiently detailed, you can obtain more information from the specialized advice services listed below. Similarly, if you are thinking of moving to a new area or emigrating, you should check with Appendix 1 for any likely pollen problems, and seek more advice if necessary.

Britain and Ireland

Pollen Research Unit
University of North London
166–220 Holloway Rd
London N7 8DB

Part of the European Aeroallergen Network (EAN) which is coordinating pollen monitoring services throughout Europe. Can offer detailed pollen information for travellers to Europe and most popular holiday destinations. Please write, enclosing a stamped, self-addressed envelope, stating what pollens cause your hayfever. (Readers outside Britain can also write to this service if there is no equivalent in their own country.)

New Zealand and Australia

Pollen Monitoring Dept
University of Otago
Dunedin
New Zealand

To the best of our knowledge, there is no service of this kind in Australia.

AIR POLLUTION

In the UK the Department of Environment runs a Pollution Helpline on freephone number 0800 556677. This gives levels of sulphur dioxide, nitrogen dioxide and ground-level ozone for different regions of the UK.

ASTHMA ADVICE

Asthma Helpline, run by the National Asthma Campaign, offers a helpline in the UK. Calls are charged at local telephone rates only, regardless of where you are calling from. The helpline is staffed by qualified nurses with counselling experience, who can give advice on how to manage asthma attacks and the best way to use medicines. They emphasize, however, that they cannot give special medical advice – that is the job of your doctor.
The helpline is open Monday–Friday, from 1pm–9pm. The number is: 0345 010203.
The line is heavily used, so you may hear the engaged tone, but keep trying. Early evening is the least busy.
The address of the National Asthma Campaign can be found on p317.

SELF-HELP GROUPS AND CAMPAIGNING ORGANIZATIONS

When writing to any of these organizations, please enclose a large, stamped, self-addressed envelope to save them time and money.

Hayfever, asthma and other allergies

Allergy Association, Australia
PO Box 298
Ringwood
Victoria 314
Australia
Tel (03) 888 1382
Fax (03) 544 2328

Can give advice to allergy sufferers of all kinds, including those with hayfever.

Allergy Recognition and Management Inc.
PO Box 2
Sandy Bay
Tasmania 7005
Australia
Tel (002) 282554
     (002) 781054

Can give advice to allergy sufferers of all kinds, including those with hayfever. Members receive discounts at certain shops.

Allergy Awareness Association
PO Box 120701
Penrose
Auckland 6
New Zealand

Asthma Society of Ireland
24 Anglesea Street
Dublin 2
Eire
Tel 01 716 551

British Allergy Foundation
St Bartholomew's Hospital
London EC1A 7BE
Tel 071-600 6127

A voluntary group launched by a number of leading medical specialists to improve the awareness, prevention and treatment of allergy. Can supply a leaflet on hayfever. Also produce a cassette tape with advice for hayfever sufferers. Organize 'National Hayfever Week' each spring.

National Asthma Campaign
Providence House
Providence Place
London N1 0NT
Tel 071-226 2260

A very active and valuable self-help group, funding research, producing an informative newsletter and organizing many activities, particularly for children and toonagers with asthma. There are local groups in many areas. Publishes a short leaflet on hayfever which may be useful to doctors seeking to inform their patients. Donations to help with their work are very welcome.

Pollution

Action on Smoking and Health (ASH)
109 Gloucester Place
London W1H 3PH
Tel 071-935 3519

Campaigns to reduce indoor pollution from tobacco smoke, and to help people stop smoking. Donations to help with this work would be appreciated.

British Lung Foundation
8 Peterborough Mews
London SW6 3BL
Tel 071-371 7704

Campaigns on behalf of those with asthma, bronchitis and other lung conditions, particularly regarding air pollution, and supports scientific research. Can give advice on pollution avoidance and sells an anti-pollution mask (see p296). Organizes the 'Breathe Easy' club for those with lung conditions.

Friends of the Earth (FoE)
26-28 Underwood Street
London N1 7JQ
Tel 071-490 1555
Fax 071-490 0881

Actively campaigning on the air pollution issue in Britain, and pressing for better monitoring. Made official complaint to the European Commission in 1989 about excessive levels of nitrogen oxides, which frequently breach World Health Organization guidelines. In 1991 they revealed that the British government had been misleading the public over air quality bulletins. As a result of pressure from FoE, the government has ensured that pollution warnings now appear on weather forecasts. Donations to help this work are welcome. There are also local groups tackling the same issues in their area; write for the name and address of your nearest group.

Breastfeeding

National Childbirth Trust
Alexandra House
Oldham Terrace
London W3 6NH
Tel 081-992 8637

Organizes a network of trained counsellors with personal experience of breastfeeding.

Nursing Mothers' Association of Australia
5 Glendale Street
Nunawading
Victoria 3131
Australia
Tel (03) 877 5011

Has many local groups all over the country offering counselling.

La Leche League New Zealand
PO Box 13383
Wellington 4
New Zealand

Part of the international La Leche League which aims to promote breastfeeding.

Parents' Centres New Zealand Inc
PO Box 17351
Wellington
New Zealand

ADVICE AND SUPPLY SERVICES FOR DOCTORS ONLY

None of these organizations can deal with enquiries from the general public – please ask your doctor to contact them.

Bio Diagnostics Ltd
Upton Industrial Estate
Rectory Road
Upton-upon-Severn
Worcs WR8 0XL
Tel 06846 2262
Fax 06846 2501

Supply a very good range of allergen extracts for skin-prick testing, the

Allergopharma range. These include extracts of pollen from individual plant species, extracts of spores from individual mould species, and dander allergens of a wide range of animals from budgerigars to camels.

Dome Hollister Stier
PO Box 3145
Terminal Annexe
North 3525 Regal Street
Spokane
Washington
USA 99220
Tel (509) 489 5656

Supply a very wide range of individual allergens for skin-prick testing.

Medical Entomology Centre at the University of Cambridge
Cambridge Road
Fulbourn
Cambs CB1 5EL

Can help doctors with particular problem cases, where allergy to insects or mites is suspected as the cause, but the species involved is not known.

Pollen Research Unit
University of North London
166-220 Holloway Rd
London N7 8DB

May be able to help if the type of pollen (or mould spore) causing a patient's hayfever is proving difficult to identify.

National Society for Research into Allergy
PO Box 45
Hinckley
Leics LE10 1JY
Tel 0455 851546

Can advise doctors on allergists offering desensitization treatments. (This society also deals directly with the public.)

FURTHER READING

The Complete Guide to Food Allergy and Intolerance by Dr Jonathon Brostoff and Linda Gamlin, published by Bloomsbury Publishing, 1992.

All About Asthma and Allergy by Dr H. Morrow Brown, published by The Crowood Press, 1990. A useful book for those who suffer from asthma.

APPENDIX 7
Air pollution

The main sources of pollution are summarized here, and suggestions for avoiding or combating them are given at the end of the appendix.

VEHICLE EXHAUST

Whereas other forms of pollution have been declining in Britain, that from traffic is steadily increasing. It may level off towards the end of the century, thanks to the introduction of catalytic converters (which remove many pollutants from the exhaust fumes), but levels of pollution will rise again in the twenty-first century as the volume of traffic continues to increase.

Of the many pollutants formed by vehicles, carbon dioxide, carbon monoxide and lead are not considered important in allergy, although they may affect health in other ways. Other pollutants which are relevant to allergic problems include diesel particulates (see p59) and nitrogen dioxide (see pp60–61). Volatile organic compounds are also important because they play a role in producing ozone which acts as an irritant to the airways (see pp61 and 70).

Nitrogen oxides

Nitric oxide (chemical formula: NO) is produced by the burning of petrol. Having left the exhaust pipe, it combines with oxygen in the air to form **nitrogen dioxide** (NO_2). The latter is a reddish-brown gas which you can actually see in the air when smogs form over busy urban areas, particularly if you are looking down on the city from a hillside or a tall building. The highest concentrations in Britain are found within the London conurbation during rush hours. However, there can also be significant levels of nitrogen dioxide in homes with gas cookers (see p321). Nitrogen dioxide is an irritant in its own right, but also plays a part in producing ozone (see below).

As nitric oxide converts to nitrogen dioxide in the air, it is more meaningful to discuss both together than to consider nitrogen dioxide separately. The abbreviation NOx is used to refer collectively to these two gases.

Volatile organic compounds

Petrol evaporates when cars are filled at a petrol station, and whenever any is spilled on the road. Oil also evaporates when it is spilled, or when it leaks from engines. These are major sources of **volatile organic compounds** or **VOCs**. (There are other sources, however, including fluids used for dry cleaning, solvents used in products such as glue and paint, spray paints used on cars, and industrial processes. Natural VOCs are described below.)

VOCs can be harmful in themselves – some are carcinogens, for example. They can also play a role in the formation of ground-level ozone (see below).

Ground-level ozone

Everyone now knows about the importance of ozone in the stratosphere (the 'ozone layer') which shields the Earth from ultraviolet radiation. Useful though it may be in the stratosphere, at ground level ozone is a menace, a serious irritant to the airways.

Ozone is not produced directly by vehicles, but through a complex interaction of nitrogen dioxide, VOCs, sunlight and the natural oxygen in the air. Ozone consists of three oxygen atoms (O_3), whereas ordinary oxygen has two (O_2). Sunlight acts as a catalyst when it shines on the polluted air of a city, the large VOC molecules begin to break down, and, with the assistance of nitrogen dioxide, they turn some oxygen molecules into ozone. The worst time for ozone formation is in summer.

These interactions create the **photochemical smogs** that now plague Los Angeles, Athens, Mexico City and, though less frequently, large British cities. Inversions, in which a layer of cooler air at ground level becomes trapped beneath a layer of warmer air above, make the smogs much worse, by preventing pollutants from escaping. Photochemical smogs can become very acidic in certain situations, which adds to the irritant effects of ozone and nitrogen dioxide.

The chemical interactions in city air are complicated, and nitric oxide in exhaust fumes can break ozone down again. Thus the highest levels of ozone are often found in the countryside downwind of a big city, which receives a stream of ozone-rich air from the urban traffic but lacks the nitric oxide concentrations needed to break ozone down again. In Britain the highest concentrations of summertime ozone are often found in the countryside to the west of London, around Swindon. Parcels of ozone-rich air can be blown about by the wind. In the summer of 1976 a smog that formed in central Europe moved westwards, reached the Atlantic Ocean and was then blown back again. It was detected moving into Ireland from the Atlantic several days after it had formed.

In addition to man-made VOCs, there are also naturally occurring VOCs, produced by plants (see p121). Trees, in particular, produce large amounts of these. When combined with nitrogen dioxide from traffic, they may contribute to the reactions of photochemical smogs and the consequent formation of ozone, but their contribution is minimal compared to synthetic pollutants. In the countryside some natural VOCs can help to break down ozone.

Diesel particulates

Diesel engines use a different type of fuel and work in a different way from ordinary petrol engines. When properly maintained and finely tuned, they are actually less polluting than petrol engines. They do not emit lead, for example, a virtue that has been made much of in car advertisements. However, the regular maintenance needed is omitted by most commercial owners, particularly those running bus fleets and lorries. The lack of tuning makes diesel engines produce large amounts of particulates (soot particles). Badly maintained diesel engines also produce sulphur dioxide, an irritant to the airways (see below). Nitrogen oxides are produced in roughly the same amounts as from petrol engines, but there are more **polycyclic aromatic hydrocarbons (PAHs)**, some of which may be irritants or carcinogens.

DOMESTIC HEATING AND POWER STATIONS

Unless very high temperatures are used, burning any fuel produces smoke – that is, a mixture of carbon particles and gases.

There are generally more particulates from coal than from oil or gas. Wood-burning stoves can also produce carbon particles, plus PAHs (see previous section).

Coal contains variable amounts of sulphur, more in the poorer grades of coal. This forms **sulphur dioxide** (SO_2) when burned, a gas that is highly irritating to the bronchi.

Carbon particulates and sulphur dioxide were the main ingredients in the 'pea-souper' fogs that once bedevilled London, Manchester, Glasgow and other large British cities. Domestic coal fires were a major cause of these pollution episodes, but industrial pollution was also a factor. The sulphur dioxide reacted within the sooty droplets of fog to form dilute sulphuric acid, probably the main cause of death among those with bronchitis and asthma.

Since the Clean Air Act of 1956, this type of pollution has been much reduced in Britain. However, there are still episodes of sulphur dioxide pollution and sulphuric acid mists in some areas. Those near coal-fired power stations or heavy industry are likely to be worst affected.

CIGARETTE SMOKE

Cigarette smoke is a major form of pollution for many people. It includes small carbon particulates, PAHs (see left) and a cocktail of other chemicals. Cigarette smoke is carcinogenic, even to those who simply inhale other people's smoke ('passive smokers'). It is also an irritant, but one which affects some people much more severely than others. The role of cigarette smoke in allergy is complex (see p45).

GARDEN BONFIRES

The smoke from a bonfire contains a similar assortment of damaging chemicals as that from a cigarette, including irritants and carcinogens. If plastics or foam rubber are added to the blaze, even more powerful irritants can be produced. The widespread idea that this form of pollution causes no harm is mistaken.

INDOOR POLLUTION

For many people the air in the home can be more polluted than that which they breathe outdoors. Tight draught-proofing in modern houses leads to poor ventilation, and if pollutants are then generated they can build up to high levels.

Tobacco smoke is one major source of pollution in the home (see p320). Another is the kitchen, where burning fats and oils create a fine blue smoke that can be highly irritating to the airways. If the cooking is done on a gas stove, some nitrogen dioxide is generated (see p61) and this can build up to significant levels if ventilation is poor. (Gas fires are provided with proper ventilation when installed, and Calor Gas heaters are designed to produce very little nitrogen dioxide, but the problem can also arise with old-fashioned paraffin heaters.)

Formaldehyde is produced by various items in the home (see p215) and can act as an irritant. Solvents from paint and household chemicals are frequently allowed to evaporate into the air within the home. Air fresheners and aerosols add to the rich cocktail of synthetic chemicals in the air.

ACTION ON POLLUTION

Reducing your own exposure

Reducing your exposure to cigarette smoke is relatively easy if you are determined about it. This applies whether you are an active or a passive smoker. Research shows that most smokers want to stop and have tried to at least once. Unfortunately, nicotine is highly addictive – more so than many 'hard drugs' such as heroin. This fact has only been realized in the past decade, and has led to the development of various aids to giving up smoking. Most supply a dose of nicotine which is gradually reduced over a period of weeks. This allows the smoker to stop cigarettes abruptly without having severe withdrawal symptoms. Ask at any chemist's shop about these products.

Kitchens with gas stoves should have some additional ventilation installed, such as a small extractor fan. Alternatively, just open the window a little when cooking. Keep ovens clean to reduce the smoke generated when they are turned on. Frying should always be done over a gentle heat, and the oil or fat watched carefully so that it does not begin to smoke.

Indoor pollution by formaldehyde can be combated by painting or varnishing all items made of chipboard, blockboard or plywood. If possible, replace veneered chipboard or plywood furniture with solid wood items. Other items that may give off formaldehyde are listed on p215. If you cannot get rid of these, store them in a well-ventilated room, garage or loft space. Air the house well to shift the lingering formaldehyde within. Where cavity wall insulation is the source of the problem, try better ventilation until all the formaldehyde has leached out. An air filter containing activated carbon may be useful for a while (see p298).

Various volatile substances (see p120) can irritate the nose, and if anything seems to make you react, it should be evicted, or sealed into an airtight container. Some bamboo furnishings, pot-holders and ornaments have a very strong-smelling varnish on the outside which can be an irritant. Felt-tip pens may give off powerful solvents – again, evict any that seem to smell unpleasant, or seal them into plastic bags. Air fresheners should also go (see p215) and aerosols kept to an absolute minimum since the droplets they produce linger in the air and are inhaled. Most things that are sold in aerosols can be found in some other type of container, or a substitute can be used. A house can be kept clean with a few simple items: washing up liquid, scouring powder and toilet cleaner. Unscented versions are preferable. Clear out all other cleaning materials, white spirit, turps, meths, dry-cleaning fluids, polish, bleach, moth balls and disinfectant. Rags or dusters with polish, window-cleaning liquid or white spirit on them should also be removed. Banish these items to a garage, shed, garden or balcony for a while. If this is impossible, store them in airtight containers such as tins or plastic bags.

Once you have reduced the level of 'pleasant' artificial odours in the house, you may begin to notice other smells. (Air fresheners actually deaden the sense of smell.) If any plastic items seem to have a strong unpleasant smell, try to replace them, or store them in a well-ventilated space. Nasty smells that were previously being covered up by air fresheners should be tackled at source if possible: these can usually be eradicated by thorough cleaning. Drains can be cleaned by pouring in boiling water that contains several large spoonfuls of washing soda, for example. Should any smells prove resistant to cleaning efforts, an air filter containing activated carbon (see p298) will eliminate them, although this is not a cheap solution to the problem.

Outdoor pollution is obviously more difficult to avoid. In Britain, the Department of the Environment runs a Pollution Helpline (see p316) giving levels of sulphur dioxide, nitrogen dioxide and ground-level ozone for different regions. In exceptionally bad conditions air pollution warnings are also given with the weather reports and on Ceefax. When levels of pollutants are high, keep away from traffic-laden streets, particularly in the afternoon and during the evening rush-hour, when pollution peaks. Don't take any strenuous outdoor exercise in the afternoon during these high-pollution periods. Stay indoors if your throat feels sore or your eyes are stinging in the outdoor air. Consider using an anti-pollution mask (see p294). Those with asthma should take particular care and increase their medication if symptoms get worse.

Unfortunately, reducing our intake of traffic fumes often means travelling by car rather than walking or cycling, so we are helping to perpetuate the problem. In the long run the pollution issue has to be tackled by legislation, better public transport and improved traffic planning, but the political will to do this in Britain is currently lacking.

The need for garden bonfires can be avoided by turning leaves and other waste into compost. Gardening books commonly advocate burning certain diseased leaves or roots in case they infect other plants. An alternative option is to wrap such material in plastic bags and put it in the dustbin, since the amounts involved are usually fairly small. Undiseased wood and prunings can be put through a shredder and used as mulch, or stacked until thoroughly dry and then burned; dry material produces far fewer pollutants, as long as you make sure air can get to the bottom of the fire. (Diseased plant material could be kept sealed in plastic until you have such a fire, then unwrapped and put on when the fire is hot.) Never light a bonfire on a damp or misty day, and remonstrate with any neighbour who does.

Environmental Health Officers from the local council can be called in if you have a particular problem with a neighbour's bonfires.

Tackling pollution on a wider scale

If you see a bus, lorry or other diesel vehicle belching black smoke, you can take down the licence number and report it to your local Traffic Area Office. The telephone numbers are:

Birmingham	021 631 3300
Bristol	0272 297221
Cambridge	0223 358922
Cardiff	0222 394027
Eastbourne	0323 21471
Edinburgh	031 225 5494
Leeds	0532 499433
London	0323 21471
Manchester	061 872 5077

Combating pollution on a broader scale requires collective action, and there are campaigning groups that you can join, or support with a donation (see p317).

APPENDIX 8
Foods that may release sulphur dioxide

Sulphur (or sulfur) dioxide is a gas that can irritate the airways of asthmatics and provoke an asthma attack. Some preservatives give off this gas in small amounts, and it is inhaled during eating. There is no need to avoid these preservatives unless you are sure they trigger off attacks.

Most dried fruits are treated with sulphur dioxide and give off the gas when chewed. *This treatment does not have to be declared on the label.* Dried fruit that has not been treated will usually be labelled 'unsulphured'.

The following preservatives give off sulphur dioxide:
    sodium sulphite
    sodium hydrogen sulphite
    sodium metabisulphite
    potassium metabisulphite
    calcium sulphite

These preservatives are widely used in wine, beer and cider, and, like other additives used in alcoholic drinks, do not have to be declared on the label. Home-made wine is no exception: Campden tablets, sold to wine-makers, contain potassium metabisulphite.

Fresh sausages may also contain these additives. Cod can be treated with sodium hydrogen sulphite to bleach and preserve it. Although sulphites are not allowed on meat, unscrupulous butchers occasionally add them to old meat to give it a 'fresh' red colour. In all these cases, the greater part of the sulphur dioxide will be driven off by the high temperatures used in cooking.

A fourth 'hidden source' of sulphur dioxide is restaurant, take-away and cafeteria food. French fries used in the catering trade have usually been dipped in a metabisulphite solution and give off significant amounts of sulphur dioxide. Prepared salads, avocado dip, shrimps, prawns and lobster are also likely to have been treated with these preservatives, and sometimes cause problems.

Fruit salad, glacé cherries, fruit juices, fruit pie fillings, dried vegetables and soup, fruit squash, pickled onions, jam, fruit jellies and custard are other possible sources of sulphur dioxide in the catering trade. It is not worthwhile avoiding these foods unless you know they trigger off your asthma attacks.

Packaged foods often contain sulphites and metabisulphites, but these are easier to avoid as they are declared on the label. Look for the names given above, or for the appropriate 'E numbers'. These are E220–E227.

APPENDIX 9
Scientific names of plants

The common names of plants vary from one part of the world to another and for clear communication it is better to use the scientific names.

These are the scientific names for the plants included in the main body of the text. The list is only intended to show which plant *we* refer to by a particular common name: some of the common names listed may be used for different species by other authors.

Common name	Scientific name	Notes
alder	*Alnus* spp.	
alfalfa	*Medicago sativa*	
amaranth family	Amaranthaceae	
ash	*Fraxinus excelsior*	
aspens	*Populus tremula* (Britain) *Populus tremuloides* (North America)	
aster	*Aster* spp.	
bald 'cypress'	*Taxodium distichum*	Not a true cypress but a relative of the redwoods.
barley	*Hordeum distichon, H. vulgare*	
bean	*Phaseolus* spp.	
begonia	*Begonia* spp.	
birch	*Betula* spp.	
bog myrtle	*Myrica gale*	
brittle bush	*Encelia* spp.	
buttercup	*Ranunculus* spp.	
cabbage	*Brassica oleracea*	
cabbage family	Cruciferae or Brassicaceae	
carrot	*Daucus carota*	
carrot family	Umbelliferae or Apiaceae	
cedar	*Cedrus* spp.	Note that Japanese red cedar is not a true cedar, but a relative of the redwoods.
'cedar'	any member of the Cupressaceae referred to as a cedar; includes species of *Thuja, Juniperus* and *Chaemaecyparis*	
chamomile	*Matricaria chamomilla, Chamaemelum nobile* and other species	The species implicated in the cross-reaction described on p166 was *M. chamomilla*; the species used for chamomile lawns is *C. nobile*.
cherry	*Prunus avium, P. cerasus*	
chicory	*Cichorium* spp.	
chrysanthemum	*Chrysanthemum* spp.	
clover	*Melilotus* spp.	
coltsfoot	*Tussilago* spp.	
couch grass	*Agropyron repens*	
cyclamen	*Cyclamen* spp.	
cypresses	*Cupressus* spp. and *Chamaecyparis* spp.	These are the true cypresses. Other trees and shrubs in the same family (Cupressaceae) commonly cross-react.

Common name	Scientific name	Notes
dahlia	*Dahlia* hybrids	
dandelion	*Taraxacum* spp.	
docks	*Rumex* spp.	Note that *Rumex* also includes a variety of species known as sorrels. These will undoubtedly cross-react with docks.
Easter lily	*Lilium* spp.	
eastern white pine	*Pinus strobus*	Also called white pine or Weymouth pine.
elder, elderberry	*Sambucus nigra*	
false oat grass	*Arrhenatherum elatius*	
fir	*Abies* spp.	
goldenrod	*Solidago* spp.	
giant ragweed	*Ambrosia trifida*	
goosefoot family	Chenopodiaceae	
grass	Gramineae or Poaceae family	
hazel	*Corylus* spp.	
heather	*Calluna* spp. and *Erica* spp.	
heather family	Ericaceae	
honeysuckle	*Lonicera* spp.	
hornbeam	*Carpinus* spp.	In the USA, *Carpinus* is called ironwood, and hornbeam means *Ostrya* spp. (called hop-hornbeams in Britain).
horse chestnut	*Aesculus* spp.	
hydrangea	*Hydrangea* spp.	
ironweed	*Vernonia* spp.	
Japanese red cedar	*Cryptomeria japonica*	Not a true cedar.
junipers	*Juniperus* spp.	
knapweed	*Centaurea* spp.	
lily	*Lilium* spp. and *Gloriosa rothschildiana*	
lucerne	*Medicago sativa*	
maize	*Zea mays*	
marigold	*Tagetes* spp.	
meadow fescue	*Festuca pratensis*	
millet	*Panicum miliaceum*	
mimosa	any species of *Albizia* or *Acacia* or *Mimosa* known as mimosa	
mugwort	*Artemisia vulgaris*	There are many other *Artemisia* spp. known as wormwoods, sagebrush, tarragon, southernwood etc.; these probably all cross-react with mugwort.
nettle	*Urtica* spp.	
oat	*Avena sativa*	
oil-seed rape	*Brassica napus*	
olive	*Olea europaea*	
orange	various *Citrus* spp., but principally *C. sinensis*	
osiers	*Salix viminalis* and other *Salix* spp.	
peach	*Prunus persica*	
pellitory-of-the-wall	*Parietaria judaica*	Can be taken to include all other *Parietaria* spp., since they will cross-react.

Common name	Scientific name	Notes
pine	*Pinus* spp.	
plantain	*Plantago* spp.	
plum	*Prunus domestica* and other *Prunus* spp.	
pond 'cypress'	*Taxodium ascendens*	Not a true cypress but a relative of the redwoods.
poplars	*Populus* spp.	
privet	*Ligustrum ovalifolium* (used for hedging) and *L. vulgare* (wild privet)	
pussy willows	*Salix caprea* and other *Salix* spp.	
rabbit brush	*Chrysothamnus* spp.	
ragweed	*Ambrosia* spp.	
ragwort	*Senecio* spp.	
redwoods	*Sequoia* and *Sequoiadendron*	
rice	*Oryza sativa*	
rose	*Rosa* spp. and hybrids	
rose family	Rosaceae	
rosinweed	*Grindelia* spp.	
rye	*Secale cereale*	
rye grass	*Lolium perenne*	
sallows	*Salix cinerea, S. caprea*	
Santa Maria feverfew	*Parthenium hysterophorus*	
sedges	Cyperaceae family	Reeds also belong to this family
she-oaks	*Casuarina* spp.	Also called 'Australian pines'.
sneezeweed	*Helenium* spp.	
sorghum	*Sorghum vulgare*	
spruces	*Picea* spp.	
sugar cane	*Saccharum officinarum*	
sunflower	*Helianthus annuus*	
swamp 'cypress'	*Taxodium distichum*	
sweet gale	*Myrica gale*	
sweet pea	*Lathyrus* spp.	
thistles	*Cirsium* spp., *Sonchus* spp.	
timothy	*Phleum pratense*	
wheat	*Triticum aestivum, T. durum, T. dicoccum*	
white cypress pine	*Callitris columellaris*	Also called Murray pine. Not a true pine but a native Australian conifer.
wild oat	*Avena fatua*	
willows	*Salix* spp.	
yew	*Taxus* spp.	
zinnia	*Zinnia* spp.	

INDEX

Numbers in italic indicate an illustration. Numbers in bold type indicate the main entry or entries on a topic, or the definition of a technical term.

For the names of individual drugs, please consult Appendix 5 on p314.

For the various regions of the world, and the plants found in them that could cause hayfever, please see Appendix 1 on p254.